Epilepsy: Current Approaches to Diagnosis and Treatment

Epilepsy: Current Approaches to Diagnosis and Treatment

Editor

Dennis B. Smith, M.D.

Director
Oregon Comprehensive Epilepsy Program
Good Samaritan Hospital & Medical Center
Professor of Neurology
Oregon Health Sciences University
Portland, Oregon

Raven Press   New York

Raven Press, 1185 Avenue of the Americas, New York, New York 10036

Made in the United States of America

Library of Congress Cataloging-in-Publication Data

Epilepsy : current approaches to diagnosis and treatment / editor,
   Dennis B. Smith.
        p.   cm.
     1. Epilepsy.   I. Smith, Dennis B.
     [DNLM: 1. Epilepsy—diagnosis. 2. Epilepsy—therapy.   WL 385

E64107]
RC372.E6634   1990   616.8′53—dc20
DNLM/DLC
for Library of Congress   89-70183
ISBN 0-88167-615-2   CIP

9 8 7 6 5 4 3 2 1

Preface

Another book on epilepsy? Within the past decade there has been no dearth of books devoted to epilepsy: Some have been highly specialized and directed toward epileptologists and clinical and basic researchers; some have been quite general in scope and have taken a more pedantic approach. This book does not attempt to provide a comprehensive overview of epilepsy but, instead, emphasizes new and evolving concepts in the diagnosis and treatment of the epilepsies.

The newer diagnostic technologies and treatment modalities are described so that their usefulness and limitations can be better understood and therefore better utilized by the patient's primary care physician. Unlike other books, it is to the primary care physician that this book is directed, whether that physician is a family practitioner, internist, emergency room physician, psychiatrist, or general neurologist.

The authors are clinicians who practice in large tertiary-care centers where the technologies described in this book are readily available. The importance of understanding contemporary concepts of classification of seizures and the epilepsies is underscored in Chapter 1, written by James Cereghino, Director of the Epilepsy Branch of NINDS. Any classification can be arduous and frequently tedious to commit to memory, but Cereghino explains the therapeutic and diagnostic importance of making as precise a classification of seizures and epilepsy as possible, and he discusses the rationale for using the terminology of the International League Against Epilepsy (ILAE) classification. In his chapter is the most comprehensive and understandable clinical description of seizure types based on location of origin one is likely to find.

To introduce the subject of diagnostic approaches, Ronald Kramer explains in Chapter 2 the limitations and misuse of routine electroencephalography (EEG), while emphasizing how to maximize its diagnostic capabilities. Don King, who developed one of the first long-term video/telemetry monitoring units, describes in Chapter 3 the clinical circumstances that may be helped by long-term monitoring and explains what kind of results a referring physician can expect from EEG/video monitoring. The clinical potential of positive emission tomography (PET) scanning is emphasized and contrasted with the anatomic imaging of magnetic resonance imaging (MRI) and computerized tomography (CT) by Chris Sackellares and Basel Abou-Khalil in Chapter 4.

All of the remaining chapters follow the pattern established in these first four chapters, and they emphasize the way in which newer diagnostic and treatment approaches can be put to best advantage by the primary care physician. Ed Dodson, Alan Troupin, David Treiman, and Svein Johannessen, and I in the next four chapters cover ground more familiar to most physicians. The latest concepts are stressed: Ed Dodson provides guidelines for the recognition of childhood epileptic syndromes, and he discusses the most effective therapeutic approaches to these

v

syndromes. My chapter stresses the rationale for selecting antiepileptic drugs (AEDs) in adults and discusses common management problems associated with AED use. Allan Troupin and Svein Johannessen then elaborate upon some of the unique problems of AED therapy in the elderly population and provide some new data about changing pharmacokinetics in this population. Lastly, David Treiman provides a unique approach to common diagnostic and treatment pitfalls.

Areas that frequently receive little attention in books on epilepsy include epilepsy surgery, psychosocial issues, and medical–legal problems. The role of surgery in the treatment of epilepsy is evolving, and surgery is no longer a treatment of last resort. Allen Wyler's chapter outlines criteria that can be used to assess the appropriateness of considering surgical therapy in individual patients, and it gives a broad overview of the evaluation process that is essential when surgery is considered. Psychosocial issues surrounding the patient with epilepsy are frequently ignored not only in textbooks but also in practice. The successful management of the patient with epilepsy may be mitigated if consideration of the psychosocial impact that the seizures and diagnosis of epilepsy have on the patient and his or her family and friends is ignored. In their chapter, Joseph Green and Rita Mercille emphasize the importance of early recognition of emotional and social problems and the effect that early intervention plays in the course of treatment. The chapter by Dietrich Blumer discusses the diagnosis and treatment of psychiatric problems associated with epilepsy. Medical–legal problems, particularly surrounding the controversy of violence associated with epilepsy, are covered by David Treiman. This is a problem that fortunately does not present frequently in clinical practice. However, when violence does occur, it can have a major impact. Thus, it is an area that needs to be understood well by anyone who treats patients with epilepsy.

We conclude this book with an overview of some of the recent advances in our understanding of the basic mechanisms of the epilepsies. The chapter by J. Kim Harris and Robert DeLorenzo explains the way in which new concepts in the treatment of epilepsy are being molded by new findings in the laboratory, and it emphasizes the clinical relevance of basic research.

The Appendix, written by Robert Gumnit, discusses the formation of the National Association for Epilepsy Centers (NAEC), and it presents the NAEC's "Recommended Guidelines for Diagnosis and Treatment."

This book, then, is not just another book on epilepsy. It is a book that emphasizes areas of diagnosis and treatment that are frequently minimized or ignored, and it attempts to demonstrate the importance and relevance to clinical practice of understanding some of the newer technologies in diagnosis and treatment—even if some of these technologies are not readily available in every community. It is our collective hope that this book will broaden the awareness of the primary care physician to the clinical usefulness of newer and less common diagnostic and treatment modalities in addition to providing a rationale for the use of contemporary treatment strategies.

Dennis B. Smith

Acknowledgments

I wish to acknowledge the contribution of Dr. Michael Wientraub to the creation of this book: It was through Dr. Wientraub's initial encouragement that the idea for this book was conceived. I also wish to thank the following people: my secretary, Ms. Bonnie Becker, for her support, skill, attention to detail, and, most importantly, patience and sense of humor, without which this book could not have been completed; Mr. Jeffrey Stier of Raven Press for his timely advice; Dr. John De-Toledo, not only for his direct contributions but also for giving me time to complete this project by helping with clinical duties; and Bonnie Smith, my wife, for support, encouragement, and for caring.

Dennis B. Smith

Section 2

1)
2)
3)
4)

Contributors

Bassel W. Abou-Khalil, M.D.   *Comprehensive Epilepsy Program, Department of Neurology, University of Michigan Medical Center, Ann Arbor, Michigan 48109*

Dietrich Blumer, M.D.   *Department of Psychiatry, University of Tennessee at Memphis, Memphis, Tennessee 38146*

James J. Cereghino, M.D.   *Epilepsy Branch, NIH NINDS DCDND, Bethesda, Maryland 20205*

Robert J. DeLorenzo, M.D., Ph.D., M.P.H.   *Department of Neurology, Medical College of Virginia, Richmond, Virginia 23298*

W. Edwin Dodson, M.D.   *Edward Mallinckrodt Professor of Neurology and Pediatrics, Division of Pediatric Neurology, Department of Pediatrics, St. Louis Children's Hospital, St. Louis, Missouri 63110*

Joseph B. Green, M.D.   *Department of Neurology, Texas Tech University Health Sciences Center, Lubbock, Texas 79430*

Robert J. Gumnit, M.D.   *National Association of Epilepsy Centers, Minneapolis, Minnesota 55416*

J. Kim Harris, M.D.   *Department of Neurology, Medical College of Virginia, Richmond, Virginia 23298*

Svein I. Johannessen, Ph.D.   *Director of Research, The National Center for Epilepsy, Sandvika, Norway*

Don W. King, M.D.   *Associate Professor of Neurology and Director, Georgia Comprehensive Epilepsy Program, Department of Neurology, Medical College of Georgia, Augusta, Georgia 30912*

Ronald E. Kramer, M.D.   *Oregon Comprehensive Epilepsy Program, Good Samaritan Hospital & Medical Center, Portland, Oregon 97210*

Rita A. Mercille, Ph.D.   *Department of Neurology, Texas Tech University Health Sciences Center, Lubbock, Texas 79430*

J. Chris Sackellares, M.D.   *Comprehensive Epilepsy Program, Department of Neurology, University of Michigan Medical Center, Ann Arbor, Michigan 48109*

Dennis B. Smith, M.D.   *Oregon Comprehensive Epilepsy Program, Good Samaritan Hospital & Medical Center, Department of Neurology, Oregon Health Sciences University, Portland, Oregon 97210*

David M. Treiman, M.D. *Neurology and Research Services, West Los Angeles Medical Center, and Department of Neurology, UCLA School of Medicine, Los Angeles, California 90073*

Allan S. Troupin, M.D. *Department of Neurology, Louisiana State University Medical School, New Orleans, Louisiana 70112*

Allen R. Wyler, M.D. *Department of Neurosurgery, University of Tennessee at Memphis, Memphis, Tennessee 38163; Semmes-Murphey Clinic, Memphis, Tennessee 38103; Director of Epilepsy Surgery, Baptist Memorial Hospital, Memphis, Tennessee 38103*

Epilepsy: Current Approaches to Diagnosis and Treatment,
edited by Dennis B. Smith,
Raven Press, Ltd., New York 1990.

1

Treatment Implications from Classification of Seizures and the Epilepsies

James J. Cereghino

Epilepsy Branch, NIH NINDS DCDND, Bethesda, Maryland 20205

Pooh looked at his two paws. He knew that one of them was right, and he knew that when you had decided which one of them was the right, then the other one was the left, but he never could remember how to begin.

> "The House at Pooh Corner"
> A. A. Milne (1)

Classification is never easy—be it right or left, big seizure or little seizure, or complex partial or absence seizure. Classification sounds simple enough—the act or result of arranging or organizing according to class or category. But the difficulty comes with the meaning of the words—how is the class or category to be defined? One must be careful not to become so preoccupied with the process of classification that the goal of using what is known about classification to help in the diagnosis and treatment of the patient is lost.

This chapter will review the available classification systems and will stress what is clinically useful from them.

HISTORICAL DEVELOPMENT OF CLASSIFICATIONS

Humans like to classify things. Just as epilepsy has been known since the beginning of recorded time, so have classification systems. Temkin (2) has documented early classification systems, which will not be reviewed here.

In 1905, William P. Spratling's presidential address to the Fifth Annual Meeting of the National Association for the Study of Epilepsy and the Care and Treatment of Epileptics (3) summarized treatment implications of seizure classification:

> It is an indisputable sign of scientific progress that the time has forever gone by when we can speak simply of "epilepsy" and particularly when we can say, "This man has epilepsy, give him some bromid."
>   We now make repeated and thorough physical, clinical and microscopic examinations of cases of epilepsy, to determine, if possible, *the cause or causes of the disease,*

1

before any treatment is applied; and we must now, perforce, speak of "the epilepsies" instead of "epilepsy," for the types and subdivisions of the disease are exceedingly numerous.

Fancy a surgeon applying a poultice to remove a splinter, or a lotion for the extraction of a piece of steel! So with epilepsy.

In Spratling's time, the epilepsies were divided into two large groups of disordered cerebral mechanisms:

1. epilepsies due to brain lesions (synonyms: symptomatic, organic, lesional, structural) and
2. epilepsies due to brain predisposition to seizures (synonyms: cryptogenic, genuine, idiopathic, essential, functional, genetic).

The distinction between these two types was on clinical grounds. Epilepsies due to brain lesions were thought to be associated with partial seizures, either alone or becoming secondarily generalized. Epilepsies due to brain predisposition were thought to be associated with generalized seizures—absence, myoclonic, or tonic–clonic without focal signs.

By the 1960s, these clinical concepts were challenged. It became recognized that epilepsies due to brain lesions could diffusely involve the brain, such as the encephalopathy of Lennox–Gastaut syndrome, rather than being restricted to focal anatomical brain lesions. Similarly, it became recognized that epilepsies due to brain predisposition could be associated with partial seizures, such as the rolandic spikes of benign childhood epilepsy, despite inability to demonstrate an anatomical brain lesion.

Merlis (4) succinctly summarized the problem:

> We can be reasonably sure that we know more about the epilepsies than was known fifty years ago, but the proliferation of nomenclature and terminology and the multiplicity of classifications of various types have made communication more and more labored and it is difficult indeed to define areas of agreement and to emerge with unifying concepts.
>
> Much of the difficulty is with language, with the meaning of words. The neurologist of today commonly speaks of "the epilepsies" rather than of "epilepsy" per se, but what is meant by this use of the plural term is frequently far from clear.

Merlis (4) listed some of the ways that had been used to classify the epilepsies:

1. seizure type and electroencephalogram (EEG),
2. etiology,
3. anatomicophysiological,
4. precipitant,
5. age of onset,
6. magnitude of seizure,
7. severity and chronicity,
8. body part,
9. sleep-waking cycle,

10. menstrual cycle, and
11. syndromes.

The need for a standardized and uniform system of grouping became apparent to both the clinician and the clinical researcher. With development of new antiepileptic drugs, better recognition of seizure patterns and epilepsy types could result in more specific, less toxic treatment. As patient populations suitable for participation in clinical research projects became more restricted, the necessity for comparability in reporting of data would be essential. Professor Henri Gastaut organized and spearheaded a movement within the International League Against Epilepsy (ILAE) to standardize terminology. Two meetings in the spring of 1964 resulted in a proposed scheme that avoided "so far as possible, both neologisms and too new or outrageous points of view" (5). The classification was published in *Epilepsia* (6) and mailed to neurologists worldwide for comment at the Joint Eighth International Neurological Congress, the Sixth International Congress of Electroencephalography and Clinical Neurophysiology, and the Tenth ILAE meeting held in Vienna in 1965. The Herculean task of summarizing the discussion from a neurophysiological basis fell to Ajmone-Marsan (7), who received instructions not "to criticize or look for possible weak aspects in the classification but rather to provide whatever 'objective bases' of a physiological nature may be available to support what has been elegantly defined as 'the product of a purely clinical cogitation by clinicians who did not want to rely on physiopathogenetic deductions.'" It is tribute to those who worked on the terminology issue that it was pushed forward and kept from being mired and discarded by debate. Further deliberation by the ILAE Commission on Terminology resulted in revised classifications of seizures and the epilepsies which were presented in September 1969 in New York at the Eleventh ILAE meeting (5,8,9) and which were subsequently published (10,11) in *Epilepsia*. Rapid development of technology for video display of seizures on magnetic tape, simultaneous recording of the electroencephalogram using hard-wired recording techniques, and radiotelemetry with split-screen display and instant replay capability then led to more objective means for studying epilepsy seizures, and two further Commissions on Classification and Terminology of the ILAE met to amend, update, and improve the classification with information obtained utilizing the new techniques. The revision was based upon the use of videotapes of simultaneously recorded electrical and clinical manifestations of epileptic seizures—the group was objective to the point of *excluding* everything on which no video documentation existed. The revised classification for epileptic seizures was published in *Epilepsia* (12) and was subsequently presented in September 1981 at the Thirteenth Epilepsy International Symposium in Kyoto, Japan. This is the currently used classification, but it must be stressed that it (a) does not represent a unanimity of views, (b) is weighted clinically, and (c) is not sacrosanct but is, instead, subject to continual revision.

Following publication of the 1981 Classification of Epileptic Seizures, the ILAE then turned its attention toward revising the earlier (11) classification of the epilepsies and epileptic syndromes. The ILAE Commission met on several occasions from

1981 to 1985, and at the September 1985 Sixteenth Epilepsy International Symposium it presented the schema, which was subsequently published in *Epilepsia* (13).

DEFINITION OF TERMS

Seizure: Attack of cerebral origin affecting a person in apparent good health or causing a sudden aggravation of a chronic pathological state. Such attacks consist of sudden and transitory abnormal phenomena of a motor, sensory, autonomic, or psychic nature resulting from transient dysfunction of part or all of the brain (14).

Epileptic seizure: A seizure resulting from an excessive neuronal discharge (14).

Consciousness: The degree of awareness and/or responsiveness of the patient to externally applied stimuli. *Responsiveness* refers to the ability of the patient to carry out simple commands or willed movement, and *awareness* refers to (a) the patient's contact with events during the period in question and (b) its recall (12).

Epilepsy: A chronic brain disorder of various etiologies characterized by recurrent seizures due to excessive discharge of cerebral neurons (epileptic seizures), associated with a variety of clinical and laboratory manifestations (14).

Epileptic syndrome: An epileptic disorder characterized by a cluster of signs and symptoms customarily occurring together. The signs and symptoms may be clinical, or findings may be detected by ancillary studies. In contradistinction to a disease, a syndrome does not necessarily have a common etiology and prognosis. Some epileptic syndromes, however, are of great prognostic importance (13).

CLINICAL APPLICATION

The classifications of epileptic seizures and epileptic syndromes are useful for diagnosing and treating the individual patient. Each epileptic seizure is a definable event—one that can be described, measured, recorded, and classified. The seizure history focuses on a description of each patient's seizure or seizures (many patients have more than one seizure type) obtained from both the patient and witnesses. Diagnosing (i.e., classifying) the patient's seizure type(s) will, in some instances, indicate whether a defined etiology will emerge, and it will provide the single largest clue in determining the correct therapeutic approach. The clinical description of the seizure and ictal and interictal electroencephalographic findings are used to determine the seizure type.

Despite the usefulness of diagnosing the seizure type, the ultimate goal is to diagnose (i.e., classify) the patient's epileptic syndrome. The syndrome delineates the cluster of signs and symptoms (e.g., etiology, age, prognosis) customarily occurring together and provides the clinician with a likelihood of the prognosis, degree of seizure control, and duration of therapy. Now that the classifications are available, the patient should benefit as physicians (a) grasp the concept of the seizure type and (b) obtain a more fundamental understanding of the syndrome in which the seizures occur.

An analogy from pulmonary medicine is used frequently by the epilepsy community to explain the differences between epilepsy and seizures. A patient presents with pneumonia. A decision must be made as to whether it is of viral or bacterial etiology and, if bacterial, which antibiotic should be selected for treatment (analogous to determining seizure type and which antiepileptic drug to select). Simultaneously, however, the patient must be explored for an underlying etiology, such as lung cancer or tuberculosis, which underlies the pneumonia (analogous to diagnosing epilepsy—the etiology determining prognosis).

CLASSIFICATION OF EPILEPTIC SEIZURES

The description of the seizure by the patient or observer is currently the most important part of patient evaluation. Our patients are routinely asked to have someone who has witnessed a seizure accompany them to the clinic and/or to ask people who have seen the seizure(s) to provide a description. Patients are asked to come prepared to discuss their seizures—when they first began, what types of seizures occur, how often the seizures occur, whether the seizures have changed since they first started, whether the seizure frequency has changed, and the medications that have been tried (the dosage, for how long, what effect they had on the seizures, and the side effects).

The seizure diagnosis can often be made from the history alone. It may require considerable time to obtain the seizure history. Particular attention should be paid to the onset, the pattern of the seizure, and the postictal state.

The first decision in the diagnosis of seizure type is whether to classify the seizure as a partial seizure or as a generalized seizure. Partial seizures have clinical and/or electroencephalographic evidence of a local onset. The abnormal discharge arises from a part of one cerebral hemisphere; however, it need not be from a discrete focus, and it may spread to involve the rest of the brain. A generalized seizure has no clinical and/or electroencephalographic evidence of a local onset, since the first clinical or electroencephalographic changes indicate initial involvement of both hemispheres.

Partial seizures are divided into three groups (see Table 1): (A) simple partial seizures, (B) complex partial seizures, and (C) partial seizures secondarily generalized.

Consciousness is *not* impaired with simple partial seizures. These seizures may be with (1) motor signs, (2) autonomic symptoms or signs (e.g., pallor, sweating, flushing), (3) somatosensory or special sensory symptoms (e.g., tingling, light flashes, buzzing), or (4) psychic symptoms (e.g., fear, déjà vu, forced thinking but *without* impairment of consciousness).

In many patients, a simple partial seizure will progress to a complex partial seizure. In most patients, only one hemisphere is involved, but there is a report of both hemispheres being involved simultaneously with sparing of consciousness (15). Postictal paralysis (Todd's paralysis) is a not infrequent accompaniment of simple partial seizures with motor signs.

TABLE 1. *Classification of seizures*

I. Partial (focal, local) seizures
   A. Simple partial seizures (consciousness not impaired)
      1. With motor signs
         a. Focal motor without march
         b. Focal motor with march (jacksonian)
         c. Versive
         d. Postural
         e. Phonatory (vocalization or arrest of speech)
      2. With autonomic symptoms or signs (including epigastric sensation, pallor, sweating, flushing, piloerection, and pupillary dilatation)
      3. With somatosensory or special-sensory symptoms
         a. Somatosensory
         b. Visual
         c. Auditory
         d. Olfactory
         e. Gustatory
         f. Vertiginous
      4. With psychic symptoms (disturbance of higher cerebral function)
         a. Dysphasic
         b. Dysmnesic (e.g., déjà vu)
         c. Cognitive (e.g., dreamy states, distortions of time sense)
         d. Affective (e.g., fear, anger)
         e. Illusions (e.g., macropsia)
         f. Structured hallucinations (e.g., music, scenes)
   B. Complex partial seizures (with impairment of consciousness)
      1. Simple partial onset followed by impairment of consciousness
         a. With simple partial features (A.1–A.4) followed by impaired consciousness
         b. With automatisms
      2. With impairment of consciousness at onset
         a. With impairment of consciousness only
         b. With automatisms
   C. Partial seizures evolving to secondarily generalized seizures
      (This may be generalized tonic–clonic, tonic, or clonic)
      1. Simple partial seizures (A) evolving to generalized seizures
      2. Complex partial seizures (B) evolving to generalized seizures
      3. Simple partial seizures evolving to complex partial seizures evolving to generalized seizures
II. Generalized seizures (convulsive or nonconvulsive)
   A. 1. Absence seizures
         a. Impairment of consciousness only
         b. With mild clonic components
         c. With atonic components
         d. With tonic components
         e. With automatisms
         f. With autonomic components (b through f may be used alone or in combination)
      2. Atypical absence
   B. Myoclonic seizures
      Myoclonic jerks (single or multiple)
   C. Clonic seizures
   D. Tonic seizures
   E. Tonic–clonic seizures
   F. Atonic seizures (astatic—combinations of the above may occur, e.g., B and F, B and D)
III. Unclassified epileptic seizures

Clinical Types of Simple Partial Seizures

1. *With motor signs.* Any portion of the body may be involved, depending on the site of origin in the motor strip. Seizures may remain relatively restricted to a part of the body, such as the arm, leg, or face, or may spread to involve the whole side of the body. If the seizure spreads to contiguous cortical areas and produces a sequential involvement of body parts (a "march"), this is then called a "jacksonian seizure." Consciousness is not impaired—the patient is aware of the seizure. Other focal motor seizures may involve (a) versive head turning to one side, (b) atonicity or sudden loss of function, or (c) speech arrest or vocalization. As a rule, partial seizures with motor signs are brief, lasting from a few seconds to a few minutes. The exception is epilepsia partialis continua, which may persist from hours to years. There may be a localized paralysis—known as Todd's paralysis—in the parts involved in the seizure which may last from minutes to hours.

2. *With autonomic symptoms.* Pupil dilatation is probably the most common autonomic phenomenon seen in partial seizures. Other phenomena include vomiting, pallor, flushing, sweating, piloerection, borborygmi, and incontinence. Recurrent abdominal discomfort and vomiting in children may be a seizure and presents a particular diagnostic dilemma. Incongruous laughter (gelastic seizures) may occur. Seizures may also present as (a) "goose bumps" or piloerection, (b) unilateral body color changes, or (c) an uncontrollable gush of saliva.

3. *With somatosensory or special-sensory symptoms.* These seizures may arise anywhere in the sensory cortex. Paresthesias (pins and needles, a feeling of numbness) are the most common symptoms. A feeling of distortion of body parts may occur. Pain as a symptom is relatively rare. The thumb, forefinger, and face are the most likely sites of origin, probably due to their larger cortical representation. These seizures may also spread or "march."

Special sensory phenomena may involve olfaction, gustation, hearing and balance, or vision. Olfactory sensations, usually described as unpleasant or disagreeable, are frequently a warning of an underlying neoplasm. These seizures may be followed by motor symptoms and frequently progress to complex partial seizures. Gustatory hallucinations are usually described as a metallic taste. Auditory seizures are usually described as crude auditory noises (e.g., hissing or high-pitched noise) or may be organized in a melody. Vertiginous seizures, while rare, have been described and include sensations of falling and floating. Visual seizures vary in elaborateness, depending on the anatomical origin. In seizures originating in the primary visual cortex, symptoms are unstructured (e.g., bright or colored scintillating lights). These seizures are commonly seen in patients with porencephaly in the distribution of the posterior cerebral artery. In seizures originating in the visual association areas, structured visual hallucinatory phenomena, such as scenes or persons, may occur.

4. *With psychic symptoms.* Psychic symptoms rarely occur without impairment of consciousness and are more commonly seen as complex partial seizures.

However, perceptual distortions and feelings of fear or other emotions may occur as the only manifestation of a seizure.

Clinical Types of Complex Partial Seizures

Complex partial seizures are divided into two categories:

1. Simple partial seizure onset followed by impaired consciousness with or without automatisms.
2. Impairment of consciousness at onset with or without automatisms.

An automatism is a more or less coordinated involuntary motor activity occurring during a state of impaired consciousness. Automatisms are not specific to a seizure type, and they may occur in partial or generalized seizures. For convenience, they will be discussed here. Penry and Dreifuss (16), studying absence seizures, have described two types of automatisms:

1. Perseverative automatisms—a continuation of activity initiated before the alteration in consciousness.
2. *De novo* automatisms—an activity started during the course of a seizure that may be regarded as "reactive" to internal or external environmental stimuli.

Automatisms have some localization significance. The following automatisms have been described:

1. Eating automatisms—a variety of oroalimentary movements, including chewing, swallowing, and lip and tongue smacking.
2. Mimicry automatisms—an expression of emotional state, usually fear but occasionally anxiety, anger, or joy.
3. Gestural automatisms—crude or elaborate movements ranging from stereotyped hand movements, such as fumbling or scratching, to quasi-purposeful activities, such as piano playing.
4. Ambulatory automatisms—includes walking, driving, or riding a bicycle. The patients may find themselves in unexpected places.
5. Verbal automatisms—may be stereotyped, repetitive utterances in response to a stimulus.

Although automatisms are frequent in complex partial seizures, they do occur in other seizure types. In recent years, the distinction between absence seizures with automatisms and complex partial seizures with automatisms has been stressed because of the ease with which the two can be clinically mistaken and because of the markedly different treatments. The EEG is of importance in the distinction, as is a precise descriptive history of the seizures, the age of the patient, the presence or absence of an aura, and the postictal behavior, which may or may not have confusion.

The ictal electroencephalographic expression of complex partial seizures is a unilateral or frequently bilateral discharge, diffuse or focal in temporal or frontotemporal regions. The interictal electroencephalographic expression of complex partial seizures is a unilateral or bilateral generally asynchronous focus, usually in the temporal or frontal regions.

Postictal amnesia usually follows the automatisms seen in complex partial seizures. The patient may be confused and make inappropriate responses to the environment and be disoriented with regard to place or time or person.

An aura is that portion of the seizure which occurs before consciousness is lost and for which memory is retained afterwards. An aura may be a simple partial seizure alone or may be the initial event described by the patient in a simple partial seizure progressing to a complex partial seizure.

Partial Seizures Evolving to Secondarily Generalized Seizures

Partial seizures may evolve to generalized seizures—tonic–clonic, tonic, or clonic. Simultaneous video and electroencephalographic recordings have documented the progression possibilities:

1. simple partial → complex partial,
2. complex partial → generalized, and
3. simple partial → complex partial → generalized.

The fragmentary partial seizures sometimes seen after a generalized tonic–clonic seizure have not been well described or classified.

Clinical Types of Generalized Seizures

Generalized seizures have clinical symptoms compatible with initial involvement of both hemispheres. Consciousness is impaired, and this may be the first manifestation of the seizure. Motor manifestations are bilateral.

The terms *convulsive* and *nonconvulsive* have been used but are not well defined. The convulsive seizures are those with tonic, clonic, tonic–clonic, or myoclonic contraction. The nonconvulsive seizures, while they may have mild clonic or tonic components, are not characterized by the muscular contractions. In the 1964 version of the classification, *nonconvulsive* referred only to absence seizures.

The major types of generalized seizures are:

1. absence,
2. myoclonic,
3. clonic,
4. tonic,
5. tonic–clonic, and
6. atonic.

The generalized tonic–clonic seizure (grand mal) is characterized by loss of consciousness, without or with only vague premonitory symptoms. There is a sudden, sharp, tonic contraction of muscles. A cry or moan may ensue as a result of involvement of respiratory muscles. The patient usually falls and lies rigid. Respiratory muscles may be in a tonic state leading to cyanosis. Tongue biting and incontinence may occur. Clonic convulsive movements follow the tonic stage—the patient usually remains cyanotic during this stage, and saliva may froth from the mouth. Deep respiration and relaxation of all the muscles occurs at the end of this stage. The patient remains unconscious for a variable period of time, may feel sore and stiff, and frequently goes into a deep sleep. On awakening, there may be complaints of a headache or muscle soreness.

Absence seizures are characterized by sudden onset. Ongoing activities may be interrupted, and there is a blank stare and possibly a brief upward rotation of the eyes. The patient will usually be unresponsive when spoken to; in some cases, however, speaking to the patient will abort the attack. The attacks are of short duration, recur many, many times during the day, and stop suddenly, almost never having a postictal change. Absence seizures may be typical or atypical.

Typical absence seizures are further subclassified as:

1. With impairment of consciousness only—a simple absence seizure.
2. With mild clonic components—varying in intensity from almost imperceptible to generalized myoclonic jerks, frequently presenting as clonic movements of the eyelids or corner of the mouth.
3. With atonic components—a diminution in tone of muscles may lead to drooping of the head, slumping of the trunk, relaxation of grip, or dropping of the arms. Falling rarely occurs.
4. With tonic components—tonic muscular contraction may occur, thereby affecting flexor or extensor muscles symmetrically or asymmetrically. The head may be drawn back, or the trunk may arch.
5. With automatisms—elaborate automatisms may occur, and these may lead to confusion with other seizure types.

Atypical absences may clinically have changes in tone that are more pronounced than in absence seizures, and the onset and/or cessation may not be abrupt. The ictal EEG may be more heterogeneous and may include irregular spike-and-slow-wave complexes, fast activity, or other paroxysmal activity. Abnormalities are bilateral but are often irregular and asymmetrical. The interictal EEG usually has an abnormal background activity. Paroxysmal activity, such as spikes or spike-and-slow-wave complexes, is frequently irregular and asymmetrical.

Myoclonic seizures are clinically seen as sudden, brief, shock-like contractions which may be generalized or confined to the face, trunk, or one or more extremities—or even to individual muscles or groups of muscles—and which, by definition, are accompanied by alteration in consciousness. They may be regularly or rapidly repetitive or may be relatively isolated. The patient may indicate in the history that they occur while going to sleep or while awakening. Myoclonic jerks exacerbated by volitional movement are called *action myoclonus*. Myoclonic jerks of myoclonus due to spinal cord disease, dyssynergia cerebellaris myoclonica, subcortical segmental myoclonus, paramyoclonus multiplex, and opsoclonus–myoclonus syndromes are not classified as epileptic seizures.

Clonic seizures lack the tonic component of generalized tonic–clonic seizures. Some generalized seizures may begin with a clonic phase; hence, the designation "clonic–tonic–clonic" seizure.

The clinical description of tonic seizures by Gowers is classic and has been chosen by the Commission (12) as a description:

> . . . a rigid, violent muscular contraction, fixing the limbs in some strained position. There is usually deviation of the eyes and of the head toward one side, and this may amount to rotation involving the whole body (sometimes actually causing the patient to turn around, even two or three times). The features are distorted; the color of the face, unchanged at first, rapidly becomes pale and then flushed and ultimately livid as the fixation of the chest by the spasms stops the movements of respiration. The eyes are open or closed; the conjuctiva is insensitive; the pupils dilate widely as cyanosis comes on. As the spasm continues, it commonly changes in its relative intensity in different parts, causing slight alterations in the position of the limbs.

Atonic seizures are clinically characterized by a sudden diminution in muscle tone—leading to a head drop, dropping of a limb, or slumping to the ground. "Drop attacks" may be extremely brief and may produce physical injury.

CLASSIFICATION OF EPILEPSIES AND EPILEPTIC SYNDROMES

To reiterate, a well-taken history—which may be lengthy and involve obtaining information from several family members—is the key factor in identifying a patient's seizure or seizure types. In reality, most patients have a relatively restricted number of seizure types, but there may be variations in the pattern of a particular seizure type. This is particularly true in patients with simple partial seizures that progress to complex partial seizures that, in turn, progress to generalized tonic–clonic seizures, where what at first may appear to be several different seizure types is in fact a part of a single seizure type. A careful history can usually determine the individual patient's pattern. In some cases the description of the seizures remains inadequate, and intensive monitoring (i.e., simultaneous video and electroencephalographic recording) will be needed to make the correct seizure diagnosis.

With the seizure type(s) defined, attention can then be turned to diagnosing (classifying) the syndrome. The ILAE Commission (13) defined a syndrome as "an epileptic disorder characterized by a cluster of signs and symptoms customarily occurring together. The signs and symptoms may be clinical (e.g., case history, seizure type, modes of seizure recurrence, and neurological and psychological findings) or findings detected by ancillary studies (e.g., EEG, x-ray, CT, and NMR). In contradistinction to a disease, a syndrome does not necessarily have a common etiology and prognosis. Some epileptic syndromes, however, are of great prognostic importance." The terminology may sound stilted in the classification of the epilepsies. In translating words from language to language, the problem of common usage or connotations occurs, and, as a result, a word with a common translation needs to be substituted.

To date, the main clinical advantage for the epilepsy classification has been that it has called to the attention of American clinicians the syndromes which have been described by our European colleagues but which have not been widely recognized in the United States. Some of the distinctions between the syndromes seem blurred; in some cases, important data are simply not present. Nevertheless, even this early identification of syndromes is providing clues with regard to improved treatment and with regard to our ability to assist the patient and their families in planning for long-term prognosis.

In classifying the epilepsies, the first step is to separate epilepsies with generalized seizures (generalized epilepsies) from epilepsies with partial or focal seizures (localization-related epilepsies). The second step is to separate epilepsies of known etiology from those that are idiopathic or cryptogenic (see Table 2).

Localization-Related Epilepsies and Syndromes

The localization-related epilepsies and syndromes (these are the ones with partial seizures) are presently divided into two categories: (i) idiopathic with age-related syndromes and (ii) symptomatic.

Idiopathic with Age-Related Onset

Two idiopathic, age-related, localization-related syndromes are currently recognized. These are clinically important to diagnose because in one of these syndromes, the seizures are subject to spontaneous remission. The two syndromes are (i) benign childhood epilepsy with centrotemporal spikes and (ii) childhood epilepsy with occipital paroxysms.

Benign Childhood Epilepsy with Centrotemporal Spikes

Seizures in this syndrome are brief partial motor seizures, frequently associated with somatosensory symptoms and not infrequently evolving to generalized tonic–clonic seizures. Seizures are often related to sleep. Onset is between 3 and 13 years of age with spontaneous remission of seizures before age 15–16. A family history and male predominance frequently occur. The EEG has blunt high-voltage centrotemporal spikes often followed by slow waves activated by sleep and tending to spread or shift from side to side.   *independent*

Case Example: Nine-year-old male with onset of numbness of right cheek followed by right facial twitching of less than a minute duration, usually occurring just before brushing of teeth in the morning. One generalized tonic–clonic seizure 6 months ago. Neurological and mental status exams normal. Paternal cousin with

TABLE 2. *International classification of epilepsies and epileptic syndromes*

1. Localization-related (focal, local, partial) epilepsies and syndromes
    1.1. Idiopathic with age-related onset
          At present, two syndromes are established, but more may be identified in the future:
          • Benign childhood epilepsy with centrotemporal spike
          • Childhood epilepsy with occipital paroxysms
    1.2. Symptomatic
          This category comprises syndromes of great individual variability, which will mainly
          be based on anatomical localization, clinical features, seizure types, and etiological
          factors (if known). Major examples are:
          • Frontal lobe epilepsies
             • Supplementary motor
             • Cingulate
             • Anterior (polar) frontal region
             • Orbitofrontal
             • Dorsolateral
             • Motor cortex
          • Temporal lobe epilepsies
             • Hippocampal (mesiobasal limbic or primary rhinencephalic)
             • Amygdalar (anterior polar–amygdalar)
             • Lateral posterior temporal
             • Opercular (insular)
          • Parietal lobe epilepsies
          • Occipital lobe epilepsies
2. Generalized epilepsies and syndromes
    2.1. Idiopathic, with age-related onset, listed in order of age
          • Benign neonatal familial convulsions
          • Benign neonatal convulsions
          • Benign myoclonic epilepsy in infancy
          • Childhood absence epilepsy (pyknolepsy)
          • Juvenile absence epilepsy
          • Juvenile myoclonic epilepsy (impulsive petit mal)
          • Epilepsy with grand mal seizures (GTCS) on awakening
          Other generalized idiopathic epilepsies, if they do not belong to one of the above
          syndromes, can still be classified as generalized idiopathic epilepsies.
    2.2. Idiopathic and/or symptomatic, in order of age of appearance
          • West syndrome (infantile spasms, Blitz–Nick–Salaam Krampfe)
          • Lennox–Gastaut syndrome
          • Epilepsy with myoclonic–astatic seizures
          • Epilepsy with myoclonic absences
    2.3. Symptomatic
          2.3.1. Nonspecific etiology
                  • Early myoclonic encephalopathy
          2.3.2. Specific syndromes
                  • Epileptic seizures may complicate many disease states
                  Included under this heading are those diseases in which seizures are a pre-
                  senting or predominant feature
3. Epilepsies and syndromes undetermined as to whether they are focal or generalized
    3.1. With both generalized and focal seizures
          • Neonatal seizures
          • Severe myoclonic epilepsy in infancy
          • Epilepsy with continuous spike waves during slow-wave sleep
          • Acquired epileptic aphasia (Landau–Kleffner syndrome)
    3.2. Without unequivocal generalized or focal features
          This heading covers all cases with GTCS where clinical and electroencephalographic
          findings do not permit classification as clearly generalized or localization-related, such
          as in many cases of sleep grand mal.
4 Special syndromes
    4.1. Situation-related seizures (Gelegenheitsanfalle)
          • Febrile convulsions
          • Seizures related to other identifiable situations such as stress, hormonal changes,
            drugs, alcohol, or sleep deprivation
    4.2. Isolated, apparently unprovoked epileptic events
    4.3. Epilepsies characterized by specific modes of seizure precipitation
    4.4. Chronic progressive epilepsia partialis continua of childhood

similar episodes. During episodes, EEG shows blunt high-voltage centrotemporal spikes. Seizure diagnosis: simple partial seizure with somatosensory symptoms and with motor signs. Epilepsy diagnosis: idiopathic localization and age-related epilepsy. The epilepsy classification will eliminate the need for further diagnostic tests and, perhaps, for antiepileptic drug therapy, and it will allow a prediction that seizures will stop as the child grows older.

Childhood Epilepsy with Occipital Paroxysms

The seizures in this syndrome often start with visual symptoms and are accompanied by motor signs and automatisms. Seizures are followed by migrainous headache in about a quarter of the cases. The EEG has paroxysms of high-amplitude spike waves or sharp waves recurring rhythmically in the occipital and posterior temporal areas of one or both hemispheres but only when the eyes are closed. During seizures, the occipital discharge may spread to the central or temporal region. Prognosis is uncertain, but the seizures frequently cease in adult life.

Case Example: Ten-year-old female with loss of vision lasting about 30 minutes. Sometimes twitching of the mouth on the left occurs during the episode. Frequently occur on bright sunny days when she has been out playing and is called back into the house by her mother. Followed by a diffuse headache. Normal neurological and ophthalmologic exams. Mental status normal. Family history of migraine. Interictal EEGs show bilateral synchronous or asynchronous occipital–posterotemporal spike waves on closure of the eyes. Psychogenic etiology considered as diagnosis prior to EEG. Seizure diagnosis: simple partial seizures with visual symptoms. Epilepsy diagnosis: idiopathic localization and age-related epilepsy. Treatment with valproate resulted in complete control of seizures. Since many of these seizures do not persist past adolescence, patient will need to be reevaluated.

Symptomatic

The symptomatic localization-related epilepsies comprise a large variety of syndromes with great individual variability. Anatomical localization, clinic features, seizure type, and known etiological factors are considered. The ILAE Commission has identified the varieties of symptomatic localization-related epilepsies according to anatomical localization. Much of the data have been collected from depth electrode studies, thus representing a highly selected minority of patients. The descriptions are useful, even though they may for an individual patient be difficult to apply. The varieties are:

1. Frontal lobe epilepsies characterized by frequent, short seizures with minimal or no postictal confusion. These are often mistaken for psychogenic seizures. Status epilepticus is particularly frequent. The seizures may be characterized by anatomical area:

a. *Supplementary motor*. Simple partial seizures with postural, simple focal tonic, phonatory (vocalization or speech arrest), fencing, and complex partial with urinary incontinence. Psychological testing may show impaired verbal fluency (dominant hemisphere) or impaired design fluency (nondominant hemisphere). Ictal EEG shows flattening, rhythmic polyspikes (16–24 Hz), and secondary generalization. Common etiologies are tumors, focal atrophy, and arteriovenous malformations.

b. *Cingulate*. Complex partial seizures with initial automatisms with sexual features, vegetative signs, change in mood and affect, and urinary incontinence. Depth electrode studies are virtually mandatory for diagnosis.

c. *Anterior (polar) frontal region*. Seizure patterns include initial loss of contact, adversive and subsequent contraversive movements of head and eyes, axial clonic jerks and falls, and autonomic signs frequently evolving to generalized tonic–clonic seizures.

d. *Orbitofrontal*. Complex partial seizure pattern with initial olfactory hallucinations or initial automatisms, autonomic signs, and urination. Ictal EEG shows flattening, rhythmic polyspikes (16–24 Hz), and secondary generalization. Common etiologies are trauma, astrocytomas, and oligodendrogliomas. Nasoethmoidal and orbital electrodes may aid in diagnosis.

e. *Dorsolateral*. Simple partial seizures with motor signs (tonic, versive, phonatory) and complex partial seizures with initial automatisms. Surface EEGs may show focus. Frequently reported psychological findings include perseveration, poor judgment, and disinhibition. Astrocytomas, trauma, or oligodendrogliomas are common etiologies.

f. *Motor cortex epilepsies*. Simple partial seizures with symptoms depending on side and topography. For example: lower prerolandic area may have speech arrest, vocalization, and contralateral tonic–clonic facial movements; paracentral lobule may have contralateral leg movements and tonic movements of ipsilateral foot; and rolandic area may have motor seizures with march.

2. Temporal lobe epilepsies are characterized by complex partial seizures, and the ILAE Commission has further characterized them by anatomical area:

a. *Hippocampal (mesiobasal limbic or primary rhinencephalic psychomotor)*. Comprises 70–80% of temporal lobe epilepsies and commonly seen with amygdalar epilepsy. Seizures occur in clusters at intervals or randomly; they may start with strange, indescribable feelings, experiential hallucinations, or interpretative illusions, followed by arrest (motionless stare) and oral and alimentary automatisms. Average duration of 2 min. May evolve to generalized tonic–clonic seizures. Interictal EEG typically may show anterior temporal sharp waves, especially during sleep. Ictal EEG typically shows initial unilateral flattening, especially in temporal lobe. Nonspecific changes of background activity or nonfocal, even nonlateralizing, surface changes may occur, as well as focal, lateralized, or bilateral 4- to 6-Hz sharp waves. Stereo EEG may reveal high-frequency (16–28 Hz) low-voltage spikes building up in one hippocampus propagating to ipsilateral amygdala and cingulate gyrus but also to contralateral mesiobasal structures. Psychological investigations may reveal impaired learning and memory (verbal or nonverbal, depending on dominant or nondominant hemisphere foci). The most common pathological finding is incisural or hippocampal sclerosis and, less frequently, gangliogliomas, hamartomas, arteriovenous malformations, astrocytomas, and oligodendrogliomas.

b. *Amygdalar (anterior polar–amygdalar).* Seizures are characterized by rising epigastric discomfort, nausea, marked autonomic signs, and other symptoms, including borborygmi, belching, pallor, fullness of face, flushing of face, arrest of respiration, pupillary dilatation, fear, panic, and olfactory–gustatory hallucinations. Onset of unconsciousness is gradual, followed by staring, oral and alimentary automatisms, and confusion. About 30% are associated with generalized tonic–clonic seizures of focal onset. Rapid eye movement (REM) sleep facilitates amygdalar spiking. Surface electroencephalographic findings are similar in hippocampal epilepsy, and stereo EEG reveals high-frequency low-amplitude 16- to 28-Hz rhythms in amygdala or amygdala and anterior temporal pole, with spread to hypothalamus, homolateral fronto-orbital regions, and hippocampal formation, as well as to contralateral homologous areas. Common etiologies are gangliogliomas, small gliomas, atypical cell layers in amygdala (and hippocampal formation), anterior temporal pole gliosis, arteriovenous malformations, hamartomas, and traumas with focal gliosis.

c. *Lateral posterior temporal.* Seizures are characterized by auras of auditory hallucinations, visual perceptual hallucinations, or language disorder when the language-dominant hemisphere is the site of the focus. These are followed by dysphasia, disturbed orientation or prolonged auditory hallucinations, head movement to one side, and sometimes staring automatisms. Surface EEG shows bilateral midtemporal or posterior temporal spikes, and stereo EEG shows low-frequency rapid spikes (16–28 Hz) building up in the supramarginal angular gyrus and posterior temporal regions. Stepwise involvement of anterior temporal and mesiobasal limbic structures is frequent. The most common etiologies are trauma with focal gliosis, gliomas, arteriovenous malformations, or as sequelae of inflammations or cerebral infarctions.

d. *Opercular (insular).* Seizures may be characterized by vestibular or acoustic hallucinations, borborygmi, belching, autonomic signs, or by unilateral face twitching or paresthesia. Olfactory–gustatory hallucinations may occur. EEG and stereo EEG reveal opercular rapid spikes (16–28 Hz), often with minimal spread. Common etiologies are arteriovenous malformations, gliomas, astrocytomas, venous angioma, and scars from cerebral infarction.

3. Parietal lobe epilepsies are characterized by simple partial sensory seizures. The patient may describe a variety of phenomena. Positive phenomena consist

of tingling and a feeling of electricity, which may be confined or may spread in a jacksonian manner. There may be a desire to move a body part, or there may be a sensation as if a part were being moved. The parts most frequently involved are those with the largest cortical representation (e.g., the hand, arm, and face). There may be tongue sensations of crawling, stiffness, or coldness, and facial sensory phenomena may occur bilaterally. Occasionally an intra-abdominal sensation of sinking, choking, or nausea may occur, particularly in cases of inferior and lateral parietal lobe involvement. Rarely, there may be pain, and this may take the form of a superficial burning dysesthesia or a vague, very severe, episodic painful sensation. Parietal lobe visual phenomena may occur as photophasias or as hallucinations of a formed variety, including colors and animal shapes. Metamorphopsia with distortions, foreshortenings, and elongations may occur; this is more frequently seen with nondominant hemisphere discharges. Negative phenomena include numbness, feeling as if a body part were absent, and a loss of awareness of a part or a half of the body (asomatognosia), particularly in right-sided attacks. Severe vertigo may indicate suprasylvian parietal lobe seizures. Posterior left parietal seizures result in a variety of receptive or conductive speech disturbances. A rare sensory disturbance with involvement of the paracentral lobule involves both lower extremities. The EEG of parietal lobe epilepsy shows appropriately localized sharp wave discharges. Seizures of the paracentral lobule area have a tendency to become secondarily generalized.

4. Occipital lobe epilepsy has simple partial seizures with visual symptoms or with psychic symptoms. The patient may describe a variety of phenomena. Elementary visual seizures are characterized by fleeting visual manifestations (paropsia), which may be either negative (scotoma, hemianopsia, amaurosis) or, more commonly, positive (sparks or flashes, phosphenes). Such sensation appears in the visual field contralateral to the discharging lesion in the specific visual cortex but can spread to the whole visual field. Perceptive illusions, in which the objects appear to be distorted, may occur, such as: polyoptic illusion (monocular diplopia); dysmetropsic illusions [a change in size (macropsia or micropsia) or change in distance (macroproxiopia or microtelepsia)]; plagiopsic illusions (inclination of objects in a given plane of space); dysmorphopsic illusion (distortion of objects); or a sudden change of shape (metamorphopsia). Visual hallucinatory seizures are occasionally characterized by complex visual perceptions (e.g., colorful scenes of varying complexity). In some cases the scene is distorted or made smaller, and in rare instances the subject sees his own image (autoscopy). Such illusional and hallucinatory visual seizures result from epileptic discharge in the temporal–occipital cortex. The initial signs may also include the following: clonic and/or tonic contraversion of eyes and head or eyes only (oculoclonic or oculogyric deviation); palpebral jerks; and forced closure of eyelids. The following may occur at the onset of seizures: sensation of ocular oscillation or of the whole body; vertiginous sensation (environment tipping); and tinnitus along with headache or migraine. The discharge may

spread to the temporal lobe, producing seizure manifestations of either lateral posterior temporal, hippocampal, or amygdalar epilepsies. When the primary focus is located in the supracalcarine area, the discharge can spread forward on the suprasylvian convexity or the mesial surface, mimicking that of parietal lobe or supplementary motor epilepsy. There is an occasional tendency to become secondarily generalized.

Generalized Epilepsies and Syndromes

The generalized epilepsies have been divided into three categories. The basic distinction at this level of the ILAE classification is between idiopathic syndromes with age-related onset and symptomatic syndromes. The third category of idiopathic and/or symptomatic generalized epilepsies includes syndromes where both idiopathic and symptomatic causes of a syndrome have been identified (e.g., West syndrome), as well as syndromes where it is unclear whether they are idiopathic or symptomatic.

Idiopathic Age-Related Onset Generalized Epilepsies

Seizures are initially generalized. Ictal EEG shows a generalized, bilateral, synchronous, symmetrical discharge. Interictal EEG usually shows normal background activity and generalized discharges. The discharges may be increased by slow sleep. The following syndromes have been identified:

1. *Benign neonatal familial convulsions.* A rare, dominantly inherited disorder of clonic or apneic seizures manifests usually on day 2 or 3 of life. No specific EEG criteria. Outcome is usually favorable, but about 14% of patients may later develop another epilepsy.

2. *Benign neonatal convulsions.* Frequently repeated clonic or apneic seizures occurring usually on the fifth day of life, with no family history. Interictal EEG may show alternating sharp theta waves (theta-pointu alternant). Psychomotor development is normal, and there is no recurrence of seizures.

3. *Benign myoclonic epilepsy in infancy.* Seizures are brief bursts of generalized myoclonus appearing in the first 2 years of life. The parents describe "spasms" or "head nodding" and frequently seek help about the time the child learns to stand or walk because of falling. EEG shows brief bursts of generalized spike waves occurring in early stages of sleep. If left untreated, the seizures may persist to midchildhood. The seizures are easily controlled with treatment—valproate is currently recommended as the drug of first choice. Generalized tonic–clonic seizures may occur in adolescence. There appears to be an unfavorable psychological prognosis, with many of these patients having (a) a relative delay of intellectual development and (b) personality disorders.

4. *Childhood absence epilepsy (pyknolepsy).* This is the best known and most frequently occurring of the absence epilepsies. Absence seizures of any type occur

before the onset of puberty (range 3–12 years, peak 6–7 years). Girls are affected more frequently, there appears to be a genetic predisposition, and the child is otherwise normal. Treatment of first choice is currently valproate, which is believed to be active for both the absence seizure and tonic–clonic seizure. The long-term prognosis is one of the most frequently asked questions by parents. Unfortunately, the answers are not yet clear-cut. There are three alternatives:

a. Patients become seizure-free. Approximately 80% of patients become seizure-free with treatment. But, with long-term follow-up, the percentage of controlled patients decreases—perhaps to as low as 30%—owing in large part to the occurrence of generalized tonic–clonic seizures that may occur many years after the end of the absence seizures.
b. Absence seizures persist. About 6% of patients have been reported to have persistence of absence seizures into adulthood. Seizures become less frequent and very short and are seldom troublesome to the patient.
c. Generalized tonic–clonic seizures develop. Forty to sixty percent of patients may develop generalized tonic–clonic seizures usually between ages 10 and 15, but some develop them at a much later time. These seizures are usually easily controlled with medication. Predisposing factors to development of generalized tonic–clonic seizures (17) are as follows:
    i. Onset after 8 years of age.
    ii. Males more often than females.
    iii. Poor initial response of absence seizure to adequate treatment.
    iv. Treatment with more than one drug. Studies suggest that patients initially treated only with an antiabsence drug (ethosuximide or oxazolidine), which does not prevent tonic–clonic seizures, or with an antiabsence drug plus a drug for generalized tonic–clonic seizures, may have a poorer prognosis. Thus, valproate is currently recommended as the drug of first choice.
    v. Abnormal EEG background activity or a photosensitive response.

5. *Juvenile absence epilepsy.* The absence seizures and EEG findings are the same as for childhood absence epilepsy, but seizures with retropulsive movements are less common. The age of onset is later—at or after puberty. The frequency of the seizures is lower (not daily), and the sex distribution is equal. Generalized tonic–clonic seizures, if present, frequently occur on awakening. (There may be an overlap with the generalized "tonic–clonic seizure on awakening" syndrome.)

6. *Juvenile myoclonic epilepsy (impulsive petit mal).* The onset of this syndrome is between 12 and 18 years. Seizures are bilateral, single or repetitive, arrhythmic, irregular myoclonic jerks, predominantly in the arms, occurring more frequently in the morning after awakening. A patient may fall from a jerk. Facial muscles are usually not involved. Consciousness appears to be retained, but patients are often in doubt about this. Both sexes are equally affected. Generalized tonic–clonic seizures and absence seizures may occur. Ictal and interictal EEGs have rapid, generalized, often irregular spike waves and polyspike waves, which may not closely correlate

with the clinical jerks. Sleep deprivation and photic stimulation may precipitate seizures. The genetics of this syndrome are being carefully explored, and a genetic locus has been suggested on chromosome 6 (18). Clinically, it is important to recognize this syndrome for proper treatment. The syndrome is responsive to valproate, but breakthrough seizures are common with carbamazepine, phenytoin, or phenobarbital (19). The electroencephalographic abnormality tends to persist throughout life, and recurrence of seizures is frequent when an effort is made to withdraw antiepileptic drugs.

7. *Epilepsy with grand mal seizures on awakening.* With a usual onset in the second decade, this syndrome is characterized by generalized tonic–clonic seizures shortly after awakening, with perhaps a second peak of occurrence in the evening drowsy period. A family history of epilepsy is common, with a slight male preponderance. Electroencephalographic findings include increased slow waves, disorganized background with sleep transients, and generalized spike-wave activity. Avoidance of precipitating factors may be an important part of therapy.

Idiopathic and/or Symptomatic, in Order of Age of Appearance

Four additional syndromes have been classified as idiopathic and/or symptomatic in order of age of appearance. These have been described by the ILAE Commission as follows:

1. *West syndrome (infantile spasms, Blitz–Nick–Salaam Krampfe).* Usually, West syndrome consists of a characteristic triad—infantile spasms, arrest of psychomotor development, and hypsarrhythmia—although one element may be missing. Spasms may be flexor, extensor, lightning, or nods, but most commonly they are mixed. Onset will peak between 4 and 7 months and will always peak before 1 year. Boys are more commonly affected, and the prognosis is generally poor. West syndrome may be separated into two groups. The symptomatic group is characterized by the previous existence of signs of brain damage (psychomotor retardation, neurological signs, radiological signs, or other types of seizures) or by a known etiology. The smaller, idiopathic group is characterized by the absence of previous signs of brain damage or of known etiology. The prognosis is partly based on early therapy with adrenocorticotropic hormones (ACTHs) or oral steroids but depends mainly on the symptomatic or idiopathic character of the syndrome. A number of idiopathic cases have had favorable prognoses without psychic impairment or later epilepsy when treated early.

2. *Lennox–Gastaut syndrome.* This syndrome is manifested in children from 1 to 8 years of age (usually before age 6). The most common seizure types are tonic–axial, atonic, and absence seizures, but other types such as myoclonic, generalized tonic–clonic, or partial may be frequently associated with this syndrome. Seizure frequency is high, and status epilepticus frequent (stuporous states with myoclonias and tonic and atonic seizures). The EEG usually has abnormal background activity, slow spike waves of less than 3 Hz, and multifocal abnormalities. During sleep,

bursts of fast rhythms (around 10 Hz) appear. Generally, there is mental retardation, the seizures are difficult to control, and the prognosis is unfavorable. In 60% of cases, the syndrome occurs in children suffering from a previous encephalopathy, but it may be primary.

3. *Epilepsy with myoclonic–astatic seizures.* Manifestation begins between 7 months and 6 years (mainly between 2 and 5 years), with (except if beginning in the first year) twice as many boys affected. There is frequently a hereditary predisposition, and development has usually been normal. The seizures are myoclonic, astatic, myoclonic–astatic, absences with clonic and tonic components, and tonic–clonic. Status frequently occurs. Tonic seizures develop late in the course of unfavorable cases. The EEG, initially often normal except for 4- to 7-Hz rhythms, may have irregular fast spike waves or polyspike waves and, during status, irregular 2- to 3-Hz spike waves. Course and outcome are variable.

4. *Epilepsy with myoclonic absences.* This syndrome is clinically characterized by absences accompanied by severe bilateral rhythmical clonic jerks, often associated with a tonic contraction. On the EEG they are always accompanied by bilateral, synchronous, and asymmetrical discharge or rhythmical spike waves at 3 Hz, similar to that of childhood absence. These seizures occur many times a day. Awareness for the jerks may be maintained. Associated seizures are rare. Age of onset is about 7 years, and there is a male preponderance. Prognosis is less favorable than in pyknolepsy as a result of resistance to therapy of the seizures, mental deterioration, and possible evolution to other types of epilepsy such as Lennox–Gastaut syndrome.

Symptomatic Generalized Epilepsies and Syndromes

These epilepsies usually have clinical, electroencephalographic, neuropsychological, and neuroradiological signs of a diffuse, specific, or nonspecific encephalopathy. To date, one syndrome has been classified as nonspecific etiology: early myoclonic encephalopathy. As described by the ILAE Commission (13), the principal features of this syndrome are (a) onset before 3 months of age and (b) initial fragmentary myoclonus—followed by erratic partial seizures, massive myoclonias, or tonic spasms. The EEG is characterized by suppression–burst activity, which may evolve into hypsarrhythmia. The course is severe: Psychomotor development is arrested, and death may occur in the first year. Familial cases are frequent and suggest the influence of one or several congenital metabolic errors, but there is no constant genetic pattern.

The symptomatic generalized epilepsies of specific etiologies are numerous and have been confined to those in which epileptic seizures are the presenting or prominent features. There are two major categories: malformation and proven or suspected inborn errors of metabolism. The malformation category includes Aicardi syndrome (absence of the corpus callosum and retinal lacunae) and lissencephaly–pachygyria. The inborn errors of metabolism can occur at any age and include nonketotic hyperglycinemia and D-glycericacidemia, phenylketonuria, Tay–Sachs, Sandhoff's disease, ceroid lipofuscinosis, pyridoxine dependency, infantile Huntington's disease, Gaucher's disease, Lafora's disease, degenerative progressive myoclonic epilepsy, dyssynergia cerebellaris myoclonica, and Kuf's disease.

Epilepsies and Syndromes Undetermined as to Whether They are Focal or Generalized

There are two categories: (i) without unequivocal generalized or focal seizures (this category includes all generalized tonic–clonic seizures where clinical and electroencephalographic findings do not permit classification as clearly generalized or localization related, such as in cases of sleep grand mal) and (ii) with both generalized and focal seizures. Neonatal seizures and three less common syndromes have been included here. The three syndromes as described by the ILAE Commission (13) are as follows:

1. *Severe myoclonic epilepsy in infancy*. Severe myoclonic epilepsy in infants is a recently defined syndrome. The characteristics include (a) a family history of epilepsy or febrile convulsions, (b) normal development before onset, (c) seizures beginning during the first year of life in the form of generalized or unilateral febrile clonic seizures, (d) secondary appearance of myoclonic jerks, and (e) a high frequency of partial seizures. EEGs show (a) generalized-spike waves and polyspike waves, (b) early photosensitivity, and (c) focal abnormalities. Psychomotor development is retarded beginning in the second year of life, and ataxia, pyramidal signs, and interictal myoclonus appear. This type of epilepsy is very resistant to all forms of treatment.

2. *Epilepsy with continuous spike waves during slow sleep*. This syndrome results form the association of (a) various seizure types (partial or generalized) occurring during sleep and (b) atypical absences when awake. Tonic seizures do not occur. The characteristic electroencephalographic pattern consists of continuous diffuse spike waves during slow-wave sleep, which is seen after the onset of seizures. Duration varies from months to years. The prognosis is guarded because of the appearance of neuropsychologic disorders, despite the usually benign evolution of seizures.

3. *Acquired epileptic aphasia (Landau–Kleffner syndrome)*. The Landau–Kleffner syndrome is a childhood disorder of acquired aphasia with multifocal spikes and spike-and-wave discharges on the EEG. Epileptic seizures and behavioral and psychomotor disturbances occur in two-thirds of the patients. There is verbal auditory agnosia and rapid reduction of spontaneous speech. The seizures are usually generalized convulsive or partial motor, and they are rare. Moreover, they remit before the age of 15 years, as do the electroencephalographic abnormalities.

Neonatal Seizures

Neonatal seizures are a significant entity affecting perhaps 0.5% of neonates (20). Neonatal seizures are a major prognostic indicator of children who will later have severe mental retardation and cerebral palsy (21). While there is agreement that neonatal seizures differ from those of older children and adults, there is a lack of conformity on terminology, classification, and clinical characterization (22). Neonatal seizures may have a consistent electroencephalographic signature or may inconsistently or not at all be associated with electroencephalographic seizure activity. Conversely, there may be electroencephalographic activity with no clinical seizure accompaniment (22). The clinical manifestations are called "subtle" because they are easy to overlook and may include swimming or pedaling movements, buccal–lingual oral movements, sucking, smacking, eyelid-jerking, and deviation of the eyes (13). It has been suggested (20) that seizures occurring during the first 3 days of life have different etiologies and prognosis than those occurring after the third day. Presumably, the advent of neonatal monitoring units to provide combined video–electroencephalographic monitoring will result in the delineation of precise types; with follow-up of these children, information on treatment response and prognosis will become available.

Special Syndromes

Included in this category are the following: (a) situation-related seizures (e.g., febrile convulsions) and seizures related to identifiable situations such as stress, hormonal changes, drugs, alcohol, or sleep deprivation; (b) isolated, apparently unprovoked epileptic events; (c) epilepsies characterized by specific modes of seizure precipitation; and (d) chronic progressive epilepsia partialis continua of childhood. Of these, the reflex epilepsies have long been recognized, and numerous precipitating events have been described in the literature (23). As an example of a situation-related seizure, there is one in the United States that is referred to as the "Spring Break Syndrome." Most American colleges and universities have a 1-week holiday in the spring. Usually, this is preceded by a week of examinations during which the students are sleep-deprived and under stress. In the typical history, the student leaves college immediately after the last exam, drives all night to a resort area, participates in strenuous physical activity such as swimming or skiing, may have unaccustomed (or accustomed) alcohol consumption, and has a first generalized tonic–clonic seizure. Also to be noted in the special syndrome category are the progressive epilepsia partialis continua syndromes of childhood where radical surgery (hemipherectomy) may alter prognosis.

Febrile Convulsions

Febrile convulsions as described by the ILAE Commission (13) are an age-related disorder almost always characterized by generalized seizures occurring during an acute febrile illness. The majority of febrile convulsions are brief and uncomplicated, but a minority may be more prolonged and followed by transient or permanent neurological sequelae, such as the hemiplegia–hemiatrophy–epilepsy (HHE) syndrome. There is a tendency for recurrence of febrile convulsions in about one-third of those affected. Controversy about the risks of developing epilepsy afterwards has largely been resolved by some recent large studies, and it seems that the overall risk is not greater than 4%. The indications for prolonged drug prophylaxis against recurrence of febrile convulsions are more clearly defined now, and it is currently thought the majority do not require treatment. Essentially, this condition is a relatively benign disorder of early childhood.

SUMMARY

Understanding the current classification is not easy. Not all patients conform to our current terminologies. There may be an underlying commonality to the epilepsies (24), or seizures may be part of a biological continuum (25). But until our knowledge increases, the physician must attempt to apply what is known to the individual patient. A number of books have provided recent reviews (26–28). Articles are beginning to appear in the archival literature showing how the classifications can be applied to large clinical populations and perhaps providing additional clues to diagnosis (29) and treatment (30). Schmidt et al. (30) present data which suggest that higher plasma concentrations of phenytoin, phenobarbital, and carbamazepine are necessary for control of epilepsy with simple or complex partial seizures as compared with epilepsy with tonic–clonic seizures alone. Thus, there are "clinical pearls" coming out of use of the classifications that can improve patient care.

A study of the classifications highlights the need for future clinical research (delineation of the precise relations of seizure type to age, genetics, etiology, response to therapy, and long-term outcomes) that is still needed to improve the goal of better patient care.

REFERENCES

1. Milne AA. The house at Pooh corner. In: *The World of Pooh*. New York: EP Dutton, 1957;260.
2. Temkin O. *The falling sickness*, 2nd ed. (revised). Baltimore: The Johns Hopkins Press, 1971.
3. Spratling WP. Presidential address. Epilepsy—the strangest disease in human history. *Transactions of the National Association for the Study of Epilepsy and the Care and Treatment of Epileptics* 1906;3:107–113.
4. Merlis JK. Treatment in relation to classification of the epilepsies. *Acta Neurol Latinoam* 1972;18:42–51.
5. Gastaut H. Clinical and electroencephalographical classification of epileptic seizures. *Epilepsia* 1969(Suppl)10:S2–S13.
6. Gastaut H, Caveness WF, Landolt H, et al. A proposed international classification of epileptic seizures. *Epilepsia* 1964;5:297–306.
7. Ajmone-Marsan C. A newly proposed classification of epileptic seizures. Neurophysiological basis. *Epilepsia* 1965;6:275–296.
8. Gastaut H. Classification of the epilepsies. *Epilepsia* 1969;(Suppl)10:S14–S21.
9. Masland RL. Comments on the classification of epilepsy. *Epilepsia* 1969;10:S22–S28.
10. Gastaut H. Clinical and electroencephalographic classification of epileptic seizures. *Epilepsia* 1970;11:103–113.
11. Merlis JK. Proposal for an international classification of the epilepsies. *Epilepsia* 1970;11:114–119.
12. Commission on Classification and Terminology of the International League Against Epilepsy. Pro-

posal for revised clinical and electroencephalographic classification of epileptic seizures. *Epilepsia* 1981;22:489–501.

13. Commission on Classification and Terminology of the International League Against Epilepsy. Proposal for classification of epilepsies and epileptic syndromes. *Epilepsia* 1985;26:268–278.

14. Gastaut H. *Dictionary of epilepsy, Part I: definitions*. Geneva: World Health Organization, 1973.

15. Weinberger J, Lusins J. Simultaneous bilateral focal seizures without loss of consciousness. *Mt Sinai Med J* 1973;40:693–696.

16. Penry JK, Dreifuss FE. Automatisms associated with the absence of petit mal epilepsy. *Arch Neurol* 1969;21:142–149.

17. Loiseau P. Childhood absence epilepsy. In: Roger J, Dravet C, Bureau M, Dreifuss FE, Wolf P, Eds. *Epileptic Syndromes in Infancy, Childhood and Adolescence*. London: John Libbey Eurotext, 1985;106–120.

18. Greenberg DA, Delgado-Escueta AV, Widelitz H, Sparkes RS, Treiman L, Maldonado HM. Is a locus related to juvenile myoclonic epilepsy and its associated abnormal EEG trait on chromosome 6? *Am J Hum Genet* 1987;41(Suppl 3):A65.

19. Delgado-Escueta A, Enrile-Bacsal F. Juvenile myoclonic epilepsy of Janz. *Neurology* 1984;34:285–294.

20. Mellits ED, Holden KR, Freeman JM. Neonatal seizures. II. Multivariate analysis of factors associated with outcome. *Pediatrics* 1981;70:177–185.

21. Nelson KB, Broman SH. Perinatal risk factors in children with serious motor and mental handicaps. *Ann Neurol* 1977;2:371–377.

22. Mizrahi EM. Neonatal seizures: problems in diagnosis and classification. *Epilepsia* 1987;28(Suppl 1):S546–S555.

23. Forster FM, Booker HE. The epilepsies and convulsive disorders. In: Baker AB, Baker LH, eds. *Clinical neurology*, vol. 2. Hagerstown, MD: Harper & Row, 1975; Chapter 24.

24. Rodin E. An assessment of current views on epilepsy. *Epilepsia* 1987;28:267–271.

25. Berkovic SF, Andermann F, Andermann E, Gloor P. Concepts of absence epilepies. Discrete syndromes or biological continuum? *Neurology* 1987;37:993–1000.

26. Dreifuss FE. *Pediatric epileptology. Classification and management of seizures in the child*. Boston: John Wright–PSG, 1983.

27. Aicardi J. *Epilepsy in children*. New York: Raven Press, 1986.

28. Roger J, Dravet C, Bureau M, Dreifuss FE, Wolf P. *Epileptic syndromes in infancy, childhood, and adolescence*. London: John Libbey Eurotext, 1985.

29. Wolf P, Goosses R. Relation of photosensitivity to epileptic syndromes. *J Neurol Neurosurg Psychiatry* 1986;49:1386–1391.

30. Schmidt D, Einicke I, Haenel F. The influence of seizure type on the efficacy of plasma concentrations of phenytoin, phenobarbital and carbamazepine. *Arch Neurol* 1986;43:263–265.

Epilepsy: Current Approaches to Diagnosis and Treatment,
edited by Dennis B. Smith,
Raven Press, Ltd., New York © 1990.

2

The Use and Misuse of Routine Electroencephalography in the Management of Seizure Disorders

Ronald E. Kramer

Oregon Comprehensive Epilepsy Program, Good Samaritan Hospital & Medical Center, Portland, Oregon 97210

When dealing with disease processes that affect the central nervous system, it is not always possible or necessary to obtain pathologic tissue to absolutely confirm a diagnosis. The prototypic example of this in clinical practice is multiple sclerosis (MS), in which the history and physical examination lead the physician, without pathologic confirmation, to the diagnosis of clinically definite MS. To obtain a "tissue diagnosis" of epilepsy outside of the neonatal age group, one must record a patient's typical paroxysmal clinical event and document a simultaneously occurring electroencephalographic (EEG) seizure pattern.[1] However as in MS, it is not always possible or necessary to obtain a "tissue diagnosis"—the clinician can use the clinical evaluation, which may (or may not) be supported by other paraclinical data. With the advent of newer neuroimaging techniques such as computed tomography (CT) and magnetic resonance imaging (MRI) scanning, the evaluation of seizure disorders is one of the few conditions that requires EEG evaluation (1). The cornerstone of the paraclinical evaluation of the patient with epilepsy is routine *interictal* electroencephalography. It is rare (and fortunate) when a typical clinical event is recorded during routine outpatient electroencephalography. The yield for recording such events dramatically increases with more invasive, prolonged, and advanced recording systems (see Chapter 3).

In this chapter, discussion centers on the use and limitations of routine interictal electroencephalography in the evaluation of a patient with a suspected seizure disorder. Emphasis is placed on (a) increasing the chances of obtaining a clinically useful result, (b) avoiding overinterpretation of the routine electroencephalogram, and (c) determining the clinical significance of specific EEG patterns and how they relate to

---

[1]The concept of what is or is not an epileptic seizure in the neonatal age group is undergoing reevaluation. For example, subtle seizures of neonates may represent epileptic events but do not always have an accompanying scalp EEG change (2). (See also Chapter 1, pp.22, 23.)

the patient with a suspected seizure disorder. As with any paraclinical data, one guiding principle is to be noted: The physician interpreting the electroencephalogram must place the results in the clinical context of the case and ultimately treat the patient and not treat the electroencephalogram.

CLINICAL REALITIES IN THE PRACTICE OF ELECTROENCEPHALOGRAPHY

The Clinical Application of Electroencephalography

The goal of the encephalographer is to extract as much useful data from a tracing as possible and to avoid overinterpretation. Overinterpretation, causing a false positive, can lead to misdiagnosis and subsequent inappropriate treatments. It is therefore desirable for the encephalographer to have a general conceptual, almost philosophical, framework about what the EEG data can reveal to the clinician.

To aid in forming this conceptual framework, it is helpful for the individual encephalographer or the entire laboratory to classify or standardize EEG abnormalities. This results in a decrease in overinterpretation and allows for easier comparison of EEG records in any one patient or groups of patients over a period of time (3,4). Of course, not every test result will fit comfortably into a standardized system, but a system will provide for a starting point for interpretation of the more difficult and atypical patterns that are always encountered in clinical practice. Once the clinical encephalographer has established the findings in the record and has classified the abnormalities, the application of these findings to the clinical situation will lead to a more focused and useful interpretation (3).

The types of abnormal EEG findings can be grouped into four major categories: slow activity; epileptogenic epileptiform patterns; patterns occurring in comatose states; and miscellaneous patterns. For the patient with a suspected seizure disorder, it is the appearance of unambiguous epileptogenic epileptiform discharges (EEDs) in the interictal electroencephalogram that is most helpful in supporting a diagnosis of epilepsy.

EEDs are associated with the appearance of spikes or sharp waves. As will be discussed below, the occurrence of spikes or sharp waves in an EEG is highly associated with the population of patients with epilepsy. The occurrence of these same discharges in the normal population is infrequent. The definition of these terms has been variable (5,6), but it is generally agreed that usage of the term implies functional pathology. There are general characteristics of these waveforms that allow them to be classified as epileptogenic. These characteristics are summarized in Table 1. Note that the term "paroxysmal" has been left out of the table. There is much confusion surrounding this term. Epileptogenic epileptiform activity is by definition paroxysmal, but there is much paroxysmal activity seen on the electroencephalogram that is not epileptogenic and is in fact normal. Examples of normally occurring paroxysmal patterns include vertex sharp waves, positive occip-

TABLE 1. *Criteria for defining epileptogenic epileptiform activity*[a]

1. The presence of spikes or sharp waves. Spikes are transients, lasting 20–70 msec; sharp waves are transients, lasting 70–200 msec.
2. A definable electrical field associated with the discharge which makes physiologic sense and which extends beyond one electrode.
3. The discharge should have a prominent surface negativity or should have as its highest component a surface negativity. A concomitant surface positivity may also be occasionally seen.
4. The discharge should occur abruptly, stand out, and disrupt the ongoing background rhythms. A subsequent slow wave is often seen, which tends to disrupt the ongoing background rhythms.
5. Nonepileptogenic epileptiform patterns can be ruled out.
6. Physiologic or nonphysiologic artifacts can be ruled out.

[a]Modified from ref. 6.

ital sharp transients of sleep, and slow-wave bursts occurring during hyperventilation.

Once an abnormal EEG pattern has been identified, it is important that localization and abundance be noted. The appearance of pathologic spikes and sharp waves supports the diagnosis of epilepsy, but it is the localization and distribution of this activity that gives insights into the patient's seizure type.

Yield of Routine Electroencephalography

When interpreting the findings of the routine electroencephalogram, several questions must be addressed. If epileptogenic epileptiform findings are seen, what does this mean in terms of formulating a diagnosis? Conversely, what does it mean if the test is normal?

The statistics found in published studies to answer these questions have remained surprisingly stable over the last several decades. In a widely quoted study (7) of 1824 electroencephalograms in over 300 epileptic patients, definite EEDs were found in 60% of the EEG records and in 83% of the patients. These were standard electroencephalograms utilizing the International 10–20 electrode placement system, occasionally performed with nasopharyngeal leads (8) and performed with routine activation procedures (see p. 31). An average of six electroencephalograms were obtained per patient to obtain this yield. Of the first electroencephalograms done in this population, 56% of the tracings revealed EEDs. The yield was highest in the patients aged less than 10 years of age and lowest in adults over the age of 40. The etiology of the seizure disorder or the presence of antiepileptic drugs (AEDs) did not alter the yield. Of the patients observed for longer than 1 year, less than 8% continued to show no evidence of EEDs. In patients with complex partial seizures observed closely, less than 2% had a negative yield for EEDs. Sundaram and Hogan (9) reported that in a population of clinically defined epileptics, the overall yield of EEDs was 50% on the first electroencephalogram. The figure was slightly higher for patients with partial seizure disorders and lower for patients with generalized seizure disorders. Statistically, AEDs played no role in altering the yield. Abnormalities were seen within the first 20 minutes of recording time, the minimum standard for performing an electroencephalogram (10). Another recent study by Salinsky et al. (11) supported these figures.

An important trend noted in previous studies is that the yield of detecting EEDs in an electroencephalogram is a function of the seizure frequency. If an electroencephalogram is obtained within several days of a seizure, there is an increase in the interictal spike activity (7). This finding has been supported by studies in patients undergoing continuous EEG monitoring utilizing computer spike detection programs (12). The rates at which spikes occurred in these studies were not a function of AED levels but were due to the occurrence of seizures. The spiking rate was especially increased after generalized tonic–clonic seizures. The duration of the postictal period was not related to the increased spiking frequency (7,12).

Equally as important as knowing the rate of occurrence of EEDs in patients with epilepsy is knowing what the false-positive rate of the electroencephalogram can be (i.e., the rate of occurrence of EEDs in the normal population). Again, the statistics on this finding have remained stable over the decades.

A study of nearly 6500 nonepileptic patients revealed that only 2.2% of that population demonstrated *potential* EEDs (13). This number may be slightly inflated, given the fact that certain nonepileptogenic epileptiform discharges (NEEDs) considered today to be normal were included in this percentage (14). EEDs in these patients were associated with acquired brain damage, brain cancers, mental retardation, prior craniotomy, and steroid or cancer chemotherapy. Only 14% of this small percentage later developed seizures. Most seizures occurred within the first 6 months after the electroencephalogram, and three of every four patients who developed seizures were less than 20 years old.

Similar results are found in studies limited exclusively to children. Petersen et al. (15) examined 1000 children aged 0–15 years and found "paroxysmal" abnormalities in close to 10% of these normal subjects. As previously stated, paroxysmal discharges do not necessarily imply an epileptogenic potential. This was an earlier study, and the 99 patients with paroxysmal findings included several NEED patterns recorded that today would be considered normal. Applying more recent EEG criteria to unequivocal EEDs was done in a group of 3726 children aged 6–13 years (16). In this population, 131 (3.5%) of the children showed an epileptogenic abnormality. The results of the study are summarized in Table 2. The EEG abnormalities in this normal population demonstrated all types of epileptogenic patterns, from unilateral focal spikes to generalized polyspike-and-wave discharges. Only seven of these 131 patients (5%) as well as only 0.2% of the total study population, subsequently developed epilepsy. The EEG abnormality was first noted in follow-up tracings in three of these seven epileptic patients, a sensitivity rate similar to that of previous studies. A longitudinal study of 189 normal adolescents over a 5-year period had similar results (17). Six percent showed possible EEDs, but if the equivocal cases were removed, then only three patients (1.5% of the study population) showed specific EEDs.

TABLE 2. *Epileptogenic epileptiform patterns found in 3726 normal children*[a]

Generalized 3-Hz spike-and-wave discharges	4	(1)[b]
Generalized spike- or polyspike-and-wave discharges	37	(4)
Unilateral focal spikes or sharp waves	79	(2)
Centroparietal	27	(1)
Temporal	50	(1)
Occipital	2	(0)
Frontal	0	(0)
Bilateral independent focal spikes and sharp waves	11	(0)
Total:	131	(7)

[a]Adapted from ref. 16.
[b]Numbers in parentheses refer to children who subsequently developed epilepsy.

The appearance of EEDs in the normal population is not surprising. As in any clinical test, there are always statistical outliers. In addition, the EEG tracing of a patient reflects underlying neuronal events that occur independently of clinical epilepsy. This has been identified particularly in patients with generalized 3-Hz spike-and-wave complexes (18). In patients with generalized epilepsy syndromes and 3-Hz spike-and-wave complexes on EEG tracings, approximately one-third of unaffected siblings and offspring and approximately 10% of unaffected parents also demonstrate the 3-Hz spike-and-wave complex on EEG tracings. It has been suggested that there is an autosomal dominant inheritance for this EEG pattern that occurs independent of the occurrence of clinical seizures (18).

There is one important EED commonly seen in clinical practice that is *not* associated with a seizure disorder in the majority of the patients in which it occurs. This is the benign focal epileptiform discharge of childhood (see below). The EEG pattern is also referred to as "benign rolandic spikes," but the location of these discharges is not necessarily limited to centrotemporal regions. Early reports and analysis of the children who demonstrate this type of discharge stated that a large percentage (40–70%) had associated seizure disorders (19,20). However, earlier reports were done on populations referred to EEG laboratories, an obvious sample bias that would weigh heavily toward patients who have suffered seizures. More recent analysis of incidence and prevalence of the EEG pattern shows that seizures occur in approximately 10% of the children with this EEG pattern (21). Therefore, the appearance of this EEG pattern in a patient referred to the EEG laboratory must be placed into the clinical context to see whether there is any clinical significance.

Activation Procedures

Several procedures have been noted to increase the yield of detecting EEDs.

Sleep deprivation for 24 hours or more has been known to increase the yield of EEDs by 40–50% or more (22–24). More important is the fact that sleep deprivation does not appear to increase the false-positive rate of EEDs in normal controls, a rate that is approximately 2% (24). The effect of sleep deprivation is independent of sleep, and both of these are known to activate either focal or generalized EEDs. Recent guidelines on the use of sleep deprivation state that it should only be used in patients suspected of having seizures whose prior electroencephalograms have been normal (24).

Hyperventilation typically results in generalized bursts of high-voltage slow waves that may appear very rhythmic. This response is much more pronounced for children. The slow activity can last up to 2 minutes after the cessation of hyperventilation in children or up to 1 minute in adults. This procedure is extremely effective in eliciting generalized 3-Hz spike-and-wave discharges. It also can elicit focal EEDs in a small percentage of patients with partial seizure disorders.

The problem with the hyperventilation response is twofold. First, the generalized rhythmic bursts may normally have a small notched component that gives the appearance of a pathologic spike-and-wave complex. Second, the hyperventilation response seen on the electroencephalogram may be associated with a mild depression in mental status. This, combined with slow bursts, may be confused with a clinical seizure with an associated EEG accompaniment.

The decreased responsiveness normally seen in the patient during hyperventilation may be due to decreased activity in the reticular formation that occurs with hyperventilation-induced hypocapnia (24). This same mechanism may be responsible for the hypersynchronous high-voltage slowing seen on the electroencephalogram. Despite assertions that hyperventilation-induced rhythmic slow activity associated with decreased responsiveness is possibly an absence seizure (25), without more prolonged recording, video monitoring, or the subsequent appearance of clear-cut EEDs, it is best to take a conservative approach and regard the response as normal.

Photic stimulation is useful in eliciting generalized bursts of spike-and-wave complexes in patients with generalized seizure disorders. Normal responses include physiologic rhythmic discharges that may be time-locked to the stimulus. More pronounced, sharper waveforms can also be seen, and if they are time-locked and occipitally dominant, they should be considered normal. The pathologic photoconvulsive response consists of generalized sharp waves or spike-and-wave complexes that are not time-locked to the stimulus and that continue after the stimulus is stopped.

The problem with photic stimulation is that it can elicit many artifacts, both physiologic and nonphysiologic (26). The most important of these is the photomyoclonic response (Fig. 1). This is a physiologic artifact that can mimic the appearance of a photoconvulsive response. It is the result of frontal and temporal muscle activity that is time-locked to the photic stimulus.

In summary, routine outpatient electroencephalography appears to have a high specificity for detecting seizure disorders. In patients with EED the false-positive rate is no more than 2%. This is not the case for benign focal (rolandic) spikes, for which a false-positive rate as high as 90% may exist. Routine outpatient electroencephalography has a variable sensitivity in showing definitive epileptogenic epilep-

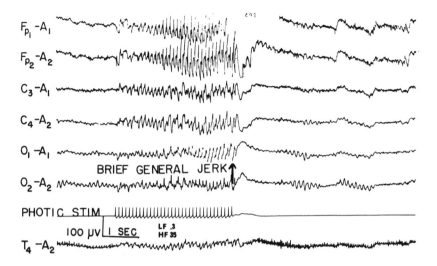

FIG. 1. Photomyoclonic response—38-year-old alcoholic found comatose after a possible seizure. Note frontal distribution and extremely short duration of the "spike" component, which is time-locked to the photic stimulus.

tiform patterns in patients with seizure disorders. This sensitivity is approximately 50% on a single electroencephalogram, but repetitive electroencephalograms can increase the yield to approximately 85% or higher. The utility of defining an EED by routine electroencephalography in a patient appears to be reached after four to five electroencephalograms. After this point, a reevaluation of the patient's diagnosis or more advanced EEG testing should be considered. The yield is higher in patients having frequent clinical events, and the yield can be highest within 3 days of a reported seizure. Having a patient report to the laboratory for an urgent electroencephalogram within 3 days of a clinical event may be very helpful in diagnosing difficult cases.

Nonepileptogenic Epileptiform Discharges

The preceding sections discussed the occurrence and meaning of the false-positive electroencephalogram in the evaluation of epilepsy—that is, the occurrence of epileptogenic potentials in a normal subject. The other source of false-positive electroencephalograms is normal EEG patterns that mimic epileptogenic discharges. Table 3 contains a list of these patterns. These are the more commonly occurring NEEDs, some of which are frequently mislabeled as having pathologic significance. Many of these patterns were initially believed to be associated with a number of nonspecific neurological symptoms as well as seizures. Studies of large control populations have shown that these paroxysmal and rhythmic patterns have no clinical significance and are not associated with the occurrence of seizure disorders.

TABLE 3. *Nonepileptiform epileptiform discharges*

---

1. Benign epileptiform transients of sleep (BETS), small sharp spikes (SSS)
2. Fourteen-and-six positive spikes (14 and 6, ctenoids)
3. Hyperventilation hypersynchrony
4. Mu-like activity from a skull defect (breach)
5. Photomyogenic response
6. Psychomotor variant (rhythmic temporal bursts)
7. Six-hertz spike-and-wave (phantom spike-and-wave)
8. Subclinical rhythmic EEG discharge of the adult (SREDA)
9. Wicket spikes

Wicket Spikes

[handwritten marginalia: probably more than 1% sleep ee... Reider (1971)]

The best description of wicket spikes (Fig. 2) comes from a study that analyzed over 4400 patients (27). This waveform is seen in approximately 1% of all electroencephalograms and tends to occur in the adult population. This activity can occur in the awake or sleep state but is seen primarily during drowsiness. The waveform occurs in the midtemporal and anterior temporal regions and may be unilateral or bilateral. There is a simple biphasic morphology that is surface-negative, and the amplitude can be as large as 120 μV. These spikes do not usually have a subsequent slow wave and do not disrupt the background.

Small Sharp Spikes (SSS) and Benign Epileptiform Transients of Sleep (BETS)

Of all the sharp transients that plague the electroencephalographer, BETS and SSS (Fig. 3) have proven to be one of the more difficult waveforms to differentiate

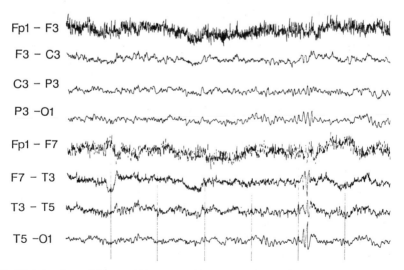

FIG. 2. Wicket spikes—38-year-old woman with recurrent headaches. Despite muscle and movement artifact, a wicket spike can be seen in the left temporal region.

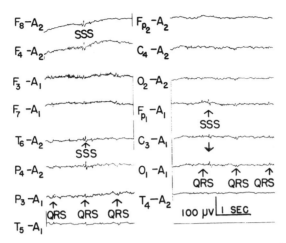

FIG. 3. Small sharp spikes (SSS or BETS)—27-year-old woman with intermittent vertigo. This small discharge, which was of short duration, appeared only when the patient was asleep. Note its similarity to the EKG artifact seen on this referential montage.

from epileptogenic spikes. BETS are seen in approximately 25% of normal controls and 20% of patients with symptomatic seizure disorders (28,29). As their name implies, they are seen exclusively in sleep and are primarily found in Stage I or Stage II sleep. They are small (i.e., 30–100 μV) discharges that usually have a simple biphasic morphology. They do not break up the ongoing background rhythms, nor are they usually associated with a subsequent slow wave. However, a detailed evaluation of these transients did reveal an occasional slow wave of up to 300 msec in duration (28). The slow wave is usually of lower amplitude than the spike component, a finding that may prove useful in identification. The distribution of these waveforms is quite extensive. These waveforms may have a widespread negativity involving the frontotemporal regions, with a rapid fall-off of the negative field. Therefore, the recording montage can greatly alter the appearance of these transients: Larger electrode distances and basal electrodes enhance their appearance.

Important points to differentiate BETS from pathologic spikes include the following (28): (a) BETS are not seen in wakefulness; (b) they are not seen in a repetitive fashion or in runs; (c) there are no associated sharp waves in the same region; (d) there is an absence of underlying pathologic slow activity in the region in which they are identified; and (e) they occur sporadically and are seen independently in each hemisphere, although one side may predominate.

Psychomotor Variant

The psychomotor variant (Fig. 4) pattern is also referred to as *rhythmic temporal bursts* and was first described by Gibbs et al. (30). It was found to occur in less than

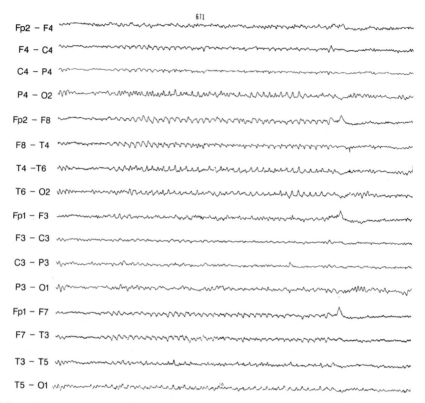

FIG. 4. Psychomotor variant—34-year-old woman with recurrent headaches. Note notched bilateral 5.5-Hz temporal discharge.

1% of 50,000 referred cases in that original study. It was described as a subclinical seizure pattern and was thought to be associated with neurovegetative symptoms (30,31). However, in a study of normal controls, its frequency was reported to be 2% (32).

The pattern is a rhythmic 4- to 7-Hz notched discharge that can be seen in brief bursts or runs lasting up to several minutes. It may be unilateral or bilateral and is seen primarily in early drowsiness or the awake state. It is located in the midtemporal region, primarily at electrodes T3 and T4. Its notched appearance is believed to represent the integration of two underlying background rhythms that, when added together, result in a single saw-toothed waveform (33).

Fourteen-and-Six Positive Spikes (14 and 6, Ctenoids)

The 14-and-6 pattern has a distinct morphology and is easily noted in EEG recordings. The waveform consists of a 14-Hz component that appears as a positive, spiky, sleep spindle. This is superimposed on an underlying, more sinusoidal 6-Hz component. It should be noted that the "14" and the "6" can be seen independent of each other. The pattern tends to come in bursts lasting under 2 seconds and is less than 100 μV in amplitude. It is usually seen as a bilateral, synchronous burst, but independent unilateral discharges are not uncommon. The spikes are located in the posterior head regions and are best seen in derivations utilizing large intraelectrode distances (i.e., referential montages). They may appear as a rhythmic train of "negative" spikes in derivations that utilize nasopharyngeal electrodes. This pattern appears in drowsiness and light sleep, and it may be seen rarely in the fully awake state.

The appearance of the 14-and-6 pattern was originally believed to be associated with nonspecific neurovegetative symptoms. Even a recent study of paroxysmal autonomic phenomena interpreted the appearance of this pattern as evidence that the patient's symptoms were a form of epilepsy (34). It is now known that this is a normal pattern and has a particularly age-dependent distribution. It appears in early childhood, has a peak incidence in the teenage years, and then subsequently decreases in older age groups. Lombroso et al. (35) reported that 58% of normal teenagers show this pattern. In a study of children from 1 to 15 years old, the incidence was approximately 16% (36).

The 6-Hz Spike-and-Wave Complex (Phantom Spike-and-Wave)

The 6-Hz spike-and-wave complex (Fig. 5) is a relatively rare pattern seen in less than 3% of all patients referred to an EEG laboratory (33). It appears primarily in young adults. The waveform consists of generalized, bisynchronous bursts of activity lasting 0.5–2 seconds with a frequency of 5–7 Hz. The spike component is small and has a magnitude of 40 μV. The pattern is seen primarily in drowsiness.

In one study (37), two subtypes of the 6-Hz spike-and-wave were proposed. One consisted of a higher amplitude, frontally dominant type, whereas the other consisted of a lower amplitude, occipitally dominant waveform. It was thought that this differentiation allowed for the identification of a 6-Hz phantom that was associated with seizures. This has not gained acceptance, and the pattern should be considered a normal variant.

Subclinical Rhythmic EEG Discharge of the Adult (SREDA)

SREDA (Fig. 6) was described in 1981 by Westmoreland and Klass. It is a very rare pattern and over a 10-year period was seen in 142 electroencephalograms obtained from 65 patients (38). It appears as a striking pattern with an acute beginning and end. Rhythmic, bilaterally synchronous 4- to 7-Hz activity is seen diffusely but appears maximally in the parietal and temporal regions. The discharges are as high as 500 μV and last an average of 60 seconds, but discharges up to 5 minutes have been reported. It was seen in patients 42 to 80 years of age, with a peak in the early

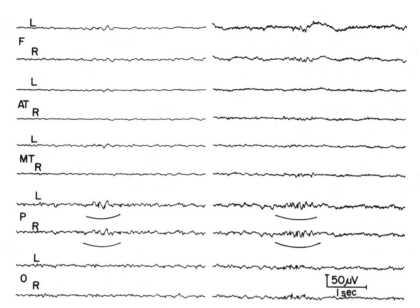

FIG. 5. Six-hertz phantom spike-and-wave. Low-amplitude posterior dominant discharge from two different patients. (From ref. 37.)

60s. It can occur in sleep or wakefulness and may occur only as an arousal response from sleep. In order to call the pattern SREDA, there should be documentation that there is no clinical change or symptomatology associated with the discharge.

K-U. associated omitted

Mu-like Activity Related to Skull Defects (Breach)

Neurosurgical procedures that create skull defects can alter the appearance of ongoing background rhythms. These may appear as a higher amplitude, spiky alpha rhythm intermixed with faster frequencies. This has been termed *breach rhythm* (39). It has no relation to seizures. Because it is related to skull defects, it may be limited to one electrode, as are many artifacts. Its relative consistent, nonreactive appearance in a tracing helps distinguish it from the commonly seen central mu rhythm (39). *but mu is reactive to movements*

The problem with this pattern is that it is seen in the neurosurgical patient population, a population that tends to have underlying structural brain lesions in the area of the breach rhythm. These underlying abnormalities can result in abnormal slow activity that admixes with the breach rhythm to give the appearance of a pathologic spike-and-wave complex. A similar misinterpretation can occur in patients with prominent beta activity with or without skull defects. Prominent frontal beta activity can intermix with normal drowsy bursts of slow activity and give the appearance of generalized, frontally dominant spike-and-wave complexes (40).

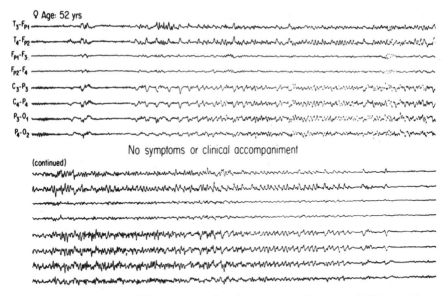

FIG. 6. Subacute rhythmic EEG discharge of adults—52-year-old woman with history of headache. (From ref. 38.)

Are There Interictal EEG Patterns That Are Epileptogenic But Not Epileptiform?

Epileptiform activity includes waveforms that contain sharp transients of either 20- to 70-msec duration (spikes) or 70- to 200-msec duration (sharp waves). The epileptiform activity can be nonpathologic or pathologic (i.e., epileptogenic). This leaves one contingency to explore: Can interictal EEG abnormalities that are not EEDs be effectively utilized in the evaluation and management of the patient with a possible seizure disorder? The most common abnormalities seen include mild diffuse background slowing, asymmetries of amplitude in background rhythms, and abnormal slow activity. The latter may be (a) focal or generalized, (b) intermittent or continuous, or (c) rhythmic or polymorphic.

As pointed out by Klass (41), any focal abnormality on the electroencephalogram may point to the site of origin of seizures in a patient with a partial seizure disorder. The absence of spikes in epileptogenic lesions can be explained because the spike-and-sharp-wave components of epileptogenic discharges do not have as widespread a scalp distribution as the slow-wave component (42). Intermittent focal slow activity may point to any type of underlying structural or physiologic disturbance. Normal slow activity such as the slow alpha variant, posterior slow waves of youth, or temporal slowing of the elderly must be considered before labeling such a record as abnormal (43,44). Focal continuous polymorphic slow activity points to a more aggressive lesion that may involve cortical or subcortical structures. Pathologic focal slow activity can be seen in the postictal state and may persist as long as 10 days, especially in children (45). Focal slow activity is also seen in migraine headache, a disease with paroxysmal clinical features that may be difficult to differentiate from seizures.

Asymmetries in amplitude of ongoing background EEG rhythms are very non-specific findings. When an asymmetry is seen, the encephalographer must determine which side is abnormal; that is, are rhythms focally increased on one side or are they focally decreased on the opposite side? Asymmetries usually indicate a focal lesion. Focal porencephalic cysts are commonly associated with suppression of EEG rhythms in the area of the cyst, but asymmetries may be related to electrical conduction differences due to extraparenchymal brain disease, as seen in the case of breach rhythm. The unexplained appearance of a new slow focus or new asymmetry in a patient's electroencephalogram may point to a more aggressive neurologic syndrome that needs evaluation.

Generalized polymorphic slow abnormalities may also be intermittent or continuous. These point to diffuse physiologic dysfunction and, like mild slowing of background activity, reflect the presence of an encephalopathy. In the epileptic patient with a noted change in mental status, the electroencephalogram may be helpful in defining the etiology of this change, a situation not uncommonly encountered in the chronic, mentally retarded patient with a difficult-to-control seizure disorder. If a decrease or change in mental status is seen in a seizure patient and these patterns are seen to emerge or worsen in the electroencephalogram, then metabolic disturbances, medication intoxication, or postictal state should all be considered as causes of the decline in mentation. Triphasic waves may also be seen in the more severe metabolic or medication-induced encephalopathies.

Intermittent rhythmic delta (IRD), also called intermittent rhythmic slow activity, is a distinct pattern that may be seen either focally or in a generalized distribution. If it has a bisynchronous, generalized, frontally dominant distribution, it is commonly referred to as a frontal IRD activity (FIRDA). In children under 10 years of age, the discharges may be more prominent occipitally and are referred to as OIRDA. The pattern consists of 2- to 4-Hz bursts of activity, usually over 70 μV and usually lasting several seconds. It is a nonspecific finding and reflects dysfunction of cortical or subcortical gray matter structures by either structural or physiologic lesions. Midline subcortical lesions or head traumas are common disorders associated with OIRDA. Focal IRD is usually associated with focal supratentorial lesions. Generalized IRD may be seen in diffuse metabolic encephalopathies and in association with triphasic waves.

Recent reports have tried to label IRD as an epileptogenic pattern. Reiher and Beaudry (46) studied the appearance of focal temporal IRD activity (TIRDA) in patients with complex partial seizures, with a control population consisting of patients without complex partial seizures. TIRDA was seen in 40 of 115 seizure patients and in none of the 115 control patients. The incidence of TIRDA in the seizure patients was one-half of the incidence of sharp waves. These investigators believed that TIRDA is as specific as epileptogenic temporal spikes and that the trains of slow waves represented spike-and-wave discharges with attenuation of the spike.

Generalized bursts of IRD were thought to represent a clinical and EEG seizure pattern in a report of seven children aged 5–11 years with presumed absence seizures (25). In this study, clinical absences were associated with generalized IRD. In three of these seven children, clear-cut interictal epileptogenic potentials were also seen. This study, therefore, showed that approximately one-half of these patients had EEDs—a yield that is to be expected after routine outpatient electroencephalography. The investigators stress that the physician must be extremely cautious in interpreting IRD as epileptogenic and that more prolonged recordings utilizing video monitoring are indicated in patients without clear-cut EEDs. Similar claims were made 30 years ago when it was noted that OIRDA may be seen in association with absence seizure (43). The IRD pattern was seen primarily during hyperventilation and was associated with decreased responsiveness.

Bursts of high-voltage, hypersynchronous IRD are commonly seen in children, adolescents, and young adults during hyperventilation (36,47,48). They can also be seen in older patients. They may be associated with a decrease in mental state or responsiveness—a reflection of the normal physiology responsible for the generation of the hyperventilation response (48).

Short of clear-cut EEDs, other abnormal findings on the routine interictal electroencephalogram are nonspecific. They can be seen in any number of structural or physiologic disease states. Their appearance in the patient with a suspected seizure disorder needs further clinical clarification. To obtain this clarification, more recordings or more advanced techniques such as ambulatory or video-monitored electroencephalography should be considered.

SPECIFIC EPILEPTOGENIC EPILEPTIFORM PATTERNS

Hypsarrhythmia

Hypsarrhythmia is a pattern whose onset is seen during the first year of life, primarily at age 4–6 months. The pattern consists of multifocal independent spikes and sharp waves superimposed on a diffusely slow, high-voltage background. Slow waves should reach an amplitude of 300 μV or higher. It may persist to as long as 4–5 years of age. In older children, it may develop into other abnormalities, specifically slow spike-and-wave complexes or multifocal independent spike discharges (see below). Over 90% of children with hypsarrhythmia have infantile spasms, and, conversely, approximately two out of three with spasms have hypsarrhythmia (49). At the onset of the infantile spasm, a relative flattening of the electroencephalogram (a so-called electrodecremental pattern) is seen. Hypsarrhythmia is an ominous pattern usually associated with diffuse bihemispheric disease and a poor prognosis. In one study, 15% of children with hypsarrhythmia had a normal intellectual outcome (49).

Slow Spike-and-Wave Complexes

Slow spike-and-wave complexes (SSWCs) (Fig. 7) are generalized discharges that occur with a frequency of repetition of less than 2.5 per second. They are usually of maximum amplitude in frontal regions and are usually associated with generalized slowing of the background rhythms. The spike component may be of a longer duration (up to 200 msec), and occasionally the discharges may be difficult to distinguish from triphasic waves. This pattern develops at 2–4 years of age and is preceded by hypsarrhythmia in a substantial percentage of patients (50). It is associated with a variety of generalized seizures, and in approximately two out of three patients, multiple seizure types are seen. Atypical absence, atonic, myoclonic, and tonic–clonic seizures are most common (51). This pattern is also associated with a poor intellectual status. Average I.Q. in hospitalized patients with SSWCs was less than 50; and less than 25% of patients overall have normal intellectual development (51,52). The electroclinical triad of SSWCs, mental retardation, and severe intractable seizures forms the Lennox–Gastaut syndrome.

Multifocal Independent Spikes

The appearance of three or more (multifocal) independent spike foci has been associated with clinical syndromes similar to SSWCs (50,51). This is not surprising

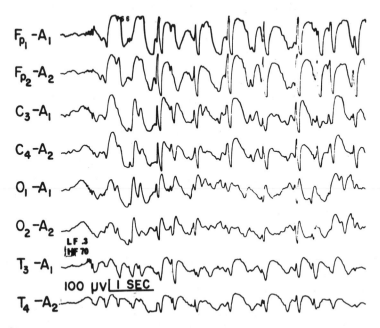

FIG. 7. Slow spike-and-wave complex—41-year-old man with severe mental retardation and intractable mixed seizure disorder. Note the irregular polyspike-and-wave morphology occurring at 1–2 Hz; also, note the disorganized background.

when one considers that this pattern is frequently seen concomitantly in patients with SSWCs. The transformation between multifocal independent spikes and SSWCs in individual patients is also reported (50). As in SSWCs, multifocal independent spikes may develop in patients previously demonstrating hypsarrhythmia. Over 80% of patients are mentally retarded or show other neurologic deficits. All types of generalized and partial seizures have been reported, with generalized tonic–clonic, atypical absence, and focal clonic seizures being most common. Over one-half of the patients have a mixed seizure disorder (53).

Three-Hertz Spike-and-Wave

The 3-Hz spike-and-wave (Fig. 8) is the pattern most often associated with typical absence seizures. Hyperventilation is a potent activator of 3-Hz spike-and-wave discharges, and in untreated children this discharge is rarely missed during this activation procedure. Its frequency may vary from 2.5 to 3.5 Hz during brief bursts. During longer bursts of 5 or more seconds, the frequency of the discharge can be 4–6 Hz at onset before slowing to 3 Hz during the major part of the discharge. This is a generalized discharge with the maximum amplitude seen in the frontal regions. Individual interictal spikes or sharp waves, usually frontal in distribution, are occasionally seen, as are generalized spike and polyspike discharges during sleep (54).

Three useful clinical points should be kept in mind: (i) The electroencephalogram can help in assessing the frequency of seizures and response to medication (55). (ii) The bursts should be considered an ictal pattern, since decreased responsiveness

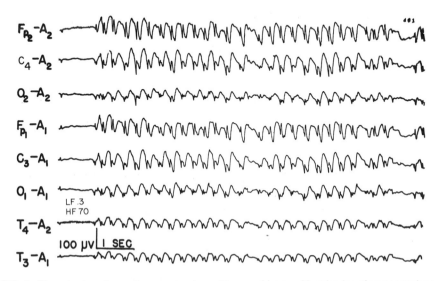

FIG. 8. Three-hertz spike-and-wave complex—19-year-old man with episodes of unresponsiveness. Note the consistent morphology.

occurs even with short bursts (45,56). (iii) The pattern can be inherited as an asymptomatic EEG finding, especially in family members of patients with documented absence seizures (18).

Generalized Spike and Spike-and-Wave Complexes

Generalized spikes, sharp waves, polyspikes, and multiple irregular spike-and-wave complexes are seen interictally which do not fit the categories described above (Fig. 9). They do not have the specificity of the other generalized discharges previously discussed and are seen in other forms of generalized epilepsies. The interictal findings are associated with all types of generalized seizures. The multiple or polyspike discharge is seen frequently in association with myoclonic seizures, but this relationship is not absolute (57). These generalized patterns are frequently accentuated during sleep, and their appearance in sleep can be seen in association with the more specific generalized patterns of discharges categorized above, such as 3-Hz spike-and-wave or slow spike-and-wave. Their appearance during sleep should not detract from or overly complicate the EEG classification or interpretation with respect to that which would be based on the awake tracing (54). As in all the generalized patterns, infrequent independent focal sharp waves or spikes may also be seen.

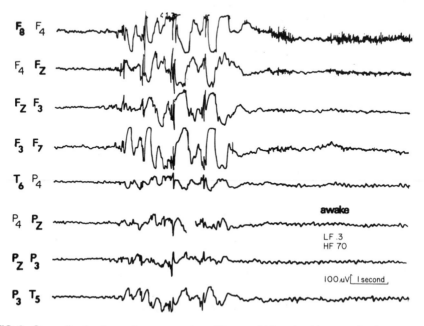

FIG. 9. Generalized spike-and-wave complex—38-year-old female with generalized myoclonic and tonic–clonic seizures. Note the irregular rate of repetition relative to that seen in Fig. 10.

The background of the electroencephalogram demonstrating such discharges can be useful in diagnosing and classifying epileptic syndromes (45). Normal background is commonly seen in idiopathic generalized epilepsies, and slowing of background with a more disorganized record is associated with the symptomatic generalized epilepsies.

Periodic Lateralized Epileptiform Discharges (PLEDs)

As their name suggests, PLEDs are discharges that occur in a periodic or pseudoperiodic fashion with a frequency of approximately 1 per second. They are usually lateralized over an entire hemisphere, although a more localized or focal distribution can also be seen. The complexes do not have a stereotyped morphology and can consist of repetitive spike, polyspike, or spike-and-wave complexes with admixed slower components. PLEDs occur in the setting of acute, aggressive lesions and are most often associated with cerebrovascular accidents, infections, or tumors. Metabolic disorders are seen in approximately one-third of the patients with PLEDs (58,59). Adults usually show a depressed level of consciousness, but in children this is not necessarily part of the electroclinical syndrome (60). Seizures are seen acutely (i.e., within 1 week) in approximately 80% of patients with PLEDs (58–61). Usually, the seizures are partial motor seizures with and without secondary generalization. Epilepsia partialis continua (i.e., repetitive focal clonic seizures) is commonly seen. PLEDs will usually persist for several weeks with or without anticonvulsant therapy and then dissipate. Persistent seizure disorders are seen in 25% or more of these patients (59,62). Although the relationship is not absolute, PLEDs within the context of encephalitis should raise the suspicion of herpes encephalitis (63).

Focal Epileptogenic Discharges

The appearance of focal spikes and sharp waves is most consistent with partial seizure disorders. The morphology of these discharges varies, and it is the location of the abnormality that usually takes on a greater significance.

Focal temporal discharges are most often associated with complex partial seizures with or without secondarily generalized seizures. These are frequently seen to occur independently over both temporal regions, and if they are clearly predominant over one area, there is the possibility that the contralateral discharges are only a reflection of the predominant focus. Frontal lobe discharges are associated with partial seizures in which motor manifestations may be the clinical hallmark. Occipital foci may give rise to unformed visual hallucinations as part of the partial seizure of occipital origin.

Secondary bilateral synchrony refers to a generalized epileptogenic discharge that has been triggered from a focal source. Such generalized discharges are often associated with a frontal focus, but other areas of the brain can generate these bursts. Strict electrographic criteria should be used to determine the presence of secondary bilateral synchrony (64). There should be an active-dominant focus that clearly precedes (by 0.5–2 sec) the generalized bursts. Clinically, generalized seizures seen in the setting of secondary bilateral synchrony raise the possibility that they are secondarily generalized seizures. Only five of 26 patients in two studies of patients with midline spikes and seizures had partial seizures, and 21 had generalized seizures (65,66). Triggering of generalized discharges from a focal source may explain the occurrence of generalized seizures in a large percentage of these patients with purely midline parasagittal spikes in the interictal electroencephalogram.

Benign focal epileptiform discharges of childhood (Fig. 10) are unique waveforms that are most often associated with a central temporal distribution. They can be found in other locations, and several foci may be seen. It is important to differentiate these from multifocal independent spikes. Electrographically, this differentia-

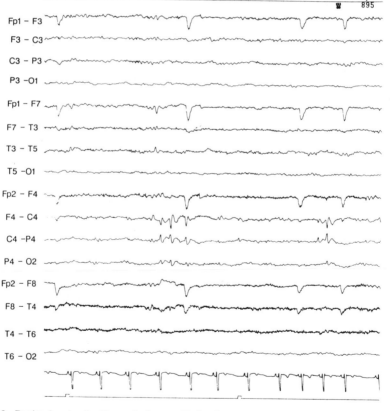

FIG. 10. Benign focal epileptiform discharges ("rolandic spikes")—8-year-old boy without a history of any seizures. Note the fairly consistent morphology of activity in right centroparietal region; also, note the independent "rolandic" discharge seen in the left temporal region.

tion is made by several points: (a) Benign focal discharges are usually sharp waves lasting 80–200 msec and not spikes lasting less than 80 msec. (b) They are activated or present only in sleep. (c) They have a stereotyped monotonous morphology. (d) No other generalized epileptogenic abnormality is seen. (e) Background activity is normal (21). Clinically, most of these children are neurologically intact, may not have seizures, or may have an easily controlled, self-limited seizure disorder.

PROGNOSTICATION, MEDICATION, AND THE ELECTROENCEPHALOGRAM

Difficult aspects of management in patients with seizures include when to start and stop medications (see Chapter 8). It would be desirable to have an objective marker to measure the patient's response to therapy. The role of routine electroencephalography in these issues is controversial, but it is safe to say that routine electroencephalography has not lived up to many of the expectations of clinicians.

The role of electroencephalography in predicting which patients who experience a single unprovoked seizure will subsequently develop recurrent seizures (i.e., epilepsy) is debated. Hauser et al. (67) reported on 244 patients of all ages who suffered one unprovoked seizure. The overall recurrence rate was 27% at 36 months. That study showed that the appearance of a generalized spike-and-wave pattern was statistically useful in prognosis. Fifty percent of the patients showing this pattern had seizure recurrence, whereas 14% had a normal or minimally abnormal record. Surprisingly, focal slow activity or focal EEDs did not affect recurrence rates when these patients were compared with patients whose electroencephalogram was normal or who showed mild abnormalities. Recent studies have shown that the electroencephalogram is not a good prognostic indicator whether the EEG abnormalities are nonspecific or epileptogenic (68–70).

The interaction between the electroencephalogram and medication in the treated epileptic can sometimes be useful in management. The best-defined relationship is between generalized 3-Hz spike-and-wave discharges and absence seizures. The rate of recurrence of the 3-Hz spike-and-wave discharge appears to be proportional to the clinical response to therapy (56,71). Other seizure types have a less-defined relationship. There is no apparent effect of oral medication on the frequency of other EEDs (12,13,71,72). Intravenous benzodiazepines and phenytoin appear to decrease EEDs. Benzodiazepines and barbiturates also accentuate fast activity, which may be of value in assessing drug compliance or drug abuse.

Medication-induced encephalopathies can be mild or severe. Slowing of background activity on the electroencephalogram may be the first objective sign of this drug effect. More severe cognitive impairment may be associated with more severe diffuse slowing on the electroencephalogram. In patients in a stuporous state resulting from medication toxicity, triphasic waves can be seen. The electroencephalogram can, therefore, be quite useful in the treated patient who has shown a precipitous decline in cognitive function. It can give the physician clues whether the patient is chronically intoxicated, in a postictal state, or in a nonconvulsive status epilepticus.

The use of routine electroencephalography as an aid in deciding when to stop medication in controlled patients has had both supporters (71,73–77) and opponents (77–80). Recent studies are summarized in Table 4. Emerson et al. (73) examined patients 6–22 years old who were seizure-free for 4 or more years. Only four of 34 patients (12%) with normal electroencephalograms relapsed, but in patients with definitely "abnormal" electroencephalogram, a classification that included all EEDs, 13 of 23 (57%) relapsed. In a study of 92 adults and children who were seizure-free for 2 or more years, 31 eventually relapsed (75). The electroencephalogram was found to be predictive in that study. Fourteen of 19 patients (74%) whose electroencephalogram was abnormal before treatment and remained unchanged at drug withdrawal eventually relapsed, whereas 15 of 66 patients (23%) with normal electroencephalograms relapsed. Despite such findings, other studies show no statistically significant relationship between (a) relapse rate in controlled epileptics withdrawn from medication and (b) EEG findings. In a study of 148 children withdrawn from antiepileptic medications after at least 4 years of being seizure-free, there was a recurrence of seizures in 41 (80). Of these 148, 116 had an abnormal electroencephalogram; of those 116, approximately 30% had seizure recurrence, a rate close to that of the total recurrence rate. However, 23 of 73 (32%) with specific EEDs and only six of 32 (19%) with normal electroencephalograms had recurrences, a trend that was not thought to be statistically significant. Other studies of controlled patients withdrawn from medications found no statistical difference between seizure recurrence and the appearance of specific epileptogenic epileptiform patterns (70,78,79).

In summary, routine electroencephalography can be helpful in managing the patient with known epilepsy in specific situations in which the clinical course is not stable and perhaps in monitoring the effects of treatment on absence seizures with 3-Hz spike-and-wave activity. It has little role in managing the patients whose seizure pattern and clinical state is stable and unchanged. With regard to antiepileptic medication initiation and withdrawal, the role of electroencephalography is evolving and is presently undefined. Therefore, for these decisions, the physician should determine beforehand how the results of electroencephalography will be applied to the clinical situation, if an electroencephalogram is to be obtained.

ADVANCED NEUROPHYSIOLOGIC TECHNIQUES

In the medical (and especially the surgical) management of seizure disorders, routine EEG studies can be complemented by advanced techniques that are already in the mainstream of clinical practice. These techniques include the use of (a) simultaneous video and EEG monitoring, (b) ambulatory EEG cassette monitoring, and (c) polysomnography. These studies require prolonged patient recording times as discussed in this chapter and in the next chapter. Scalp recorded evoked potentials

TABLE 4. *Usefulness of electroencephalogram in deciding medication withdrawal in controlled patients: recent studies*

Study	N	Age (in years) at time of withdrawal	Minimum years seizure free	Relapse rate (%)	Electroencephalogram helpful (yes/no)	Comments
Emerson et al. (73)	68	6–22	4	26	Yes	Five of 41 (12%) relapsed if electroencephalogram was normal or "minimally abnormal."
Sofijanov (81)	46	18–60	3	63	No	No statistically significant difference.
Holowach et al. (82) and Holowach-Thurston et al. (80)	148	5–18	4	28	No	19% relapsed if electroencephalogram was normal; 30% if EEG was abnormal—not a significant difference.
Todt (83)	473	3–16	2*	34	Yes	26% relapsed if electroencephalogram was normal at time of withdrawal; 59% relapsed if there was "paroxysmal activity" on electroencephalogram.
Shinnar et al. (84)	88	2–24	2	25	Yes	84% with normal record were seizure-free; 5% with spikes and abnormal slowing were seizure-free.
Bouma et al. (85)	116	3–20	2	81	No	Improvements in electroencephalogram at time of withdrawal, when compared with previous electroencephalograms; had trend toward good prognosis.
Callaghan et al. (75)	92	Average of 24	2	34	Yes	23% relapsed with normal electroencephalograms compard with 74% with abnormal electroencephalograms showing no improvement during treatment.
Arts et al. (77)	146	3–20	2	25	Yes	If electroencephalogram is normal at withdrawal, then other variables can be used to predict prognosis.

*One year for absence seizures.

(i.e., auditory, visual, or somatosensory evoked potentials) are not useful in the routine management of epileptic patients. Newer technologies are presently being researched which extract information from ictal and interictal electrical brain activity that may prove useful in patient management. Like routine interictal electroencephalography, they do not necessarily require prolonged recording time in a hospital or laboratory setting.

Magnetoencephalography (MEG) is the measurement of the extracranial magnetic fields of the brain that are produced from the intracranial electrical currents. These signals are quite small—the earth's magnetic field is approximately one billion times larger than the measured fields of the brain.

The MEG instrumentation consists of placing a sensing coil perpendicular to and near the source of electrical currents to measure the induced magnetic field. This sensing coil is part of a superconducting quantum interference device (SQUID). The SQUID converts weak magnetic fields to an electrical signal that can then be amplified and ultimately printed out by pen writing systems similar to that used for EEG signals.

The major advantage of MEG is that it gives three-dimensional localization of spike foci as opposed to the "two-dimensional" electrode array of standard scalp electroencephalography. It does this by using the assumption that the MEG source is an electrical dipole. This assumption has been shown to be a good first approximation of an epileptic spike source (86,87). Given the measured magnetic field and the assumption of a dipole source, one may apply several mathematical techniques that will solve the "inverse problem" of where that source must be located in the skull to generate the measured magnetic fields.

Despite the encouraging data obtained by MEG, it has several disadvantages and limitations. The magnetic fields of the brain are very small, and contamination by magnetic fields in the environment can happen easily. Therefore, shielded rooms are necessary and sometimes quite costly. At present, there is a limitation to the number of sensors that are available for each magnetometer. This leads to the need to do sequential recordings over several sites; consequently, it may take several hours to obtain adequate interictal data for an epileptic patient. Obtaining precise ictal recordings is even more difficult, given the need to have exact positioning of the sensors over a patient's head and a need to do sequential recording. MEG may prove to be an effective method for noninvasive recordings in epileptic patients once the number of "channels" recorded increases and, more importantly, once its cost effectiveness can be improved.

Within the realm of routine EEG recordings has been the development of a great number of quantitative EEG (QEEG) techniques that attempt to extract more information from the routine EEG recording. It is hoped that more sensitive and specific data will emerge by applying QEEG techniques than by using routine electroencephalography. One such technique has been the dipole localization method (DLM) (88). The generator of an interictal spike or a focal EEG seizure pattern onset can be assumed to be, for a first approximation, a dipolar source (86,87). By measuring the electrical field of an event on the scalp, a mathematical model very similar to that used in MEG can be applied to solve the "inverse problem"—that is, given the recorded electric potentials on the scalp, where would a dipolar source have to be located to generate such potentials? This technique allows for a three-dimensional localization in the skull based on scalp recorded EEG data. Unlike the MEG, the mathematical computations must take into account the differences in resistance between the brain, skull, and scalp. This technique has been confirmed with intracranial recordings as well as with clinical data and magnetic resonance imaging (MRI) scans (89). DLM and similar techniques have the advantage of using standard recording equipment; therefore it is potentially very cost effective, unlike MEG.

The QEEG technique of topographic mapping (TM) has received much clinical and research attention. Most probably, this interest is a reflection of the appearance of these maps which gives the clinician the sense that he or she is looking at an "electrical computed tomography (CT) scan." This is not the case. TM attempts to quantify the EEG or evoked potential signal at each recording electrode and then attempts to construct from these a complete electrical field map of the brain. In addition to voltage topography, many different interpolated maps can be constructed. Common ones include: (a) a *power* spectrum, usually expressed as microvolts squared (μV^2), at a fixed frequency for the entire electrode array; (b) a *frequency* map, which can be constructed at a given time or at a given power; or (c) a *statistical* map, which can demonstrate how a certain variable (e.g., power or frequency) may deviate from given normative or group data or from a given baseline for an individual patient.

These maps do not represent actual EEG signals occurring across the skull but represent a mathematical construct of what they *may* look like. The maps are constructed on grids of data points; for example, an entire TM may be constructed from a 32 × 32 display grid. The resulting map gives 1024 points that are displaying data, but only 16 or 32 of these points may represent real data while the other 992 "electrical pixels" represent interpolated display. This is very different from CT or MRI scanning, where each pixel of the display represents an actual point of data acquisition.

Despite this limitation, there are some clear advantages to TM, the primary one being the significant amount of data reduction a TM allows. This is of even greater importance when larger numbers of channels are used. By quantifying the electroencephalogram, the signal can be processed and stored by computer for future analysis. TM is a very objective method of displaying brain electrical activity that in some instances could be interpreted by clinicians without rigorous EEG training. An objective display also allows a comparison of EEG data from research center to research center. As will be discussed, TM is bringing into focus the importance and usefulness of looking at background EEG signals and not just the epileptogenic waveforms. TM is showing changes in patients with epilepsy with apparent normal background that are not always seen in the normal population.

TM may develop into a useful test in the evaluation of the patient with a seizure disorder, but at this time it is still only a research tool (90). There are many aspects of TM that need definition prior to full clinical utilization. Indeed, to interpret TM at this time requires one to be familiar with all aspects of routine EEG recording. No TM can be interpreted without having the routine EEG signal properly evaluated. The reasons for this are clear. There must be a completely artifact-free portion of electroencephalogram analyzed; otherwise, irrelevant maps and false interpretations could occur. The TM represents a brief snapshot of electroencephalogram, and no more than several seconds are usually analyzed at a time; consequently, intermittent abnormalities may be completely missed. In other words, variations over time are not always taken into account with each individual map. It is debated as to which recording technique is best for obtaining data, and the amount of data collected is so voluminous that clinically significant variables have not been totally defined. A whole series of new TM artifacts are now being found, and the extent and characteristics of these TM artifacts awaits definition (91). Finally, it should be noted that color displays of TM can be deceiving to the eye. Large color differences may represent small changes in frequency or voltage, and again many of the points of

TABLE 5. *Electroclinical syndromes*

Interictal EEG finding	Frequently associated seizure type	Frequently associated epilepsy syndrome[a]
Hypsarrhythmia	Generalized tonic and myoclonic (infantile spasms)	West syndrome
Slow spike-and-wave complexes	Mixed	Generalized epilepsies; Lennox–Gastaut syndrome
Multifocal independent spike	Mixed	Generalized epilepsies
Three-hertz spike-and-wave complexes	Absence	Adolescent and juvenile absence epilepsy
Generalized spikes, sharp-wave or irregular spike-and-wave complexes	Generalized	Generalized epilepsies
Benign focal epileptiform discharges	Partial with or without secondarily generalized	Benign childhood epilepsy with centrotemporal spikes; childhood epilepsy with occipital paroxysms
Focal spikes or sharp waves and secondary bilateral synchrony	Partial with or without secondarily generalized	Localization related symptomatic (partial) epilepsies
PLEDs	Focal motor with or without secondarily generalized (epilepsia partialis continua)	Localization related symptomatic (partial) epilepsies

[a]Syndromes are from the International Classification of Epileptic Syndromes (93).

color change are interpolated data. For this reason, black-and-white displays are better for objectively analyzing results.

At some point, TM may emerge as a useful adjuvant to the evaluation of the seizure patient who is undergoing video–EEG analysis of his or her seizure disorder. In many ictal recordings, nonspecific, nonfocal changes may occur prior to a definitive EEG seizure pattern, and the EEG seizure pattern can lag behind the time the patient clearly has started his or her clinical seizure. Defining an abnormality at or prior to the clinical onset of a clinical seizure is the most desirable result when evaluating a patient for seizure surgery or when trying to clearly diagnose a patient's seizure disorder. Ictal recordings have been examined, and preliminary reports show that TM can help identify localized abnormalities at clinical onset of seizures which are not clearly evident by routine electroencephalography. One study showed that when maps of the theta frequency were analyzed, five of five patients with complex partial seizures of temporal lobe origin had properly localized TM when compared to standard and advanced localization techniques such as positron emission tomography (PET) scanning, intracranial recordings, and routine scalp EEG data (92). In one of these five patients the scalp electroencephalography was falsely localizing, but the mapping data converged with the other techniques.

TM may prove to help increase the yield of EEG data in the interictal recordings of seizure patients—especially that 8–10% of patients whose electroencephalograms repeatedly never show definitive epileptogenic abnormality. But the interictal abnormalities defined by TM at this time are still nonspecific, and specific epileptogenic markers need definition. After proper evaluation and research, TM may prove helpful in identifying ambiguous ictal and interictal foci in the epilepsy patient. For the patient with seizures, TM may also help define epilepsy syndromes based on (a) field analysis of spikes, (b) interictal background analysis, and (c) evoked potential characteristics.

CONCLUSION

Normal records and abnormal nonspecific findings are commonly seen in patients with seizures as well as other disorders. Therefore, all EEG reports can include the phrase "the record is consistent with seizures." The appearance of clearly epileptogenic epileptiform patterns supports the diagnosis of a seizure disorder, but even this finding has to be applied to the clinical situation.

Certain EEG findings are associated with clinical syndromes as summarized in Table 5, but no association holds across all cases. If conflicts arise between clinical, laboratory, and interictal EEG data or, more importantly, if therapeutic strategies are not meeting with success, it may be a signal to the clinician to pursue more advanced or more intensive testing.

REFERENCES

1. Engel J. A practical guide for routine EEG studies and epilepsy. *J Clin Neurophysiol* 1984;1;109–142.

2. Mizrahi EM, Kellaway P. Characterization and classification of neonatal seizures. *Neurology* 1987;37:1837–1844.
3. Torres F, Ellingson RJ, Klass DW, Mattson RH. Committee on guidelines for writing EEG reports. American EEG Society guidelines in EEG and evoked potentials. *J Clin Neurophysiol* 1986;3 (Suppl):34–37.
4. Ochs RF, Cayaffa J, Ho S, Olson S. A method for the standardization of EEG interpretation. *J Clin Neurophysiol* 1987;4(3):279–280.
5. Chatrian GE, Bergamni L, Dondey M, et al. A glossary of terms most commonly used by clinical electroencephalographers. *Electroencephalogr Clin Neurophysiol* 1974;37:538–548.
6. Maulsby RL. Some guidelines for assessment of spikes and sharp waves in EEG tracings. *Am J EEG Technol* 1971;11(1):3–16.
7. Ajmone-Marson CA, Zivin LS. Factors related to the occurrence of typical paroxysmal abnormalities in the EEG records of epileptic patients. *Epilepsia* 1970;11:361–381.
8. Jasper HH. The 10–20 electrode system of the international federation. *Electroencephalogr Clin Neurophysiol* 1958;10:371–373.
9. Sundaram M, Hogan T. First standard EEG in epilepsy. *J Clin Neurophysiol* 1987;4(3):284.
10. Lesser RP. American EEG Society guidelines in EEG and evoked potentials. *J Clin Neurophysiol* 1986;3(Suppl 1):1–7.
11. Salinsky M, Kanter R, Dasheiff RM. Effectiveness of multiple EEG in supporting the diagnosis of epilepsy: an operational curve. *Epilepsia* 1987;28(4):331–334.
12. Gotman J, Marciani MG. Electroencephalographic spiking activity, drug levels and seizure occurrence in epileptic patients. *Ann Neurol* 1985;17:597–603.
13. Zivin L, Ajmone-Marson CA. Incidence and prognostic significance of "epileptiform" activity in the EEG of non-epileptic subjects. *Brain* 1968;91:751–778.
14. Klass DW, Westmoreland BF. Nonepileptogenic epileptiform electroencephalographic activity. *Ann Neurol* 1985;18:627–635.
15. Petersen I, Eeg-Olofsson O, Selldin U. Paroxysmal activity in EEG of normal children. In: Kellaway P, Peterson I, eds. *Clinical electroencephalography of children*. Stockholm: Almquist and Wiksell, 1968;167–188.
16. Cavazzuti GBC, Cappella L, Nalin A. Longitudinal study of epileptiform EEG patterns in normal children. *Epilepsia* 1980;21:43–55.
17. Eeg-Olofsson O. The development of the electroencephalogram in normal adolescents from the age of 16 through 21 years. *Neuropadiatrie* 1971;3:11–45.
18. Metrakos JD, Metrakos MD. Genetic factors in the epilepsies. In: *The epidemiology of epilepsy*. A workshop NINDS monograph, no. 14, 1972;99–102.
19. Engel M, Luders H, Chatrian AM. The significance of focal EEG spikes in epileptic and non-epileptic children who are otherwise normal. *Ann Neurol* 1977;2(3):157.
20. Smith JMB, Kellaway P. Central (Rolandic) foci in children: an analysis of 200 cases. *Electroencephalogr Clin Neurophysiol* 1964;17:451–472.
21. Luders H, Lesser RP, Dinner DS, Morris HM. Benign focal epilepsy of childhood. In: Luders H, Lesser RP, eds. *Epilepsy: electroclinical syndromes*. Heidelberg: Springer-Verlag, 1987.
22. Mattson RH, Pratt KL, Calverley JR. Electroencephalograms of epileptics following sleep deprivation. *Arch Neurol* 1965;13:310–315.
23. Pratt KL, Mattson RH, Weikers NJ, Williams R. EEG activation of epileptics following sleep deprivation: a prospective study of 114 cases. *Electroencephalogr Clin Neurophysiol* 1968;24:11–15.
24. Ellingson RJ, Wilken K, Bennett DR. Efficacy of sleep deprivation as an activation procedure in epilepsy patients. *J Clin Neurophysiol* 1984;1:83–101.
25. Lee SI, Kirby D. Absence seizure with generalized rhythmic delta activity. *Epilepsia* 1988;29:262–267.
26. Tyner F, Knott JR, Mayer WB. *Fundamentals of EEG technology, vol 1: basic concepts and methods*. New York: Raven Press, 1983.
27. Reiher J, Lebel M. Wicket spikes: clinical correlations of a previously undescribed EEG pattern. *Can J Neurol Sci* 1977;4:39–47.
28. White JC, Langston JW, Pedley TA. Benign epileptiform transients of sleep. *Neurology* 1977;27:1061–1068.
29. Reiher J, Lebel M, Klass DW. Small sharp spikes: reassessment of electro-encephalographic characteristics and clinical significance. *Electroencephalogr Clin Neurophysiol* 1977;43:775.

30. Gibbs FA, Rich CL, Gibbs UL. Psychomotor variant type of seizure discharge. *Neurology* 1963;13:991–998.
31. Lipman LJ, Hughes JR. Rhythmic mid-temporal discharges. *Electroencephalogr Clin Neurophysiol* 1968;27:43–47.
32. Maulsby RL. EEG patterns of uncertain diagnostic significant. In: Klass DW, Daley DD, eds. *Current practice of clinical electroencephalography.* New York: Raven Press, 1979;27–36.
33. Pedley TA. EEG pattern that mimics epileptiform discharges that have no association with seizures. In: Henry CE, ed. *Current clinical neurophysiology: update on EEG and evoked potentials.* Amsterdam: Elsevier/North-Holland, 1980;307–336.
34. Kimura T, Hatta T, Fujimoto Y, et al. Cyclic vomiting as an autonomic seizure. *Yonago Acta Med* 1975;19:160–169.
35. Lombroso CT, Schwartz JH, Clark DM, et al. Ctenoids in healthy youths. Controlled study of 14- and 6-per-second positive spiking. *Neurology* 1966;16:1152–1158.
36. Eeg-Olofsson O. The development of the electroencephalogram in normal children from the age of 1 through 15 years: 14- and 6-Hz positive spike phenomena. *Neuropadiatrie* 1971;2:405–427.
37. Hughes JR. Two forms of the 6 per sec spike-and-wave complex. *Electroencephalogr Clin Neurophysiol* 1980;48:535–550.
38. Westmoreland BF, Klass DW. A distinctive rhythmic EEG discharge of adults. *Electroencephalogr Clin Neurophysiol* 1981;51:186–191.
39. Cobb WA, Guiloff RJ, Cast J. Breach rhythm: the EEG related to skull defects. *Electroencephalogr Clin Neurophysiol* 1979;47:251–271.
40. Kubichi S, Holler L, Pastelak-Price C. Subvigil beta activity: a study of fast EEG patterns in drowsiness. *Am J EEG Technol* 1987;27:15–31.
41. Klass DW. Electroencephalographic manifestations of complex partial seizures. In: Penry JK, Daly DD, eds. *Advances in neurology,* vol. II. New York: Raven Press, 1975;113–140.
42. Abraham K, Ajmone-Marson CA. Patterns of cortical discharges and their relationship to routine scalp electroencephalography. *Electroencephalogr Clin Neurophysiol* 1958;10:447–461.
43. Aird RB, Gastaut Y. Occipital and posterior electroencephalographic rhythms. *Electroencephalogr Clin Neurophysiol* 1959;11:637–656.
44. Arenas AM, Brenner RP, Reynolds CF. Temporal slowing in the elderly revisited. *Am J EEG Technol* 1986;26:105–114.
45. Pedley TA. Interictal epileptiform discharges: discriminating characteristics and clinical correlations. *Am J EEG Technol* 1980;20:101–119.
46. Reiher J, Beaudry M. Temporal interictal rhythmic delta activity: specificity and predictive value. *J Clin Neurophysiol* 1987;4:272–273.
47. Petersen I, Eeg-Olofsson O. The development of the EEG in normal children from the age of 1 through 15 years. *Neuropadiatrie* 1971;2:247–304.
48. Patel VM, Maulsby RL. How hyperventilation alters the electroencephalogram: a review of controversial viewpoints emphasizing neurophysiologic mechanisms. *J Clin Neurophysiol* 1987;4:101–120.
49. Jeavons PM, Bower BD, Dimitrakoudi M. Long term prognosis of 150 cases of "West syndrome". *Epilepsia* 1973;14:153–164.
50. Noriega-Sanchez AL, Markand ON. Clinical and electroencephalographic correlation of independent multifocal spike discharges. *Neurology* 1976;26:667–672.
51. Blume WT, David RB, Gomez MR. Generalized sharp and slow wave complexes: associated clinical features and long term followup. *Brain* 1973;96:289,306.
52. Gastaut H, Roger J, Soulayrol R, et al. Childhood epileptic encephalopathy with diffuse slow spike-waves (otherwise known as "petit mal variant") or Lennox syndrome. *Epilepsia* 1966;7:139–179.
53. Blume WT. Clinical and electroencephalographic correlates of the multiple independent spike foci pattern in children. *Ann Neurol* 1978;4:541–547.
54. Luders H, Lesser RP, Dinner DS, Morris HH. Generalized epilepsies: a review. *Cleve Clin Q* 1984;51:205–226.
55. Brown TR, Dreifuss FE, Penry JK, Porter RJ, White BG. Clinical and EEG estimates of absence seizure frequency. *Arch Neurol* 1983;40:469–472.
56. Browne TR, Penry JK, Porter RJ, Dreifuss FE. Responsiveness before, during, and after spike-wave paroxysms. *Neurology* 1974;24:659–665.
57. Delgado-Escueta AV, Enrile-Bascal F. Juvenile myoclonic epilepsy of Janz. *Neurology* 1984;34:285–294.

58. Chatrian GE, Shaw C, Leffman H. The significance of periodic lateralized epileptiform discharges in EEG: an electrographic, clinical and pathological study. *Electroenceph Clin Neurophysiol* 1964;17:177–193.
59. Young GB, Goodenough P, Jacono V, Schieven JR. Periodic lateralized epileptiform discharges (PLEDS): electrographic and clinical features. *Am J EEG Technol* 1988;28:1–13.
60. PeBenito R, Cracco JB. Periodic lateralized epileptiform discharges in infants and children. *Ann Neurol* 1979;6:47–50.
61. Markand ON, Daly DD. Pseudoperiodic lateralized paroxysmal discharges in electroencephalogram. *Neurology* 1971;21:975–981.
62. Schrader PL, Singh N. Seizure disorders following periodic lateralized epileptiform discharges. *Epilepsia* 1980;27:647–653.
63. Lai C, Gragasin E. Electroencephalography in herpes simplex encephalitis. *J Clin Neurophysiol* 1988;5:87–103.
64. Blume WT, Pillay N. Electrographic and clinical correlates of secondary bilateral synchrony. *Epilepsia* 1985;20:636–641.
65. Nelson KR, Brenner RP, De La Paz D. Midline spikes: EEG and clinical features. *Arch Neurol* 1983;40:473–476.
66. Pedley TA, Tharp BR, Herman K. Clinical and electroencephalographic characteristics of midline parasagittal foci. *Ann Neurol* 1981;142–149.
67. Hauser WA, Anderson VE, Loewenson RB, McRoberts ST. Seizure recurrence after first unprovoked seizure. *N Engl J Med* 1982;307:522–528.
68. Elwes RDC, Johnson AL, Shovon SD, Reynolds EH. The prognosis for seizure control in newly diagnosed epilepsy. *N Engl J Med* 1984;311:944–947.
69. Hopkins A, Garman A, Clarke C. The first seizure in adult life. *Lancet* 1988;1:721–726.
70. Beghi E, Tognoni G. Prognosis of epilepsy in newly referred patients: a multicenter prospective study. *Epilepsia* 1988;29:236–243.
71. Duncan JS. Antiepileptic drugs and the electroencephalogram. *Epilepsia* 1987;28:259–266.
72. Theodore WH, Sato S, Porter RJ. Serial EEG in intractable epilepsy. *Neurology* 1984;34:863–867.
73. Emerson R, D'Souza BJ, Vining E, et al. Stopping medication in children with epilepsy. *N Engl J Med* 1981;304:1125–1129.
74. Chadwick D, Reynolds EH. When do epileptic patients need treatment starting and stopping medications. *Br Med J* 1985;290:1885–1888.
75. Callaghan N, Garrett A, Goggin T. Withdrawal of anticonvulsant drugs in patients free of seizures for two years. *N Engl J Med* 1988;318:942–946.
76. Pedley TA. Discontinuing antiepileptic drugs. *N Engl J Med* 1988;318:982–984.
77. Arts WFM, Visser LH, Loones MCB, et al. Followup of 146 children with epilepsy after withdrawal of antiepileptic therapy. *Epilepsia* 1988;29:244–250.
78. Janz D, Sommer-Burkhardt EM. Discontinuation of antiepileptic drugs in patients with epilepsy who have been seizure free for more than two years. In: *Epileptology proceedings, 7th international symposium of epilepsy*. Stuttgard: G. Thieme 1975;228–234.
79. Overweg J, Rowan AJ, Binnie CD, Oosting J, Nagelkerke NJD. Prediction of seizure recurrence after withdrawal of antiepileptic drugs. In: Dom M, Gram L, Penry JK, eds. *Advances in epileptology: XIIth epilepsy international symposium*. New York: Raven Press, 1981.
80. Holowach J, Thurston DL, Hixon BB, Keller AJ. Prognosis in childhood epilepsy additional followup of 148 children 15 to 23 years after withdrawal of anticonvulsant therapy. *N Engl J Med* 1982;306:831–836.
81. Sofijanov NG. Clinical evolution and prognosis of childhood epilepsies. *Epilepsia* 1982;23:61–69.
82. Holowach J, Thurston DL, O'Leary J. Prognosis in childhood epilepsy: follow-up study of 148 cases in which therapy had been suspended after prolonged anticonvulsant control. *N Engl J Med* 1972;286:169–174.
83. Todt H. The late prognosis of epilepsy in childhood: results of a prospective followup study. *Epilepsia* 1984;25:137–144.
84. Shinnar S, Vining EPG, Mellites, ED, et al. Discontinuing antiepileptic medication in children with epilepsy after two years without seizures. *N Engl J Med* 1985;313:976–980.
85. Bouma PAD, Peters ACB, Marts RJH, Stijen Th, Van Rossum J. Discontinuation of antiepileptic therapy: a prospective study of children. *J Neurol Neurosurg Psychiatry* 1987;50:1579–1583.
86. Rose DF, Smith PD, Sato S. Magnetoencephalography and epilepsy research. *Science* 1987;238:329–335.

87. Ricci GB, Romani GL, Salustri C, et al. Study of focal epilepsy by multichannel neuromagnetic measurements. *Electroencephalogr Clin Neurophysiol* 1987;66:358–368.
88. Smith DB, Sidman RD, Flanigin H, et al. A reliable method for localizing deep intracranial sources of the EEG. *Neurology* 1985;35:1702–1707.
89. Lee L, Smith DB, Sidman R, Kramer RE. Intracranial localization of epileptic spikes using DLM. *J Clin Neurophysiol* 1988;5:336.
90. Nuwer MR. American Electroencephalographic Society statement on the clinical use of quantitative EEG. *J Clin Neurophysiol* 1987;4:197.
91. Nuwer MR, Jorden SE. The centrifugal effect and other spatial artifacts of topographic EEG mapping. *J Clin Neurophysiol* 1987;4:321–326.
92. Naylor DE, Lieb JP, Risinger M. Computer enhancement of scalp sphenoidal ictal EEG in patients with complex partial seizures. *Electroencephalogr Clin Neurophysiol* 1988;70:205–219.
93. Commission on Classification and Terminology of the International League Against Epilepsy. Proposal for classification of epilepsies and epileptic syndromes. *Epilepsia* 1985;26:268–278.

Epilepsy: Current Approaches to Diagnosis and Treatment,
edited by Dennis B. Smith,
Raven Press, Ltd., New York © 1990.

3

Prolonged Monitoring in the Management of Patients with Epilepsy

Don W. King

Department of Neurology, Medical College of Georgia, Augusta, Georgia 30912

Epilepsy is a paroxysmal disorder characterized by intermittent episodes of altered behavior separated by periods of normal behavior. Because of their intermittent and usually unpredictable occurrence, seizures are rarely observed by the physician caring for the patient with epilepsy. The workup of patients with epilepsy generally consists of a history and physical examination, metabolic and imaging studies to search for an underlying cause, and standard electroencephalography (EEG) to document "epileptiform" abnormalities that show a strong correlation with epilepsy. In most patients, standard evaluation is adequate. In a number of patients, however, additional information is needed before appropriate treatment can be initiated.

In an attempt to gain more definitive information, methods have been developed to record simultaneously the clinical behavior and electroencephalogram during clinical seizures. In the 1950s, Ajmone-Marson and Ralston (1) photographed the clinical behavior and recorded the electroencephalogram during seizures precipitated by the injection of pentylenetetrazol. During the past 10–15 years, techniques have been developed to continuously monitor the clinical and EEG phenomena in order to capture spontaneous seizures (2–5). This chapter will include an overview of techniques used for continuous monitoring, a brief review of the types of data obtained during monitoring, and a discussion of the indications and uses of prolonged monitoring in clinical practice. For more detailed information, readers may consult refs. 2 and 3.

METHODS AND EQUIPMENT

There are a wide variety of systems used for prolonged monitoring. This is due both to the rapidly changing technology and to the different clinical needs of the centers that perform monitoring. It should be emphasized that there is not one ideal system for monitoring. Systems should be adapted to the clinical needs, technical personnel, and resources available at an individual center.

Equipment for Prolonged EEG Recording

Electrodes

Depending on the clinical application, scalp, basal, or intracranial electrodes may be used. Standard scalp electrodes are used for all major clinical applications. Basal electrodes, either nasopharyngeal or sphenoidal, are used to record activity from the mesial temporal regions. Because they are better tolerated for long periods of time, sphenoidal electrodes are more useful than nasopharyngeal electrodes for prolonged monitoring. Intracranial electrodes, either depth or subdural, are used in selected patients who are being evaluated for ablative surgery. In general, they are appropriate for patients in whom localization is inadequate using noninvasive scalp and sphenoidal recording.

Amplification, Transmission, and Storage of EEG Data

Multiple methods have been developed for the amplification, transmission, and storage of EEG data. The four most commonly used types of systems are: (i) "hard-wired" recording using a standard EEG machine; (ii) cable telemetry; (iii) radio-telemetry; and (iv) ambulatory cassette recording.

A "hard-wired" system uses standard electrode connector pins, an EEG jack box, a cable transmitting EEG data from the jack box to the EEG machine, and a standard EEG machine for amplification of the signal (Fig. 1). The EEG signals may be written out on-line and stored on paper as in routine EEG, or they may be recorded onto tape using the output jacks of the EEG machine. Each channel of data may be stored individually onto tape, or up to 16 channels of EEG activity may be multiplexed into a single signal before recording onto tape. One advantage of a hard-wired system is that much of the equipment is readily available to all EEG laboratories. In addition, montage selection and amplifier adjustment are easily accomplished using the standard controls of the EEG amplifiers. Disadvantages include (a) limited mobility of the patient and (b) excessive amounts of paper if the data are stored on paper. To allow more patient mobility, some manufacturers have recently developed single cables up to 20 feet connecting the patient electrodes with the EEG jack box.

Cable telemetry uses small amplifiers placed near the electrodes for initial amplification (Fig. 2). The amplifiers are placed in a box secured to a platform on the patient's head or in a pouch on the upper chest. The amplified EEG signals from up to 64 channels are multiplexed near the source and transmitted by cable for storage onto tape. The stored, multiplexed signal is replayed through a demultiplexor before paper writeout through an EEG machine. Recording characteristics of cable telemetry are usually excellent, and cable telemetry allows freedom of movement up to the length of the cable, usually about 50 feet. Cable systems have become the most commonly used form of prolonged monitoring in centers evaluating patients for

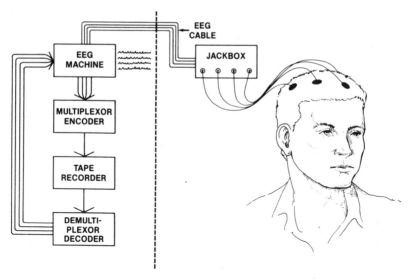

FIG. 1. Schematic diagram of "hard-wired" EEG monitoring system. This system uses the amplifiers of standard EEG machines for initial amplification. The EEG signals may be played directly onto paper or may be multiplexed into a single signal and recorded onto tape for storage. It is replayed through a multiplexor/decoder before playback through the EEG machine.

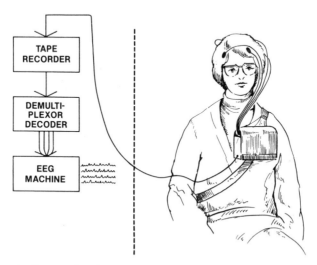

FIG. 2. Schematic diagram of cable telemetry system. In cable telemetry, the EEG signals are amplified and multiplexed within the box attached to the patient, and the multiplexed signal is transmitted to the tape recorder by a long cable that allows patient mobility up to the length of the cable. The signal is replayed through the multiplexor/decoder before playback through the EEG machine.

epilepsy surgery. Previous disadvantages of cable telemetry were as follows: Montage selection was limited to preset montage boards placed in the telemetry box, and amplifier adjustment during recording was not possible. Recent improvements in technology, however, now permit "reformatting" and changes in amplification and filter settings "off-line."

As with cable telemetry, radiotelemetry provides for initial amplification and multiplexing of EEG signals near the recording electrodes (Fig. 3). The amplified/multiplexed signal is transmitted by radiofrequency to antennas/receivers which then transmit the signal; this signal is replayed through a demultiplexor before EEG paper writeout. Radiotelemetry allows complete freedom of movement up to the distance allowed by the radiotransmitter, usually approximately 50 ft. One disadvantage is that there is usually more amplifier blockage with radiotelemetry than with cable telemetry.

Ambulatory cassette recording is the most common form of prolonged monitoring in general use (Fig. 4). In early cassette recording systems, initial amplification was adjacent to the electrodes, and the amplified signal was transmitted by a short cable for storage onto a cassette tape that rested in a pouch at the patient's waist. In some of the newer systems, amplification is achieved within the box at the patient's waist. In general, the quality of ambulatory cassette recording is excellent, and cassette recording allows complete freedom of movement inside or outside the

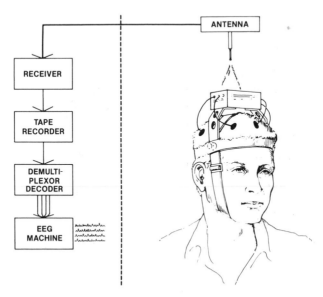

FIG. 3. Schematic diagram of radiotelemetry system. The EEG signals are amplified and multiplexed within the box near the electrodes, and the multiplexed signal is transmitted by radiofrequency to antennas in the ceiling. The multiplexed signal is recorded onto the tape recorder as with cable telemetry. The signal is replayed through the multiplexor/decoder before replay through the EEG machine.

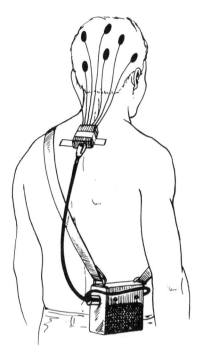

FIG. 4. Schematic diagram of ambulatory cassette recorder system. EEG signals are amplified adjacent to the electrodes and recorded onto a cassette tape within a pouch at the patient's side. This system allows maximal patient mobility. The EEG signals can be replayed through a scanner for visual and auditory scanning or through the EEG machine for paper writeout.

hospital. One disadvantage is that, at present, only eight channels of continuous EEG activity can be stored on the cassette tapes. Because of the mobility allowed with these systems, cassette recording is usually used for outpatient monitoring and not for combined EEG and video/audio monitoring. However, video and audio systems can be used with cassette recording, providing simultaneous EEG and video/audio data. Montage selection is limited, and amplifier adjustment is not possible during recording.

Playback and Review of Stored EEG Data

Review of a standard paper EEG writeout is the most common method for reviewing EEG data obtained during prolonged monitoring. If the EEG activity has been stored as a single multiplexed signal, paper writeout requires replaying the stored data through a demultiplexor/decoder before entry into the EEG machine. A number of manufacturers have developed devices for visually scanning the data on screen as it is being replayed. This has proven to be very helpful in analyzing large amounts of EEG data.

Reformatter

A reformatter takes 8, 16 or more channels of EEG data and electronically records the data in analog form onto video tape. This allows one to observe continuous EEG activity on the video screen. A reformatted electroencephalogram on the video screen is very helpful for technicians monitoring the electroencephalogram at the time of recording. However, reviewing the electroencephalogram on a video screen is, in general, not adequate for precise interpretation such as in the localization of seizure onset during evaluation for surgery.

Equipment for Prolonged Video/Audio Recording

There are four major components of a video/audio monitoring system: cameras, audio equipment, video cassette recorders (VCRs), and television monitors. Since it is often necessary to record during sleep, high-quality cameras specifically designed for low-light-level recording should be employed. Although not essential, two cameras allow greater flexibility than one. A zoom lens is helpful for close-up monitoring of the face, and a "fish eye" lens which covers an entire room allows the patient to move about during the recording.

The audio portion of the monitoring system should allow two-way communication between the patient and the technician or nurse monitoring the patient. This can be accomplished by employing microphones and amplifier/speakers in both the patient room and the control room. The microphone in the control room must be easily activated so that instructions to the patient and questioning during seizures are transmitted to the patient, but ongoing conversation within the control room is not transmitted to the patient. Sound from both the patient and control room microphones is recorded onto one audio channel of the video tape for correlation with the video data at the time of replay.

The video image and audio data are recorded onto a VCR for storage and later playback. Initially, most centers used industrial-grade ³/₄-inch VCRs for prolonged monitoring, and these remain the standard from the standpoint of video quality. However, high-quality ¹/₂-inch beta and VHS VCRs have become available and are now used in most centers.

Television monitors are used by the technician or nurse to continuously monitor patient behavior. This is an important aspect of the system, both to check for quality of the video and EEG signals (see reformatter) and to detect otherwise undiscovered clinical episodes.

Synchronization Between Video and EEG Signals

Synchronization between the EEG and video/audio data is usually accomplished by means of a time code generator that places the time (either analog or digital) onto both video and EEG tapes. Another excellent method for synchronization is to record the multiplexed EEG signal onto the second audio channel of the video tape so that only one tape stores all of the data. This allows precise synchronization and easy simultaneous replay of EEG and video/audio data.

TYPES OF DATA OBTAINED

There are three major types of useful data obtained during prolonged monitoring: interictal EEG data, ictal EEG data, and behavioral manifestations of clinical episodes.

The most useful interictal EEG data are paroxysmal sharp waves and spikes, referred to as "epileptiform discharges" (Figs. 5 and 6). Both clinical and experimental data show a strong correlation between interictal epileptiform discharges and clinical epilepsy (6). In clinical practice, interictal discharges are used for confirmation of epilepsy in patients with an appropriate history, for assistance in the determination of seizure type in certain patients, and for localization of an abnormal brain area responsible for seizures in patients being evaluated for surgery. If interictal discharges are present on standard recordings, prolonged monitoring for interictal activity adds little useful information. However, in patients with suspected epi-

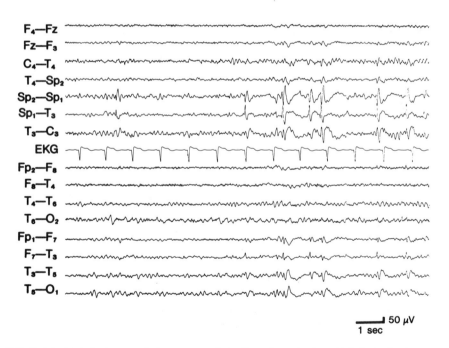

FIG. 5. Interictal electroencephalogram recorded with scalp and sphenoidal electrodes in a patient with complex partial seizures. There are frequent spikes and sharp waves ("epileptiform discharges") from the left temporal region, maximal from the left mesial temporal region, with phase reversals at the Sp$_1$ electrode.

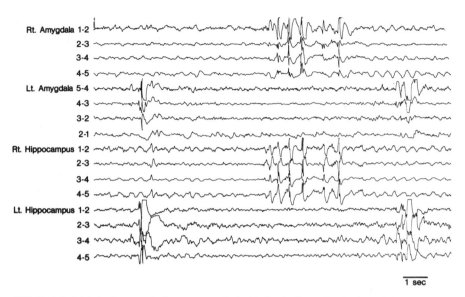

FIG. 6. Interictal electroencephalogram recorded with depth electrodes implanted from a vertex approach (15) into the amygdala and hippocampus in a patient with complex partial seizures. Numbers refer to contact points. Number 1 is the deepest contact for each electrode, and subsequent points are more superficial. Contact points are separated by 5 mm. There are frequent bilaterally independent "epileptiform discharges" from the mesial temporal regions.

lepsy and no epileptiform activity on standard EEG, prolonged monitoring in search of interictal epileptiform discharges may be helpful in confirming the diagnosis of epilepsy. Basal electrodes are especially valuable in detecting interictal discharges from mesial temporal structures in patients with suspected complex partial seizures.

The "ictal" electroencephalogram refers to EEG activity that occurs at the time of a clinical seizure. There are a wide variety of EEG abnormalities that occur during seizures (Figs. 7 and 8). The ictal pattern is dependent on the age of the patient, the type and severity of the seizure, the area of brain involved in the seizure, the type and location of recording electrodes, and other factors. In general, the hallmark of an EEG seizure is rhythmic activity. The most common EEG patterns seen during an EEG seizure include: attenuation of EEG activity; rhythmic "sinusoidal-appearing" activity; and rhythmic sharp waves, spikes, or spike-and-wave discharges (Figs. 7 and 8). Seizures that occur in structures at a distance from the recording electrodes may show either nonrhythmic slow activity or no EEG change during a seizure. Thus, negative scalp electroencephalograms during an episode do not rule out the possibility that the episode was a seizure. Either attenuation of activity or nonrhythmic slow activity is characteristic of the postictal state, and, at times, postictal slowing may be the only finding suggestive of a seizure.

The behavioral manifestations of a clinical episode are the third major type of data obtained with prolonged monitoring. Behavioral manifestations include: subjective phenomena experienced by the patient; adversive, tonic, and clonic motor

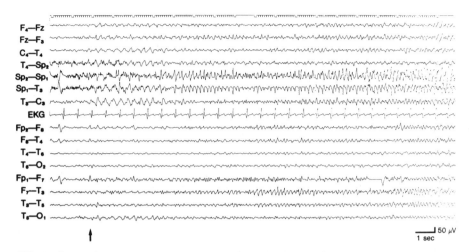

FIG. 7. Onset of complex partial seizure recorded with scalp and sphenoidal electrodes. The arrow denotes the onset of the EEG seizure. There is initially a burst of unlocalized rhythmic delta activity that is followed (in approximately 4 sec) by rhythmic theta activity, maximal from the left mesial temporal region as recorded by the Sp$_1$ electrode.

phenomena; various forms of automatisms; and various levels of responsiveness. Certain phenomena are suggestive of specific seizure types or central nervous system (CNS) localization. Generalized seizures are characterized by impaired responsiveness and, in most instances, symmetric motor phenomena. The clinical phenomena during generalized tonic–clonic seizures, absence attacks (7), and infantile spasms (8) are well described. Auras and lateralized motor phenomena at seizure onset suggest a focal onset (i.e., a partial seizure). The ictal manifestations of the seizure may provide evidence as to the location of seizure onset. Recent data suggest that partial seizures of frontal onset exhibit different clinical manifestations from those of temporal lobe onset (9,10). Pseudoseizures may also have characteristic clinical patterns (11).

CLINICAL APPLICATIONS

In general, prolonged monitoring is indicated when standard evaluation leaves unanswered questions that may be resolved by prolonged monitoring. For this chapter, clinical applications are classified into four basic categories: differentiation of epileptic seizures from nonepileptic episodes; determination of types of seizures in patients with known epilepsy; better characterization of seizures in patients with known epilepsy; and localization of an epileptogenic focus in patients who are candidates for surgery.

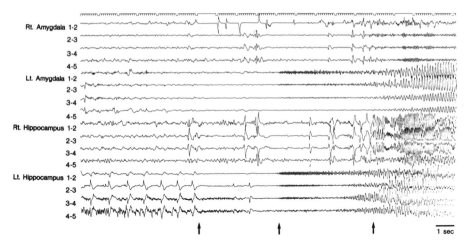

FIG. 8. Onset of complex partial seizure originating in the left mesial temporal region recorded with depth electrodes implanted into the amygdala and hippocampus bilaterally (see Fig. 6 for details of electrodes). This figure shows a number of EEG seizure patterns. At the first arrow, there is attenuation of activity from the left amygdala (channels 5–8) and left hippocampus (channels 13 and 14). At the second arrow, there is the development of high-frequency rhythmic activity in the left amygdala (channels 5–7) and left hippocampus (channels 13–16). The rhythmic activity gradually increases in amplitude and decreases in frequency. At the third arrow, there is spread of the EEG seizure from the left to the right mesial temporal region.

Differentiation of Epileptic Seizures from Nonepileptic Episodes

"Spells" of uncertain mechanism represent a common clinical problem seen by most physicians. The differential diagnosis may include seizure, reflex or cardiac syncope, vestibular dysfunction, focal cerebral ischemia, and pseudoseizure. In many patients, there is a question concerning the nature of all of the patient's episodes. In this group, interictal epileptiform discharges are very helpful; that is, in a patient with a single type of episode suggestive of seizures, interictal epileptiform discharges provide strong confirmatory evidence that the episodes are epileptic. If standard and sleep-deprived electroencephalograms reveal no epileptiform activity, prolonged monitoring may be used to detect interictal epileptiform events.

In a second group of patients—namely, those with known seizures and additional episodes of uncertain mechanism—interictal epileptiform discharges are of less value in determining the nature of the uncertain episodes. Behavioral and EEG data during an episode are usually necessary to make a diagnosis. An EEG seizure during a typical clinical episode is conclusive that the episode is epileptic. However, the lack of an EEG seizure must be interpreted with caution. Muscle and movement artifact often obscure EEG seizures. In addition, seizures often arise in deep structures that may be distant from the recording electrodes. On the other hand, most seizures with *loss of consciousness* show some form of EEG change with 16-channel recording (i.e., an EEG seizure, focal slowing, or diffuse slowing). A normal

16-channel EEG during prolonged unresponsiveness suggests that the episode is not epileptic. The diagnosis of pseudoseizure should be reserved for episodes with no EEG change and behavioral manifestations during the episode suggestive of a pseudoseizure (11).

Each of the systems previously described may provide useful information in determining the nature of an episode of uncertain mechanism. Ambulatory cassette monitoring is often helpful in documenting interictal and ictal epileptiform activity in patients with negative standard electroencephalograms (12). When positive, ambulatory cassette monitoring may obviate the need for hospitalization. However, if ambulatory recordings provide equivocal data or if observation of the event is important for the diagnosis, simultaneous video/audio and EEG monitoring must be performed. Even when episodes are recorded during prolonged monitoring, a definite diagnosis may not be possible in some patients.

At the Medical College of Georgia, we use prolonged inpatient video/audio and EEG monitoring to differentiate epileptic seizures from nonepileptic episodes. Patients are usually admitted to the hospital for up to 1 week of daytime monitoring or continuous 24-hr monitoring. In patients without EEG evidence of epilepsy, medications may be gradually withdrawn. In 90 consecutive patients who underwent daytime monitoring for up to 1 week because of episodes of uncertain mechanism, episodes were recorded in 66: 21 were determined to be epileptic, 43 were determined to be nonepileptic, and for two patients a determination could not be made. Ten additional patients had interictal epileptiform abnormalities allowing us to make a presumed diagnosis of epilepsy without actually recording an event. In 14 patients, no events were recorded, and no diagnosis was made.

Determination of Types of Seizures in Patients with Known Epilepsy

Patients with known seizures often have "minor" episodes that are difficult to diagnose based on history alone. These episodes may be absence seizures, complex absence seizures, simple partial seizures, complex partial seizures, tonic seizures, or, occasionally, myoclonic seizures. In many cases, differentiation is important for prescribing appropriate treatment. Interictal discharges recorded during standard EEG may strongly suggest a specific type of seizure. However, if standard EEG is not helpful, prolonged monitoring to record a clinical episode may be required. In most cases, both the clinical manifestations of the seizure and the ictal electroencephalogram are helpful in determining the type of seizure. Characteristic EEG patterns include: generalized three-per-second spike-and-wave activity in patients with absence attacks; generalized attenuation or high-frequency rhythmic activity in patients with tonic seizures; and generalized spike-and-wave or polyspike-and-wave discharges during myoclonic jerks. Partial seizures may be characterized by focal or diffuse rhythmic activity, or by focal or diffuse slowing, during the clinical episode. Rhythmic theta activity recorded with basal electrodes is a common EEG pattern seen in patients with complex partial seizures of mesial temporal origin (Fig. 7).

Any of the systems described may provide useful information in determining the type of epileptic seizure. Ambulatory cassette recording may demonstrate interictal activity and EEG seizures which are characteristic of a specific seizure type. When EEG coverage broader than eight channels is required or when observation of the episode is important, complete video/audio and EEG monitoring is required.

In 138 consecutive epileptic patients evaluated for seizure type with video/audio and EEG monitoring, we were able to firmly classify seizures in 119. Classification was based on recorded episodes in 74 patients and on interictal epileptiform discharges in 45 patients. Seizures remained unclassified in 19 patients. This included 10 patients in whom we were able to record episodes but whose seizure phenomena were not easily classified according to the International Classification of Epileptic Seizures.

Characterization of the Seizure Disorder in Patients with Known Epilepsy

There are a number of instances in which proper management requires a better understanding of the seizure disorder than can be obtained by standard evaluation procedures. For example, it may be important to determine the frequency of episodes before and after medication change in order to determine the effectiveness of a specific medication. This is most easily accomplished in patients with multiple seizures per day, such as absence attacks or infantile spasms (7,8). Prolonged monitoring may also help clarify the relationship between clinical seizures and the sleep/wake cycle or specific precipitating events. Documentation of a specific type of reflex epilepsy may allow one to recommend measures to prevent seizures. Prolonged monitoring may also assist in determining the effect of seizures on clinical behavior or cognition. This may be helpful in providing counseling for patients, families, school officials, and others.

Localization of an Epileptogenic "Focus" in Patients Who Are Candidates for Epilepsy Surgery

Localization of the "epileptogenic" region responsible for the patient's seizures requires the integration of a number of types of data. These include: the clinical phenomena of the seizures; neuropsychological data; imaging study data; and interictal and ictal EEG data. When a structural lesion is present in an appropriate location, EEG is used to confirm that the seizures arise in the vicinity of the structural lesion. When a structural lesion is not present, EEG investigation becomes the primary means for localization. Scalp electrodes are used in all patients being evaluated for surgery, and basal electrodes are used to detect interictal discharges and electrographic seizures from the mesial temporal regions. Implanted electrodes are necessary for (a) patients with bilateral or poorly localized interictal discharges or (b) patients with unlocalized EEG seizure onset precipitated by scalp and sphenoidal electrodes (6,13–16).

Consistently localized interictal discharges provide important information concerning the site of seizure origin (6). In the early years of epilepsy surgery, interictal discharges were the primary means of localization; improvement in a large percentage of patients following surgery proved the value of this method. However, because interictal discharges may be poorly localized, multifocal, or falsely localizing (17), the electrographic onset of a patient's habitual seizure is generally considered the most reliable criterion for localizing the epileptogenic region prior to surgery. Most centers now require prolonged monitoring in order to record at least three of the patient's habitual seizures before recommending surgery (13–16).

Correlation of clinical seizure phenomena with electrographic onset is especially important in the work-up of patients for epilepsy surgery. A localized electrographic seizure onset that precedes the clinical onset provides evidence that the seizure originated in the area recorded by the involved electrode. Since scalp and sphenoidal electrodes may not record the onset of a seizure arising from deep mesial temporal structures, a scalp- or sphenoidal-recorded onset that follows soon after clinical onset may still have localizing value. In our experience, if all interictal and ictal abnormalities are localized to one temporal region, a localized, sphenoidal-recorded EEG seizure onset that follows soon after clinical onset can still be used for recommending surgery (18). On the other hand, a depth-recorded electrographic seizure that follows clinical onset suggests the seizure arose in a location distant to the recording electrode.

Since both clinical seizure phenomena and detailed ictal EEG data are required, only combined video/audio and EEG monitoring with at least 16 channels is adequate for presurgical evaluation.

Of 79 consecutive patients admitted to the Medical College of Georgia for evaluation for ablative surgery, localization was obtained in 55. This included 47 patients with unilateral anterior/midtemporal seizure onset, three with bilaterally independent temporal seizure onset, and five with extratemporal seizure onset. In 16 patients we were unable to localize seizure onset adequate to recommend surgery; two patients had recorded pseudoseizures, and six patients did not complete the evaluation.

ADDITIONAL CONSIDERATIONS

Prolonged monitoring is a diagnostic technique that is an excellent procedure for answering specific questions that cannot be answered by traditional diagnostic techniques. However, it should be emphasized that prolonged monitoring is an expensive procedure, and by itself it will not improve seizure control. There are many patients with uncontrolled seizures in whom prolonged monitoring is not of value. In addition, inpatient monitoring in an attempt to record an episode is of relatively little value in patients with infrequent seizures. For these reasons, prolonged monitoring should be used only in patients in whom there is a specific indication and whose episodes occur frequently enough that there is a reasonable chance of benefit.

A second consideration deals with the withdrawal of medications. In general, if it is important to record an episode and episodes do not occur frequently while the patient is on medication, medications should be gradually tapered during the period of monitoring. This applies to patients with episodes of uncertain mechanism and to those being evaluated for epilepsy surgery. One must always be aware that seizures that occur during medication withdrawal may not be identical to the patient's habitual seizures. Despite this possibility, medication withdrawal is often a valuable adjunct to prolonged monitoring.

CONCLUSION

Prolonged monitoring has proven to be a valuable procedure in selected patients with epilepsy and suspected epilepsy. It has become a commonly used procedure in most epilepsy centers, and it is rapidly becoming available to many community hospitals. However, caution in the selection of centers for the referral of patients is advised (see Appendix). Because of the present shortage of data, we cannot make a reasonable estimate of the number of people who may benefit from prolonged monitoring; however, long waiting lists for inpatient monitoring at most epilepsy centers suggest that the demand is presently much greater than the ability to meet the demand. Improvements in technology plus more widespread application of monitoring should continue to improve the diagnosis and treatment of selected patients with epilepsy.

REFERENCES

1. Ajmone-Marson C, Ralston B. *The epileptic seizure. Its fundamental morphology and diagnostic significance.* Springfield, IL: Charles C Thomas, 1957.
2. Engel J, Ebersole JS, Burchfield JL, et al. American Electroencephalographic Society guidelines for long-term neurodiagnostic monitoring in epilepsy. *J Clin Neurophysiol* 1985;2:419–452.
3. Gotman J, Ives JR, Gloor P. *Long-term monitoring in epilepsy (Supplement 37 to EEG Clin Neurol).* Amsterdam: Elsevier, 1985.
4. Ives JR, Thompson CJ, Gloor P. Seizure monitoring: a new tool in electroencephalography. *EEG Clin Neurol* 1976;41:422–427.
5. Porter RJ. Methodology of continuous monitoring with video tape recording and electroencephalography. In: Wada JA, Penry JK, eds. *Advances in epileptology: the tenth epilepsy international symposium.* New York: Raven Press, 1980;35–42.
6. Gloor P. Contributions of electroencephalography and electrocorticography to neurosurgical treatment of the epilepsies. In: Purpura D, Penry K, Walter R, eds. *Advances in neurology,* vol 8. New York: Raven Press, 1975;59–105.
7. Penry JK, Porter RJ, Dreifuss FE. Simultaneous recording of absence seizures with video tape and electroencephalography: a study of 374 seizures in 48 patients. *Brain* 1975;98:427–440.
8. Kellaway P, Hrachovy RA, Frost JD, Zion T. Precise characterization and quantification of infantile spasms. *Ann Neurol* 1979;6:214–218.
9. Walsh GO, Delgado-Escueta AV. Type II complex partial seizures: poor results of anterior temporal lobectomy. *Neurology* 1984;34:1–13.
10. Williamson PD, Spencer DD, Spencer SS, Novelly RA, Mattson RH. Complex partial seizures of frontal lobe origin. *Ann Neurol* 1985;18:497–504.
11. Gulick TA, Spinks IP, King DW. Pseudoseizures: ictal phenomena. *Neurology* 1982;32:24–30.
12. Bridgers SL, Ebersole JS. The clinical utility of ambulatory cassette EEG. *Neurology* 1985;35:166–173.

13. Delgado-Escueta AV, Walsh GO. The selection process for surgery of intractable complex partial seizures: surface EEG and depth electrography. In: Ward AA, Penry JK, Purpura D, eds. *Epilepsy*. New York: Raven Press, 1983;295–326.

14. Engel J, Crandall PH, Rausch R. The partial epilepsies. In: Rosenberg RN, ed. *The clinical neurosciences*, vol. 2. New York: Churchill Livingstone, 1983;1349–1380.

15. Flanigin H, King D, Gallagher B. Surgical treatment of epilepsy. In: Pedley TA, Meldrum BS, eds. *Recent advances in epilepsy*, vol. 2. Edinburgh: Churchill Livingstone, 1985;297–339.

16. Rasmussen TB. Surgical treatment of complex partial seizures: results, lessons, and problems. *Epilepsia* 1983;24(Suppl 1):S65–S76.

17. Engel J, Rausch R, Lieb JP, Kuhl DW, Crandall PH. Correlation of criteria used for localizing epileptic foci in patients considered for surgical therapy of epilepsy. *Ann Neurol* 1981;9:215–224.

18. King DW, Flanigin HF, Gallagher BB, et al. Temporal lobectomy for partial complex seizures: evaluation, results, and 1-year follow up. *Neurology* 1986;36:334–339.

Epilepsy: Current Approaches to Diagnosis and Treatment,
edited by Dennis B. Smith,
Raven Press, Ltd., New York © 1990.

4

Advanced Neuroimaging Techniques as Diagnostic Tools in Epilepsy

J. Chris Sackellares and Bassel W. Abou-Khalil

*Comprehensive Epilepsy Program, Department of Neurology,
University of Michigan Medical Center,
Ann Arbor, Michigan 48109*

The introduction of x-ray computed tomography (CT) brain scanning in the early 1970s ushered in a new era of noninvasive techniques for imaging the brain. With this new tool, clinicians could, for the first time, generate pictures of the brain parenchyma, including structural abnormalities within (a) the soft tissue of the brain, (b) the surface of the brain, or (c) the ventricles. Over the years, improved scanners were introduced, resulting in a diagnostic tool that has proven to be highly effective in detecting small structural lesions. Since CT scans can be performed with very little risk to the patient, the threshold for employing the x-ray CT scan as a diagnostic screening examination is much lower than that for older imaging techniques such as pneumoencephalography and angiography.

The utility of x-ray CT scanning in the diagnostic evaluation of patients with primary generalized epilepsy has been limited. This finding was not unexpected, since primary generalized seizures are not due to structural lesions. However, the x-ray CT scan has proven to be an important diagnostic tool for the partial epilepsies because partial seizures are often associated with focal abnormalities of the cerebral cortex. Although x-ray CT brain scanning is extremely useful for early detection of tumors causing partial seizures, it is of more limited value in cases where the seizure focus is associated with mesial temporal sclerosis. Even small tumors such as low-grade gliomas may not be detectable with x-ray CT scanning.

More recently, newer imaging techniques have been added to the diagnostic armamentarium. Magnetic resonance imaging (MRI) is now available in most major medical centers. The MRI scan provides an image of the brain which is of even higher resolution than that of the x-ray CT brain scan. Because of its recent introduction, we have only limited experience with the MRI scan in the evaluation of patients with partial seizures. However, MRI scanning may be even more sensitive than the x-ray CT brain scan in detecting focal lesions in patients with partial epilepsy. The MRI technique has the added advantage that the patient is not subjected to radiation exposure.

75

The use of both x-ray CT scanning and MRI scanning in the diagnostic evaluation of patients with partial epilepsy is limited by the nature of the disorder. An epileptic focus can occur as a result of very small structural lesions that may not be detectable by either technique. The most striking feature of partial epilepsy is not the structural abnormality but, instead, the focal disturbance in brain function. Until recently, electroencephalography was the only diagnostic tool capable of detecting the physiological disturbances of partial epilepsy. The advent of positron emission tomography (PET) introduced a new tool for detecting disturbances in brain function.

PET scanning involves the injection of biologically active substances that have been labeled with positron-emitting radioisotopes. PET scans using ^{18}F-fluorodeoxyglucose (^{18}F-FDG) have proven to be sensitive in detecting local disturbances in glucose metabolism in the interictal, ictal, and postictal states. The use of ^{18}F-FDG PET scans has already proven to be of clinical utility. This technique is currently employed as a means of confirming the location of a seizure focus in the workup for epilepsy surgery.

The potential use of PET scanning for clinical purposes is limited by the fact that most hospitals lack the facilities and personnel required for generating the isotopes and synthesizing the radiopharmaceuticals employed in the technique. Current PET scanners do not produce the degree of spatial resolution provided by x-ray CT and MRI scans. However, the potential of PET scanning for the study of brain processes associated with epilepsy is unprecedented. For example, PET techniques have been used to reflect metabolic and blood-flow changes that occur during seizures, and techniques for imaging neurotransmitter receptors are currently under development.

The use of these new imaging techniques in the diagnostic evaluation of patients with epilepsy is best understood in the context of what we know about (a) the pathological processes underlying the disorder and (b) the treatment modalities available. Since the clinical value of these techniques appears to be in the diagnostic evaluation of patients with partial epilepsy, the underlying pathology of the partial epilepsies will be reviewed in this chapter.

PATHOLOGY OF PARTIAL EPILEPSY

Partial epilepsy is a chronic condition in which seizures are caused by focal disturbances of neuronal excitability. In many cases, these physiological disturbances are associated with focal structural abnormalities. These structural abnormalities include: the residual effects of brain abscesses, meningitis, and encephalitis; vascular malformations; infarctions; gliosis and tumors. The incidence of specific types of lesions varies with a variety of factors, including (a) age of the patient when the seizures began and (b) anatomical location of the lesion (1).

Seizures of temporal lobe origin are most commonly associated with mesial temporal sclerosis (1). Mesial temporal sclerosis consists of localized neuronal loss and gliosis (2,3). Neurons that remain in the area often have reduced arborization of dendrites, irregularities in the dendritic spines, and irregularities in small vessels

(4). The causes of mesial temporal sclerosis have not been determined conclusively. However, neuronal loss and gliosis have been shown to occur as a result of a variety of insults to the nervous system, including hypoxia and ischemia and profound hypoglycemia. Mesial temporal sclerosis also has been associated with a history of status epilepticus and prolonged febrile convulsions in childhood.

Neoplasms represent another common cause of focal seizures of temporal lobe origin. In most instances, the tumors are low-grade gliomas. However, a variety of other tumor types have been reported in patients with medically refractory temporal lobe seizures. Low-grade gliomas may be quite small when seizures first occur, and they may progress very slowly over months, years, or even decades. As a result, they often produce little in the way of focal neurological signs and may not be detectable by conventional imaging techniques such as x-ray CT brain scans or angiography. Tumors most commonly involve the frontal and temporal lobes. Other lesions that may be associated with extratemporal seizure foci include: vascular malformations; gliotic scars secondary to trauma or infection; tuberous sclerosis; ulegyria; and hamartomas (1).

IMAGING TECHNIQUES EMPLOYED IN PARTIAL EPILEPSY

X-Ray CT Scan

X-ray CT scanning is performed by sending a series of x-ray beams at various angles through the target organ and measuring x-ray transmission. Computerized analysis of these transmission values is used to produce an image based upon the mass density of regions within the brain slice. X-ray CT scans have the highest yield of abnormalities in patients with new onset partial seizures. For example, patients whose first seizure was a simple partial seizure have had up to 62% incidence of focal CT abnormalities (5,6). When considering chronic complex partial epilepsy, the incidence of CT abnormalities may decrease to 22% (7). Even then, reported abnormalities have included mild diffuse atrophic changes or localized dilatation of a section of the lateral ventricle. Such abnormalities may have little relevance to the seizure disorder and do not necessarily assist in the localization of the epileptic focus (8).

The main role of CT scanning in epilepsy is in the detection of brain tumors, vascular malformations, focal atrophic lesions, and congenital malformations. Calcified lesions are readily detected by x-ray CT scans. Figure 1 shows an example of multiple calcified lesions in a patient with tuberous sclerosis. While large focal atrophic lesions are easily detectable by x-ray CT scanning, the more common lesion of mesial temporal sclerosis is usually not detectable by this technique. Aside from the problem that many lesions underlying partial epilepsy may be similar in density to surrounding brain, these lesions often occur in the floor of the middle cranial fossa. Because of this close proximity to thick bone, the area of interest may be obscured by artifact. Modified CT scanning techniques such as changing the angle of the tomographic plane or the use of intrathecal metrizamide or quantified

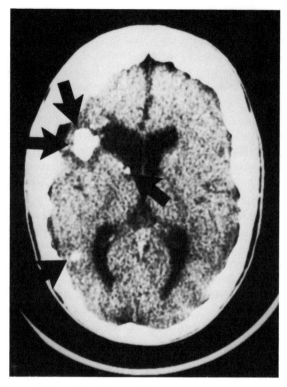

FIG. 1. X-ray CT scan performed in a 22-year-old woman with tuberous sclerosis. Multiple focal calcifications are seen as areas of high attenuation (*arrows*).

measures of contrast enhancement have been suggested as a means of increasing the sensitivity of this technique for finding focal abnormalities such as mesial temporal sclerosis in patients with chronic partial seizures being evaluated for surgical therapy (9–11). These techniques provide a modest contribution to basic x-ray CT scanning.

X-ray CT scans currently are employed routinely as a screen for tumors or other structural lesions such as vascular malformations in patients with partial seizures. For this purpose, x-ray CT scanning is significantly more suitable than the more invasive imaging techniques such as angiography and pneumoencephalography. Noncontrasted x-ray CT scans subject the patient only to the risks of radiation. Contrast enhanced scans may be useful for picking up vascular malformations and vascular tumors. The use of contrast involves the additional risk of allergic reactions to the contrast material.

Magnetic Resonance Imaging

Magnetic resonance imaging (MRI) utilizes nuclear magnetic resonance (NMR) technology. In this technique, a large fixed magnetic field causes alignment of the spin axes of the atomic nuclei. This results in alignment of the magnetic moments. A radiofrequency field is then applied (excitation). This causes the aligned atomic nuclei for a given nuclear species to precess around the axis of the static magnetic field. The resonance frequency required for excitation depends upon the nuclear species and the strength of the magnetic field. When the radiofrequency field is switched off, the precessing atomic nuclei emit high-frequency electromagnetic radiation of specific frequencies. The amplitude of the emitted high-frequency field decreases with time constants referred to as *relaxation times*. The amplitude of this electromagnetic signal depends upon (a) the density of the atomic species in the region (e.g., hydrogen) and (b) properties of the chemical environment. The chemical properties of the region also affect the relaxation times. The relaxation times relevant to imaging are called T_1 and T_2. By varying the excitation and measurement parameters, images can be produced which emphasize different properties of the tissue being imaged. There are a number of good reviews on the physical principles and technical aspects of MRI scanning (12–14).

Multiple studies have indicated that MRI is more sensitive than x-ray CT scan for detecting low-grade gliomas, focal atrophic lesions, and, possibly, mesial temporal sclerosis (15–22). However, there have been exceptions: MRI does not detect calcifications and may miss lesions with altered blood–brain barrier that the CT scan can detect through contrast enhancement (18,20). Moreover, the sensitivity of the x-ray CT scan in detecting small tumors of low vascularity, such as low-grade gliomas, has been disappointingly low. Unfortunately, this is just the type of tumor that is not uncommonly associated with chronic partial epilepsy.

Factors that may contribute to the sensitivity of the MRI scan include the absence of bone artifact and the ability to vary the technique to emphasize various properties of the tissue (T_1 and T_2 relaxation times and proton density). Another important feature of MRI is that it allows imaging the brain in various planes. Coronal images have improved the structural representation of the temporal lobes (17).

McLachlan et al. (17) identified focal findings in the MRI scan that are of value in localization of the epileptic focus in patients with temporal lobe epilepsy. These findings include small temporal lobe, small mesial temporal structures, small hemisphere, and focal increase in T_2 (increased signal on T_2 weighted scans) in the mesial aspect of one temporal lobe. In our series of patients with medically refractory partial seizures (15), the most common focal abnormality found on MRI scans was a focal area of increased signal in the mesial or basal temporal lobe. In every case, the location of these focal signal abnormalities corresponded to the location of the epileptogenic focus detected by electroencephalography (EEG).

Whether or not mesial temporal sclerosis can be detected by MRI scanning has been a controversial issue (17,23,24). Sperling et al. (23) found normal MRI studies in all their patients with pathologically proven mesial temporal sclerosis. Other investigators found gliosis and cell loss in areas corresponding to increased T_2 on MRI scans. However, the same histopathology (gliosis and cell loss) was found in areas without increased T_2 on MRI scans or in patients with no MRI signal abnormalities (17,22). Berkovic et al. (25) found focal areas of increased MRI signal localized to the hippocampus. In their group of patients, surgical pathologic speci-

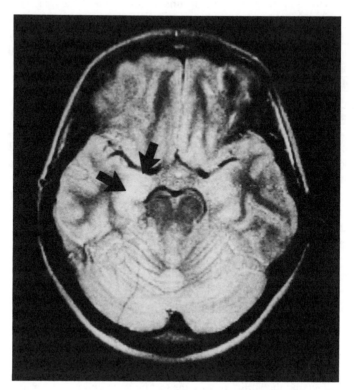

FIG. 2. Transverse and coronal sections of an MRI scan in a 24-year-old woman with complex partial seizures of right temporal origin. There is an area of increased signal in the right mesial temporal region (*arrows*). Seizure control was achieved following excision of this lesion. Histological examination of the surgical specimen revealed gliosis and neuronal loss.

mens showed neuronal loss and gliosis, features characteristic of mesial temporal sclerosis. All but one of these patients had a history of prolonged febrile convulsion in infancy, and one had a history of childhood encephalitis. Berkovic et al. (24,25) have suggested that with close attention to anatomy using coronal image sections, mesial temporal sclerosis may be detected by MRI. The hippocampus has a normally high signal relative to surrounding tissue. Therefore, comparison between the two hippocampi in the coronal plane may be necessary to detect the presence of relatively increased signal in one hippocampus. Transverse sections may not be suitable for this purpose. In those patients from our series (15) in whom temporal lobectomies have been performed, we have found signal abnormalities that corresponded to gliosis and cell loss as well as to low-grade astrocytomas.

Several examples of MRI abnormalities found in patients with partial epilepsy are shown in Figs. 2 through 5. These cases were selected to illustrate the sensitivity of MRI scanning in detecting lesions which are not seen (or which are poorly seen) with x-ray CT scans.

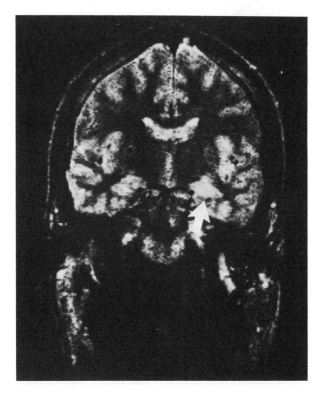

FIG. 3. Coronal MRI of a 22-year-old man with a left mesial temporal focus. An increased signal in the hippocampus (*arrow*) corresponds to the epileptogenic focus. Histological studies revealed mild neuronal loss and gliosis.

Figure 2 shows an example of a focal signal abnormality seen on MRI scanning in a 24-year-old woman with medically refractory complex partial seizures of right mesial temporal origin as a result of encephalitis. The x-ray CT scan in this patient was normal. Following surgical removal of the focus, the pathological finding was mesial temporal sclerosis. Examination revealed mild neuronal loss and gliosis in the hippocampus. Figure 3 shows a focal signal abnormality seen in the coronal plane in a patient with a prior history of prolonged febrile convulsions.

Figure 4 shows a right temporal lesion in a 29-year-old woman with refractory complex partial seizures. This lesion was found to be a thrombosed vascular malformation. The same lesion was present on her x-ray CT scan (not shown), but it had not been detected because of the relatively poor resolution of the CT image.

An example of a low-grade astrocytoma in the left temporal lobe of an 18-year-old boy with complex partial and simple partial seizures of left temporal origin is shown in the MRI slice depicted in Fig. 5. This lesion was detected by previous x-ray CT scans (not shown), but the quality of the image was not nearly as clear as that of the MRI scan.

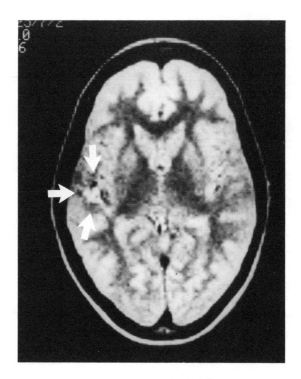

FIG. 4. MRI scan performed in a 29-year-old woman with complex partial seizures of right temporal origin. The area of mixed intensity signal in the right temporal lobe (*arrows*) corresponds to a thrombosed vascular malformation found at the time of surgery.

Positron Emission Tomography

Positron emission tomography (PET) scanning provides a means for measuring local cerebral blood flow (LCBF), local cerebral rate of oxygen uptake (LCRO$_2$), or local cerebral metabolic rate for glucose (LCMRG). Methods for imaging neurotransmitter receptors are currently under development. PET imaging is performed by injecting ligands tagged with positron emitters such as fluorine-18 (^{18}F), carbon-11 (^{11}C), or oxygen-15 (^{15}O). These isotopes emit positrons. When a positron collides with an electron in brain tissue, the positron annihilates the tissue, emitting two gamma rays at a 180° angle. The scanner is designed to detect these gamma rays and to determine the source of gamma emission.

PET scans of LCMRG have been shown to be useful for confirming the location of an epileptogenic focus in partial epilepsy. LCMRG PET scans usually are performed using a glucose analogue, deoxyglucose, labeled with ^{18}F (26–29). [^{18}F]fluorodeoxyglucose ([^{18}F]FDG) is injected intravenously while serial blood samples are taken from the radial artery. The arterial blood samples are assayed to

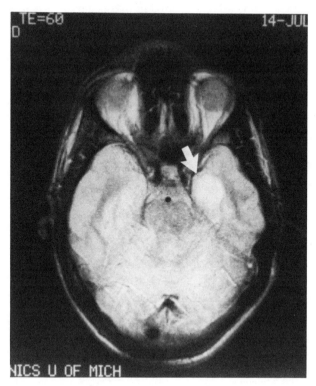

FIG. 5. MRI scan showing an area of increased signal in the left temporal lobe (*arrow*) of an 18-year-old boy with complex partial and simple partial seizures. The signal abnormality corresponded to a low-grade astrocytoma.

yield a curve of arterial ^{18}F concentration versus time. After an uptake period of approximately 30 minutes, the brain is scanned and the concentration of ^{18}F in various regions of the brain is calculated. Using computerized modeling based on Sokoloff's model (30), the local concentration of glucose is calculated for various brain regions. These calculated values are converted to images using either a gray scale or a color scale. The color or brightness of each pixel forming the image correlates with the calculated glucose metabolic rate in that part of the image. An example of an ^{18}F]FDG PET scan performed in a normal adult volunteer is shown in Colorplate 1.

The ^{18}F]FDG PET scan provides a visual display of the local metabolic rate for glucose. Image processing software allows one to isolate regions of interest within the image and to calculate the LCMRG. The metabolic rate for any given region of the brain will depend upon normal as well as abnormal physiological processes in that part of the brain. For example, when the eyes are closed, the LCMRG in the visual cortex is lower than when the eyes are open.

It should be emphasized that the ^{18}F]FDG PET scan technique reflects the metabolic activity in the brain during the period of isotope uptake. Therefore, in partial epilepsy, the findings on the [^{18}F]FDG PET scan depend upon the state of the patient at the time of the scan. [^{18}F]FDG PET studies have been performed during the interictal state in a fairly large number of patients with partial seizures. Because of the difficulty with timing the injection of [^{18}F]FDG to coincide with the onset of a seizure, there are fewer examples of ictal [^{18}F]FDG studies.

In the interictal state, the LCMRG in the area around a seizure focus is usually reduced relative to the LCMRG in the homologous region of the contralateral hemisphere. Local hypometabolism occurs in 70–80% of patients with medically refractory partial seizures (18,31–34). Interestingly, there is a wide range of normal values for LCMRG in the temporal lobe. In normal adult volunteers, we found a mean LCMRG in the lateral temporal cortex of approximately 6.0 mg glucose/min/100 g of brain tissue (1.25 S.D.) (31). Even the area of relative hypometabolism associated with a seizure focus may fall within two standard deviations of the mean for normals. Thus, measurement of absolute values for LCMRG is not a sensitive technique for identifying the location of a seizure focus. However, when the degree of asymmetry between the left and right temporal lobes (asymmetry index) is calculated in scans from patients with refractory partial seizures, the asymmetry will be beyond two standard deviations of the mean for normals in 81% of these patients (31).

Engel et al. (32,35) found that the anatomical location of the zone of relative hypometabolism correlates well with the EEG seizure focus as determined by EEG recordings. This finding has been confirmed by several other investigators (18,31–34). However, the exact location and anatomical extent of the hypometabolic region varies from patient to patient (36). The area of local hypometabolism is consistently much larger than the area of structural damage found in surgical specimens (36). In a study of 10 patients with medically refractory seizures with EEG evidence of epileptogenic foci of mesial temporal origin, we found that the area of hypometabolism consistently involved the lateral temporal cortex. In contrast, the mesial temporal region ipsilateral to the focus was less often hypometabolic (37).

Colorplate 2 is an example of an interictal [^{18}F]FDG scan taken in the same patient whose MRI is shown in Fig. 2. This scan illustrates a relatively hypometabolic zone of the right temporal region (area of the seizure focus) as compared to that of the left.

For patients in our series in whom EEG studies reveal a well-defined unilateral seizure focus, the interictal [^{18}F]FDG PET scan showed an area of hypometabolism corresponding to the EEG focus in 79% of cases (31). However, in two cases (10.5%) with unilateral EEG foci, the relative hypometabolic area was present in the contralateral hemisphere. In five of the seven patients with diffuse or shifting EEG foci, the [^{18}F]FDG PET scans showed no areas of relative hypometabolism. These results indicate that hypometabolic regions in the interictal [^{18}F]FDG PET scans usually correspond to the EEG focus, but this correlation is not perfect. Furthermore, when scalp-recorded EEG studies do not identify a clear epileptogenic focus, the PET studies may not yield definitive information regarding the site of the seizure focus.

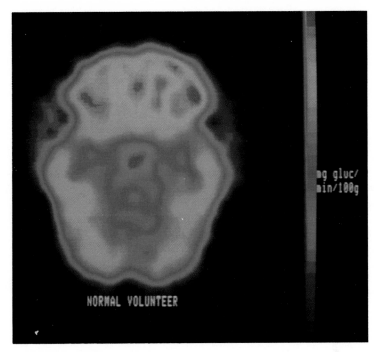

Colorplate 1. [18F]FDG PET scan performed in a 30-year-old normal male volunteer. The color bar at right indicates calculated LCMRG in mg/min/100 g tissue.

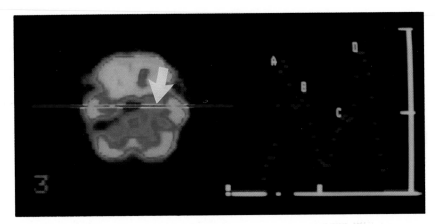

Colorplate 2. [18F]FDG PET scan performed during an interictal period in the same patient described in Fig. 2. The arrow indicates an area of relative reduction in the LCMRG involving the right mesial temporal lobe. The area of hypometabolism on the PET image corresponds to peak C on the histogram. The neocortical peaks (A and D) and the left mesial temporal peak (B) reveal normal local metabolic rates for glucose for those areas.

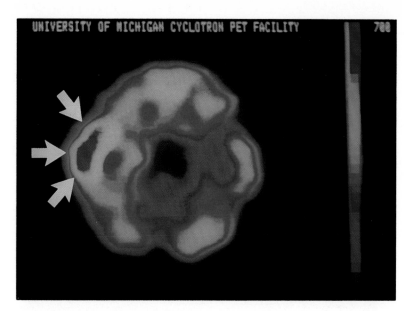

Colorplate 3. [18F]FDG PET scan performed during a complex partial seizure of left temporal origin. Marked increase in local cerebral metabolic rate occurs in the left hemisphere, most prominently in the left temporal lobe (*arrows*). Red areas in the image represent a rate of approximately 7 mg glucose per 100 g tissue per minute.

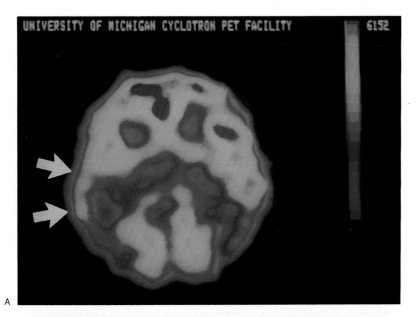

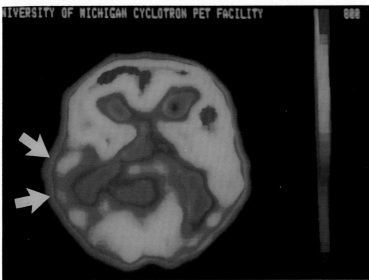

Colorplate 4A: Interictal [^{15}O]H$_2$O PET scan showing an area of reduced cerebral blood flow in the left temporal lobe (*arrows*). The color bar indicates calculated local cerebral blood flow in ml/min/g tissue. **B**: Interictal [^{18}F]FDG PET scan of the same patient showing an area of hypometabolism (*arrow*) which corresponds roughly with the area of reduced blood flow. At surgery, this patient was found to have mesial temporal sclerosis.

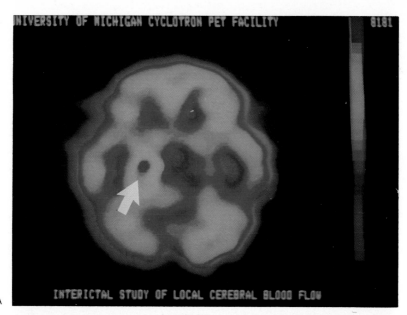

UNIVERSITY OF MICHIGAN CYCLOTRON PET FACILITY 8181

INTERICTAL STUDY OF LOCAL CEREBRAL BLOOD FLOW

A

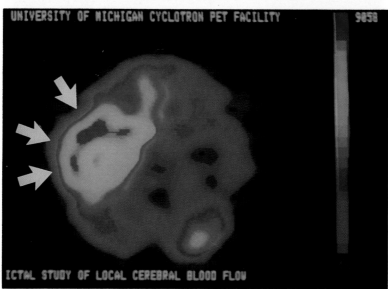

UNIVERSITY OF MICHIGAN CYCLOTRON PET FACILITY 9858

ICTAL STUDY OF LOCAL CEREBRAL BLOOD FLOW

B

Colorplate 5. A series of [¹⁵O]H₂O PET scans showing the changes in blood flow which occur during the transition from the interictal (**A**) to the ictal (**B**) states. Note that there is a small area of increased blood flow in the left mesial temporal region (*arrow*) in the interictal state (**A**) even though there was no clinical or EEG evidence of seizure activity at the time. During the seizure (**B**), there is markedly increased blood flow in left temporal lobe (*arrows*). The reduced blood flow in the right hemisphere probably results from hyperventilation performed to induce the seizure. Compare this figure to the ictal [¹⁸F]FDG scan in the same patient which is shown in Fig. 8.

Ictal [^{18}F]FDG PET scans have shown a variety of metabolic patterns that vary from patient to patient (31,38,39). During a seizure, there may be an increase in LCMRG in the region of the epileptogenic focus as well as in other sites near the focus. Ictal scans may show a variety of metabolic patterns (31,39). The areas in which this increase in metabolism is seen depend upon the timing of the glucose injection with respect to the onset of the seizure. The PET image reflects glucose metabolic activity during the approximately 10–20 minutes of uptake time following the injection. However, partial seizures usually last from 1–5 minutes. As a result, in most cases, "ictal" [^{18}F]FDG PET scans actually represent a composite picture of the ictal and postictal states. Thus, the ictal [^{18}F]FDG PET scan is of limited value for identifying the site of a seizure onset. Furthermore, the temporal resolution of the FDG technique is not sufficient for the study of the dynamic changes in metabolism which occur during the transition from the interictal to the ictal and then to the postictal state. The images obtained during seizures are among the most dramatic and interesting in the PET literature. Colorplate 3 illustrates a focal increase in the LCMRG in the left hemisphere in a patient experiencing a complex partial seizure of left temporal origin.

PET scanning has also been used to study local cerebral blood flow in patients with partial seizures. Kuhl et al. (38), using [^{13}N]NH$_3$ to image local cerebral blood flow, found that areas of interictal hypometabolism often were associated with relative hypoperfusion. Another PET technique for measuring local cerebral blood flow involves the injection of [^{15}O]H$_2$O followed by concomitant sampling of arterial ^{15}O concentrations. The images are obtained over approximately 2–4 minutes. The short time required for scanning and the short half-life of ^{15}O provide the opportunity for performing serial scans in the same patient at intervals as small as 10 minutes. This approach is particularly suited to the study of dynamic changes that occur in the transition from the interictal to the ictal and then to the postictal state (40).

An example of an [^{15}O]H$_2$O PET scan of LCBF in a patient with partial seizures of left temporal origin is shown in Colorplate 4A. This scan, performed in the interictal state, shows relatively reduced blood flow in the left hemisphere in an area corresponding roughly to the area of hypometabolism shown in the FDG scan illustrated in Colorplate 4B. An example of the dramatic changes in LCBF which occur during the transition from the interictal to the ictal state is illustrated in Colorplate 5.

IMAGING TECHNIQUES EMPLOYED IN GENERALIZED EPILEPSY

Primary generalized epilepsies usually are responsive to medical therapy and often have a good prognosis for spontaneous remission. As a result, little is known about the microscopic pathology of these epileptic syndromes. They have generally been considered to have normal microscopic pathology. Meencke and Janz (41) found abnormalities of microdysgenesis in 15 patients with primary generalized epilepsy. However, the significance of the findings has been a point of controversy (42,43). Gastaut and Gastaut (6) reported normal CT in 89% of 80 patients with primary generalized epilepsy. Eleven percent had "atrophic lesions," with no further specification. The authors did not further characterize these atrophic lesions.

Secondary or symptomatic generalized epilepsy, on the other hand, may occur as a consequence of a variety of pathologic processes. Gastaut and Gastaut (6) found CT abnormalities in 77% of 30 patients with West syndrome and in 52% of 94 patients with Lennox–Gastaut syndrome. Fifty-three percent of a total of 160 patients with secondary generalized epilepsy had an abnormal CT. In the vast majority of these patients, the abnormalities were those of atrophy or malformations.

Little data are available on MRI in generalized epilepsy. The MRI scan is likely to follow the CT scan in showing a high incidence of abnormalities with secondary generalized epilepsies.

PET was applied by Engel et al. (44) to the study of four patients with petit mal absences. The pattern of LCMRG was normal, but there was a 2.5- to 3.5-fold diffuse increase in LCMRG in hyperventilation studies that induced seizures when compared with the LCMRGs in control hyperventilation studies.

Theodore et al. (45) studied nine patients with absence or generalized tonic–clonic seizures. Interictal scans showed no apparent abnormalities. Ictal scan in two patients showed diffuse increases in LCMRG similar to what was described by Engel's group (44). One patient in "atypical" absence status, however, had a diffuse decrease in LCMRG when compared to the LCMRGs in the interictal study.

PET studies have also been performed in patients with Lennox–Gastaut syndrome. Gur et al. (46) reported unilateral temporal lobe hypometabolism in two patients with this syndrome. Chugani et al. (47) found four metabolic patterns in 15 children with the Lennox–Gastaut syndrome: (a) unilateral focal hypometabolism; (b) unilateral diffuse hypometabolism; (c) bilateral diffuse hypometabolism; and (d) normal. The utility of this subdivision with respect to diagnosis, treatment, and prognosis remains to be determined. Theodore's group also studied 10 patients with the Lennox–Gastaut syndrome and found diffuse reductions in LCMRG (48).

In summary, the yield of CT imaging studies is low in patients with primary generalized epilepsy but appears to be high in secondary generalized epilepsy. Since the classification of the epilepsy or epileptic syndrome based on clinical and EEG criteria may not be possible in some patients, the presence of pathology on CT scan may help in that classification. PET remains an investigational tool whose clinical value for generalized epilepsy is largely a matter of speculation. Since defects in inhibitory or excitatory neurotransmitters have been proposed as possible mechanisms underlying the generalized epilepsies, PET studies that image neurotransmitter receptors may provide some interesting new insights into generalized epilepsies in humans.

CLINICAL APPLICATIONS

The recent technological advances in neuroimaging are no less than revolutionary. However, the impact of this new technology on the care and treatment of patients with epilepsy has yet to be fully realized. As with other technological advances, the clinical significance will be measured in terms of how they affect treatment and the outcome of that treatment. Already, x-ray CT scanning has been established as an important tool for early detection of cerebral neoplasms in patients with partial epilepsy. Because x-ray CT scanning is noninvasive, it has come to be used routinely as a screen for neoplasms in essentially every patient presenting with partial seizures.

Experience has shown that, in some cases, small tumors or low-grade gliomas can defy detection by the x-ray CT scan. Since the introduction of MRI scanning, we have discovered that many lesions which are not detectable by x-ray CT scans are detectable with MRI scanning. However, like the x-ray CT scan, the MRI scan can reveal the presence of a focal lesion, but it cannot tell the clinician whether that lesion is a static lesion or a neoplasm. Early detection of a tumor offers the chance for therapeutic intervention at a point when the lesion is smaller. It remains to be seen how much this earlier intervention will affect the clinical course in terms of morbidity and mortality. The role of PET scanning in detecting neoplasms in patients with partial epilepsy has not been defined.

In many patients, partial seizures cannot be adequately controlled with antiepileptic drugs. When medical therapy fails, surgical excision of the epileptogenic focus reduces or abolishes seizures in 60–80% of selected patients (39). Successful excision of the epileptogenic focus depends upon reliable identification and localization of the focus. Localization of the focus depends upon EEG techniques supported by other clinical data such as clinical manifestations of the seizures, x-ray CT scans, and neuropsychological tests. A focal x-ray CT scan abnormality that corresponds anatomically to the EEG focus provides important confirmatory evidence regarding the location of the seizure focus. Unfortunately, focal x-ray CT abnormalities are not present in the majority of cases.

The increased sensitivity of the MRI scan can now provide confirmatory evidence for localizing the seizure focus in a substantial number of those patients in whom the x-ray CT does not reveal focal abnormalities. This may be particularly important in epileptogenic foci associated with mesial temporal sclerosis. However, the sensitivity, specificity, and reliability of the MRI scan in detecting mesial temporal sclerosis are not clear at the present time. It does appear, though, that when focal MRI abnormalities are detected, the location of focal MRI signal abnormalities correlates highly with the location of EEG and PET abnormalities. Thus, in cases where the MRI lesion corresponds with the location of an EEG seizure focus, invasive procedures such as depth electrodes may not be required prior to surgical excision of the focus. Therefore, the MRI scan may play a role in reducing the morbidity and costs of the presurgical evaluation.

The interictal [^{18}F]FDG PET scan is even more sensitive than the MRI in detecting local functional disturbances in the region of the seizure focus. As a result, the PET scan has been incorporated into the presurgical workup of patients at several centers. Of course, hypometabolic areas may not be epileptogenic. Therefore, demonstration of the seizure focus by EEG techniques remains essential. However, if surface and sphenoidal EEG recordings demonstrate a single clearly defined epileptogenic focus and the interictal PET scan reveals hypometabolism in the same area, depth electrode studies may be avoided (31,50). In cases where scalp and sphenoidal EEG findings and PET data reveal conflicting evidence regarding the location of the seizure focus, depth electrode or subdural EEG recordings may be required. Interictal [^{18}F]FDG PET studies have been disappointing in cases where scalp and sphenoidal EEG recordings fail to reveal clear unilateral epileptogenic foci. In the majority of these cases, PET studies have failed to show focal areas of hypometabolism (31).

In a relatively brief period of time, clinical utility of the advanced neuroimaging techniques reviewed in this chapter has already been demonstrated. Each of these techniques has been usefully employed in the diagnostic evaluation of patients with partial epilepsy. MRI and PET techniques are still undergoing rapid technological advances that should enhance their sensitivity and spatial resolution. These advances should even further enhance the diagnostic power of these procedures. The use of contrast enhancement in MRI scanning is being evaluated. It may increase the sensitivity of MRI, but it may result in morbidity (51). Sodium MRI has now become possible (52). It has not yet been evaluated in epilepsy. Phosphorus magnetic resonance spectroscopy has been used to study brain metabolism, particularly in cerebrovascular disease. With the advent of more powerful magnets, phosphorus MRI may become available (53).

Newer tracers being developed for PET scanning may provide a means for studying other metabolic processes such as protein synthesis and neurotransmitter receptors. These techniques may result in more powerful diagnostic tools. But even more exciting is the possibility that they could lead to a better understanding of the mechanisms underlying human epilepsy.

REFERENCES

1. Mathieson G. Pathological aspects of epilepsy with special reference to the surgical pathology of focal cerebral seizures. In: Purpura D, Penry J, Walter R, eds. *Advances in neurology, vol. 8: Neurosurgical management of the epilepsies.* New York: Raven Press, 1975;107–138.
2. Penfield W. Epileptogenic lesions. *Acta Neurol Psychiatr Belg* 1956;56:75-88.
3. Falconer MA. Mesial temporal (Ammon's horn) sclerosis as a common cause of epilepsy: etiology, treatment, and prevention. *Lancet* 1974;2:767–770.
4. Scheibel ME, Scheibel AB. Hippocampal pathology in temporal lobe epilepsy. A golgi survey. In: Brazier MAB, ed. *Epilepsy: its phenomena in man.* New York: Academic Press, 1973.
5. Ramirez-Lassepas M, Cipolle RJ, Morillo LR, Gumnit RJ. Value of computed tomographic scan in the evaluation of adult patients after their first seizure. *Ann Neurol* 1984;15:536–543.
6. Gastaut H, Gastaut JL. Computerized axial tomography in epilepsy. In: Penry JK. *Epilepsy, the eighth international symposium.* New York: Raven Press, 1977.
7. Jabbari B, Huott AD, DiChiro G, Martins AN, Coker SB. Surgically correctable lesions detected by CT in 143 patients with chronic epilepsy. *Surg Neurol* 1978;10:319-322.
8. Blom RJ, Vinuela F, Fox AJ, Blume WT, Girvin J, Kaufmann JCE. Computed tomography in temporal lobe epilepsy. *J Comput Assist Tomogr* 1984;8(3):401–405.
9. Wyler AR, Bolender NF. Preoperative CT diagnosis of mesial temporal sclerosis for surgical treatment of epilepsy. *Ann Neurol* 1983;13:59–64.
10. Oakley J, Ojemann GA, Ojemann LM, Cromwell L. Identifying epileptic foci on contrast-enhanced computerized tomography scans. *Arch Neurol* 1979;36:669–671.

11. Gammal TE, Adams RJ, King DW, So EL, Gallagher BB. Modified CT techniques in the evaluation of temporal lobe epilepsy prior to lobectomy. *AJNR* 1987;8:131–134.
12. Gademann G. *NMR–tomography of the normal brain.* New York: Springer-Verlag, 1984.
13. Young S. *Nuclear magnetic resonance imaging—basic principles.* New York: Raven Press, 1984.
14. Oldendorf WH. The use and promise of nuclear magnetic resonance imaging in epilepsy. *Epilepsia* 1984;25(Suppl 2):S105–S117.
15. Latack JT, Abou-Khalil BW, Siegel GJ, Sackellares JC, Gabrielson TO, Aisen AM. Patients with partial seizures: evaluation by MR, CT, and PET imaging. *Radiology* 1986;159:159–163.
16. Laster DW, Penry JK, Moody DM, Ball MR, Witcofski RL, Riela AR. Chronic seizure disorders: contribution of MR imaging when CT is normal. *AJNR* 1985;6:177–180.
17. McLachlan RS, Nicholson RL, Black S, Carr T, Blume WT. Nuclear magnetic resonance imaging, a new approach to the investigation of refractory temporal lobe epilepsy. *Epilepsia* 1985;26(6): 555–562.
18. Theodore WH, Dorwart R, Holmes M, Porter RJ, Di Chiro G. Neuroimaging in refractory partial seizures: comparison of PET, CT, and MRI. *Neurology* 1986;36:750–759.
19. Baker HL, Berquist TH, Kispert DB, et al. Magnetic resonance imaging in a routine clinical setting. *Mayo Clin Proc* 1985;60:75–90.
20. Ormson MJ, Kispert DB, Sharbrough FW, et al. Cryptic structural lesions in refractory partial epilepsy: MR imaging and CT studies. *Radiology* 1986;160:215–219.
21. Jabbari B, Guderson CH, Wippold F, et al. Magnetic resonance imaging in partial complex epilepsy. *Arch Neurol* 1986;43(9):869–872.
22. Lesser RP, Modic MT, Weinstein MA, et al. Magnetic resonance imaging (1.5 tesla) in patients with intractable focal seizures. *Arch Neurol* 1986;43:367–371.
23. Sperling MR, Wilson G, Engel J Jr, Babb TL, Phelps M, Bradley W. Magnetic resonance imaging in intractable partial epilepsy: correlative studies. *Ann Neurol* 1986;20:57-62.
24. Berkovic SF, Ethier R, Olivier A, et al. Magnetic resonance imaging of the hippocampus. I. Normal anatomy. *Epilepsia* 1986;27(5):611.
25. Berkovic SF, Ethier R, Robitaille Y, et al. Magnetic resonance imaging of the hippocampus. II. Mesial temporal sclerosis. *Epilepsia* 1986;27(5):000–000.
26. Reivich M, Kuhl DE, Wolf A, et al. The [^{18}F]fluorodeoxyglucose method for the measurement of local cerebral glucose utilization in man. *Circ Res* 1979;44:127–137.
27. Phelps ME, Huang SC, Hoffman EJ, Selin C, Sokoloff L, Kuhl DE. Tomographic measurement of local cerebral glucose metabolic rate in humans with (F-18)2- fluoro-2-deoxyglucose: validation of a method. *Ann Neurol* 1979;6:371–388.
28. Huang SC, Phelps ME, Hoffman EJ, et al. Noninvasive determination of local cerebral metabolic rate of glucose in man. *Am J Physiol* 1980;238:E69–E82.
29. Hichwa RD. Positron production and PET scanning. *IEEE Trans Nucl Sci* 1983; NS-30:1688–1692.
30. Sokoloff L, Reivich M, Kennedy C, et al. The [^{14}C]deoxyglucose method for the measurement of local cerebral glucose utilization: theory procedure and normal values in the conscious and anesthetized albino rat. *J Neurochem* 1977;28:897–916.
31. Abou-Khalil BW, Siegel GJ, Sackellares JC, Gilman S, Hichwa R, Marshall R. Positron emission tomography studies of cerebral glucose metabolism in patients with chronic partial epilepsy. *Ann Neurol* 1987;22:480–486.
32. Engel J Jr, Kuhl DE, Phelps ME, Mazziotta JC. Interictal cerebral glucose metabolism in partial epilepsy and its relation to EEG changes. *Ann Neurol* 1982;12:510–517.
33. Gloor P, Yamamoto L, Ochs R, et al. Regional cerebral metabolism measured by positron emission tomography in patients with partial epilepsy: correlation with EEG findings. In: Porter RJ, Mattson RH, Ward AA, et al. eds. *Advances in epileptology: XVth epilepsy international symposium.* New York: Raven Press, 1984;99–103.
34. Theodore WH, Newmark ME, Sato S, et al. [^{18}F]Fluorodeoxyglucose positron emission tomography in refractory complex partial seizures. *Ann Neurol* 1983;14:429–443.
35. Engel J Jr, Kuhl DE, Phelps ME, Crandall PH. Comparative localization of epileptic foci in partial epilepsy by PCT and EEG. *Ann Neurol* 1982;12:529–537.
36. Engel J Jr, Brown WJ, Kuhl DE, et al. Pathological findings underlying focal temporal lobe hypometabolism in partial epilepsy. *Ann Neurol* 1982;12:518–528.
37. Abou-Khalil BW, Siegel GJ, Hichwa RD, Sackellares JC, Gilman S. Topography of glucose hypometabolism in epilepsy of mesial temporal origin. *Ann Neurol* 1985;18(1):151–152.
38. Kuhl DE, Engel J Jr, Phelps ME, Selin C. Epileptic patterns of local cerebral metabolism and

perfusion in humans determined by emission computed tomography of ^{18}FDG and ^{13}NH$_3$. *Ann Neurol* 1980;8:348–360.

39. Engel J Jr, Kuhl DE, Phelps ME. Patterns of human local cerebral glucose metabolism during epileptic seizures. *Science* 1982;218:64–66.
40. Sackellares JC, Abou-Khalil BW, Siegel GJ, et al. PET studies of interictal, ictal and postictal changes in local cerebral blood flow in temporal lobe epilepsy. *Neurology* 1986;36(Suppl 1):338.
41. Meencke HJ, Janz D. Neuropathological findings in primary generalized epilepsy: a study of eight cases. *Epilepsia* 1984;25(1):8–21.
42. Lyon G, Gastaut H. Consideration of the significance attributed to unusual cerebral histological findings recently described in eight patients with primary generalized epilepsy. *Epilepsia* 1985;26(4):365–367.
43. Meencke HJ, Janz D. The significance of microdysgenesia in primary generalized epilepsy: an answer to the considerations of Lyon and Gastaut. *Epilepsia* 1985;26(4):368–371.
44. Engel JR, Lubens P, Kuhl DE, Phelps EM. Local cerebral metabolic rate for glucose during petit mal absences. *Ann Neurol* 1985;17:121–128.
45. Theodore WH, Brooks R, Margolin R, et al. Positron emission tomography in generalized seizures. *Neurology* 1985;35:684–690.
46. Gur RC, Sussman NM, Alavi A, et al. Positron emission tomography in two cases of childhood epileptic encephalopathy (Lennox–Gaustaut syndrome). *Neurology* 1982;32:1191–1194.
47. Chugani HT, Mazziotta JC, Engel J Jr, Phelps ME. The Lennox–Gastaut syndrome: metabolic subtypes determined by 2-deoxy-2[^{18}F]-fluoro-*d*-glucose positron emission tomography. *Ann Neurol* 1987;21:4–13.
48. Theodore WH, Rose D, Patronas N, et al. Cerebral glucose metabolism in the Lennox–Gastaut syndrome. *Ann Neurol* 1987;21:14–21.
49. Ward AA Jr. Surgical management of epilepsy. In: Browne, Feldman, eds. *Epilepsy: diagnosis and management*. Boston: Little, Brown, 1983.
50. Engel J Jr, Rausch R, Lieb JP, Kuhl DE, Crandall PH. Correlation of criteria used for localizing epileptic foci in patients considered for surgical therapy of epilepsy. *Ann Neurol* 1981;12:518–528.
51. Brasch RC. Work in progress: methods of contrast enhancement for NMR imaging and potential applications. *Radiology* 1983;147:781–788.
52. Hilal SK, Maudsley AA, Ra JB, et al. *In vivo* NMR imaging of sodium-23 in the human head. *J Comput Assist Tomogr* 1985;9(1):1–7.

Epilepsy: Current Approaches to Diagnosis and Treatment,
edited by Dennis B. Smith,
Raven Press, Ltd., New York © 1990.

5

Special Problems in the Diagnosis and Treatment of Epilepsy in Childhood

W. Edwin Dodson

*The Edward Mallinckrodt Department of Pediatrics and the
Department of Neurology and Neurological Surgery (Neurology),
Washington University School of Medicine,
St. Louis, Missouri 63110; and
Division of Pediatric Neurology, St. Louis Children's Hospital,
St. Louis, Missouri 63110*

In evaluating children with epilepsy there are two levels of diagnosis. First, the patient's seizure type is defined. Second, the type of epilepsy is diagnosed if possible. This chapter addresses the more common types of epilepsy in children. However, before a long-term commitment is made to symptomatic therapy with antiepileptic drugs, a careful search must be conducted for specifically treatable causes of seizures.

In patients of any age, seizures are a symptom of abnormal brain function. Although the cause of seizures cannot be identified in a majority of children, this does not negate the need for a careful search for an etiology. The failure to recognize potentially encephaloclastic causes of seizures (such as hypoglycemia or infections) keeps the patient at risk for progressively severe brain damage. This is especially important to very young patients, among whom treatable etiologies are most prevalent.

In children, like in adults, focal brain lesions must be excluded when there are focal signs or focal seizures. However, even when there are focal indicators, a focal brain lesion is found in less than half of these patients. In childhood, the developmental state of the brain influences the types of seizures that the brain produces. For example, infantile spasms are a type of seizure that is limited to early childhood. These seizures usually disappear by age 5 years, being replaced by other seizure types when the epilepsy persists. Newborns usually have focal or multifocal fragmentary ictal spread as compared to children and adults, even when there is a metabolic cause (1). Age-related seizure types thus reflect the changing patterns of functional connections and pharmacology of the developing nervous system (2). Nonetheless, focal brain pathology must still be excluded in newborns or older children when there are focal seizures, focal electroencephalographic (EEG) abnormalities, or focal neurological deficits.

As Cereghino has emphasized in Chapter 1, a classification of epileptic syndromes (the epilepsies) (3) should be distinguished from the International Classification of Epileptic Seizures (4). The latter classification of seizure types is based on the patient's subjective experience and ictal behavior and the ictal electroencephalogram. The specific type or types of seizures that a patient has is but one aspect of the total picture that is considered when diagnosing an epileptic syndrome. Other aspects that contribute to the definition of epileptic syndromes include precipitating factors, response to specific antiepileptic drugs, inheritance pattern, and natural history. Furthermore, many children with epilepsy have more than one type of seizure.

Generalized tonic–clonic seizures are said to be the most common type of seizure in children and occur in all of the epileptic syndromes considered here (5). However, in epilepsy clinics these are rarely the sole seizure type in primary epilepsy. Many patients who are initially diagnosed as having generalized seizures are subsequently found to have partial seizures on closer inspection. For example, in one series of infants initially diagnosed as having generalized tonic–clonic seizures, all were found to have partial seizures when video–EEG documentation was obtained (6). Sometimes the focal origin of generalized seizures is not recognized until the patient is treated with antiepileptic drugs and the ictal progression becomes apparent. During the midchildhood years, partial seizures are the most common type of seizure in some series (7). Thus the prevalence of primary epilepsy with generalized tonic–clonic seizures has probably been overestimated.

The most consistent feature of epilepsy that is caused by genetic disorders (including inborn errors of metabolism) is the age of onset. The observation that some of the primary epilepsies have a high prevalence of positive family histories for epilepsy has led to the speculation that primary epileptic syndromes might have distinctive biochemical and pharmacological epileptic mechanisms (8). However, there are no proven examples that substantiate this theory thus far. In fact, when a given inborn error of metabolism or other genetic disorder such as tuberous sclerosis causes epilepsy, each of these conditions typically produces multiple epileptic syndromes, but the age of onset is a fairly consistent feature. Thus, age of onset is emphasized in this chapter as elsewhere (9) (Table 1). Only the more common syndromes from Table 1 are considered here.

NEONATAL SEIZURES

Neonatal seizures are usually caused by identifiable metabolic or infectious causes, many of which are associated with perinatal complications (1,10). Asphyxia, hypoglycemia, electrolyte disorders, intracranial hemorrhage, septicemia, and meningitis are common causes. Less common causes include brain malformations, inborn errors of metabolism, drug abstinence syndromes (neonatal drug withdrawal), and drug intoxication (caffeine, theophylline, and local anesthetics). Be-

TABLE 1. *Selected epileptic syndromes of childhood grouped by age of onset[a]*

Newborns
Benign neonatal convulsions (fifth-day fits)
Familial benign neonatal convulsions
Early myoclonic encephalopathy
Early infantile epileptic encephalopathy with suppression–burst

Infants and Young Children
Febrile convulsions
Infantile spasms (West syndrome)
Benign myoclonic epilepsy in infants
Severe myoclonic epilepsy in infants
Myoclonic–astatic epilepsy of early childhood
Lennox–Gastaut syndrome

Children
Childhood absence epilepsy (pyknolepsy)
Epilepsy with myoclonic absences
Epilepsy with generalized convulsive seizures
Benign partial epilepsies
Landau–Kleffner syndrome
Epilepsy with continuous spikes and waves during sleep
Epilepsy with photosensitivity

Older Children and Adolescents (Juveniles)
Juvenile absence epilepsy
Juvenile myoclonic epilepsy (JME)
Epilepsy with grand mal on awakening (GMA)
Benign partial seizures of adolescence
Progressive myoclonus epilepsies

[a]From ref. 9.

cause treatable causes are prevalent, the initial management of the convulsing newborn is directed at diagnosing metabolic and infectious causes.

Less often, neonatal seizures are idiopathic or genetically determined. These primary disorders include benign familial neonatal convulsions and benign idiopathic neonatal convulsions (fifth-day fits). The epilepsy is long-lasting in 14% of the familial cases, as opposed to less than 1% of the nonfamilial cases (11).

Newborns do not have generalized tonic–clonic seizures. Instead they have either focal tonic, focal clonic, or multifocal clonic seizures (seizures with fragmentary ictal spread), which do not occur in children and adults (1). Subtle patterned behaviors (automatisms) usually are not associated with paroxysmal EEG discharges in newborns even though they have been classified traditionally as seizures. Similarly, generalized tonic movements are only rarely associated with epileptic EEG discharges and usually represent decerebrate posturing.

Treatment of Neonatal Seizures

The initial steps in treating neonatal seizures are closely associated with diagnostic measures. First, one must estimate the blood glucose with a blood glucose test tape (Dextrostix) and draw blood for the laboratory determination of glucose and electrolytes, including calcium and magnesium. If the Dextrostix is not available or if it suggests hypoglycemia (less than 40 mg/dl), glucose should be given intravenously as 25% dextrose in a dose of 2–4 ml to provide 0.5–1.0 g of glucose per kilogram of body weight, followed by the continuous infusion of solution containing 10% dextrose (10). Follow-up measurements of blood glucose are necessary to ensure that the blood glucose is adequate.

Hypocalcemia and hypomagnesemia are treated only after they are documented by the chemistry laboratory (10). Hypocalcemia is treated by giving 5% calcium gluconate [4 ml/kg (200 mg/kg)] intramuscularly. Hypomagnesemia is treated by giving 50% magnesium sulfate (0.2 ml/kg) intramuscularly.

Pyridoxine dependency is a rare cause of continuous neonatal seizures or refractory seizures in older infants (12,13). When status is occurring, the disorder is diagnosed and treated by giving pyridoxine (50–100 mg) intravenously. Seizures caused by pyridoxine dependency sometimes respond to antiepileptic drugs. Thus, temporary control or reduced seizure frequency while taking anticonvulsants does not exclude this disorder. A thoughtfully designed clinical trial of pyridoxine is currently the only way to make this diagnosis.

Continuous neonatal seizures that are not reversed by glucose should be treated with anticonvulsant drugs. The drugs used most often include phenobarbital, phenytoin, diazepam, and lorazepam. Diazepam is short-acting because it is redistributed from the brain into other tissues. Lorazepam theoretically is longer-acting and is increasingly being used in situations where diazepam is indicated (14,15). When diazepam is used, it must be followed by a longer-acting anticonvulsant.

The first drug is either phenobarbital, lorazepam, or diazepam. Experience with lorazepam is limited. The initial recommended dose of lorazepam is 0.05 mg/kg, but doses as high as 0.23 mg/kg have been reported (16). Traditionally, phenobarbital has been used first (17).

Phenobarbital is given in two doses of 10 mg/kg separated by 15–20 minutes (total dose of 20 mg/kg) (18). If these doses are ineffective, additional doses can be given, but respiratory depression is expected. Phenobarbital should be given intravenously to provide the most rapid and certain dosage, but it can be given intramuscularly if a slower onset of action is tolerable. If seizures are controlled by the first 10 mg/kg, the additional 10 mg/kg should still be given to produce therapeutic drug concentrations after the drug redistributes into tissues.

When phenobarbital in doses of 20 mg/kg is ineffective, the next option is either additional phenobarbital or phenytoin. Phenytoin must be given intravenously because it is too slowly absorbed from muscle. The phenytoin loading dose is 20 mg/kg given slowly, no more than 3 mg/kg/min, preferably while observing an electrocardiographic monitor (18). Infusing phenytoin too rapidly can cause hypotension, bradycardia, or asystole.

When convulsions continue after both phenobarbital and phenytoin loading doses, my preference is to give additional doses of phenobarbital, 5–10 mg/kg per dose, every 20 minutes until the seizures cease. At these doses, apnea is expected and mechanical ventilation is required. Hypotension limits the maximal phenobarbital dosage. When this occurs, fluid should be administered to expand the plasma volume.

After neonatal seizures are controlled acutely, maintenance therapy should be given with either phenobarbital or phenytoin. The recommended phenobarbital maintenance dose is 3.5 mg/kg/day in neonatal seizures (19). The maintenance phenytoin dose varies widely, but the usual initial dose of phenytoin is 6 mg/kg/day. However, phenytoin dosage requirements often increase drastically in the first few weeks of life.

The capacities of newborns with seizures to eliminate drugs change dramatically over the first weeks of life (17,20). Because phenobarbital has a very long half-life, phenobarbital levels change slowly even though phenobarbital elimination accelerates considerably. On the other hand, the apparent half-life of phenytoin is shorter, and changes in phenytoin elimination usually make it necessary to readjust the dose several times during the neonatal period if stable levels are required for seizure control. Although it was previously suspected that newborns malabsorb phenytoin, they absorb orally administered phenytoin completely but slowly. However, newborns have nonlinear phenytoin elimination kinetics, which causes dosage requirements to vary widely. Maturing hepatic drug-eliminating mechanisms and slow absorption cause phenytoin levels to decline when it is administered orally to older newborns (21).

Only 10% of newborns who have seizures require prolonged therapy with antiepileptic drugs. Usually these patients are distinguished by their obvious and severe neurological abnormalities. Newborns who have seizures due to metabolic causes, who develop normally, and who have normal electroencephalograms usually require anticonvulsant therapy only briefly. Most authorities recommend withdrawing the anticonvulsants by age 3 months or sooner when the newborns are doing well and developing normally (10).

INFANTILE SPASMS (WEST'S SYNDROME)

The term "infantile spasms" is confusing because it connotes both a seizure type and an epileptic syndrome, infantile myoclonic epilepsy. Other names for this seizure type include blitz–nick–salaam–krampfe, massive myoclonic spasms, lightning spasms, flexion spasms, and jackknife convulsions. The combination of infantile spasms with developmental arrest and an EEG pattern of hypsarrhythmia is known as *West's syndrome*. Rarely, children present with movements that are similar to infantile spasms but have normal interictal and ictal electroencephalograms (22). This last condition is benign and does not require treatment.

"Infantile spasms" is an age-dependent epilepsy with primary and secondary forms. The electroencephalogram is almost always abnormal here, with two-thirds of patients having a pattern of hypsarrhythmia (23). Eighty-five percent of the children who develop this begin to manifest spasms by the age of 12 months. Similarly, most patients who have infantile myoclonic epilepsy stop having spasms by age 5 years, but half of these persist with other forms of epilepsy (24–26). Other types of convulsive and absence seizures occur in about half of the infants with this syndrome.

The most common types of spasms are mixed flexion and extension or purely flexor (23,27). Flexor spasms, sometimes termed *salaam fits*, cause brief flexion of the neck and trunk with adduction of the outstretched arms and leg flexion. Spasms vary from subtle to dramatic in intensity; these occur in clusters, most commonly on awakening.

The etiology of infantile spasms is diverse. In 60% of patients the disorder is a symptom of an identifiable brain disease, usually of prenatal or perinatal origin. Only 17% have postnatal etiologies. Patients who lack an identifiable cause and who are neurologically normal are classified as "cryptogenic." This group has the best prognosis (27).

In older studies, hypoxic–ischemic disease was the most common cause of infantile spasms. In more recent studies, tuberous sclerosis usually is most common. Among the patients with tuberous sclerosis, periventricular and parenchymal calcifications on computed tomography (CT) brain scan may be the first indicators of the actual etiology because more than half of newborns with tuberous sclerosis lack hypopigmented skin macules (28). CT brain scans are abnormal in a majority of children with infantile myoclonic epilepsy. Atrophic lesions are most common, followed by malformations, atrophy plus calcification, calcifications, and porencephaly. Aicardi's syndrome, a rare cause of infantile spasms, consists of agenesis of the corpus callosum, chorioretinitis, vertebral anomalies, and cortical heterotopias and occurs almost exclusively in females (29,30).

The prognosis in infantile spasms is related both to etiology and to therapy. Patients with the cryptogenic variety have the best prognosis (27). The optimal therapy of infantile myoclonic epilepsy appears to be adrenocorticotropic hormone (ACTH) administered within 1 month of the onset of the spasms (27,31). Treatment with conventional anticonvulsants alone has been inferior to ACTH in immediate and long-term seizure control and in later intellectual development. Patients with structural brain disorders have the worst prognosis. Unfavorable prognostic features include (a) onset before 3 months of age, (b) abnormal development or neurological examination, (c) presence of multiple seizure types, (d) hypsarrhythmia, and (e) a delay of more than 1 month before ACTH is given. Although infantile spasms is noted for an ominous prognosis, any epilepsy that begins in the first year of life tends to be severe (32).

The optimal doses and duration of ACTH therapy have not been established, but recommended doses consistently cause potentially lethal side effects (33). Doses of 40–80 IU of ACTH gel daily are most common. ACTH is preferable to oral corticosteroids. The recommended duration of therapy ranges from 10 days to 3 months or more. Of the patients who respond, most do so within a few days after initiating treatment. Prolonged treatment increases the risk of severe side effects. In large studies, ACTH therapy is associated with a 5% mortality rate. When ACTH is ineffective, conventional anticonvulsants are used, most often a benzodiazepine.

MYOCLONIC–ASTATIC EPILEPSY OF INFANCY
AND EARLY CHILDHOOD (DOOSE'S SYNDROME,
LENNOX–GASTAUT SYNDROME)

These disorders have several subtypes, and variable nomenclature is used by different authorities (8,9,34,35). A consistent feature is the association of multiple types of seizures including atonic or astatic drop attacks. The subtypes include a relatively benign, rare idiopathic variant that consists of multiple seizure types and that involves normal development, a generalized epileptiform EEG pattern, and a good response to valproic acid. This is most widely known as *benign myoclonic epilepsy of infancy*, although some workers refer to this benign variant as *Doose's syndrome*. Others use the term Doose's syndrome to label the idiopathic but encephalopathic group (35). When these patients first begin to have seizures, classification may be impossible until sufficient time has transpired for evolution of the patient's full clinical profile.

The most severe variant is called the *Lennox–Gastaut syndrome* (36–38). Some workers reserve this label for symptomatic and encephalopathic form; others use the term independent of etiological considerations. This syndrome consists of the combination of (a) multiple types of seizures (including atonic seizures, absence seizures, and partial or generalized tonic–clonic seizures with either mental retardation or progressive encephalopathy) and (b) an EEG pattern of slow (<2.5 Hz) spike-and-wave (36,37). The EEG pattern of slow spike-and-wave, the so-called petit mal variant, is a variable feature that comes and goes (38). During seizures, the slow spike-and-wave pattern sometimes attenuates with diffuse depression of brain electrical activity or there may be no change in the EEG pattern at all.

This syndrome, like infantile spasms, is age-dependent (5). In a majority of cases the atonic seizures abate with maturation but are replaced by partial, partial complex, and secondarily generalized convulsions. The usual age of onset is between 1 and 5 years. Characteristically, these patients have more than one type of seizure usually including drop attacks and generalized tonic–clonic seizures. Absence or atypical absence seizures also are common, but they usually appear after convulsive seizures are well established (39). Among the patients with infantile spasms who have persistent epilepsy, half evolve into the Lennox–Gastaut syndrome. With advancing age, mental retardation is found in an increasing percentage of these patients such that by age 6 years, most children with Lennox–Gastaut syndrome are mentally subnormal (5). In certain patients, intellect dramatically deteriorates at times when the epilepsy is uncontrolled.

As with infantile spasms, any disorder that causes severe cortical dysfunction can be manifest as Lennox–Gastaut syndrome. The lists of etiologies causing both of these syndromes overlap considerably (5). Prenatal and perinatal causes predominate; fewer than one-fourth of cases result from postnatal causes. In various studies, the etiology is unidentified in 30–70% of patients. Overall, the prognosis in Lennox–Gastaut syndrome is poor. Features that indicate a bad prognosis include prior infantile spasms, onset before 2 years of age, and the presence of either tonic seizures or minor motor, nonconvulsive status.

Typically, Lennox–Gastaut syndrome is difficult to treat. Because patients usually present with partial or generalized tonic–clonic seizures, they are often begun on an anticonvulsant such as phenobarbital, carbamazepine, or phenytoin, thereby resulting in the appearance of drop attacks and absence seizures. When this occurs, valproic acid should be added and the initial anticonvulsant should be withdrawn. This maneuver occasionally controls both seizure types, but most patients require multiple drug therapy. ACTH is also used to treat progressive juvenile myoclonic epilepsy, but the benefits here are not as impressive as in infantile spasms. As with the infantile form, a good response is most likely when ACTH is initiated soon after the seizures appear (40). Benzodiazepines, especially clonazepam, are frequently required here despite their side effects. Prior to the use of valproic acid, the ketogenic diet was an important and primary therapy in this disorder. This is used less frequently now but is worth a try if other therapies fail.

FEBRILE SEIZURES

Febrile seizures occur among children aged 3 months to 5 years old who have fever and no evidence of another cause (41). Thus, febrile seizures represent a diagnosis of exclusion. Approximately 4% of children are affected (42,43). A history of febrile seizures is present in 8–22% of parents and in 9–17% of patients' siblings. Offspring of patients with febrile seizures have an 11% chance of being plagued by febrile seizures.

For many years there was controversy about the significance of febrile seizures (44), but population-based studies indicate that the disorder is usually benign and not associated with later epilepsy in a majority of children. Typically, neurological and neurosurgical studies indicated that febrile seizures were associated with a variety of serious neurological sequelae, including intractable temporal lobe epilepsy, hemiplegia, mental retardation, and other encephalopathies. Most of these studies were retrospective and involved highly selected patients, with a bias toward the neurologically abnormal. Among Falconer and Taylor's 40 patients with mesial temporal sclerosis, 33 had histories of prolonged febrile convulsions in childhood (45).

The largest population-based investigation of febrile seizures is the Collaborative Perinatal Project conducted by the National Institutes of Health between 1959 and 1972 (40,43). That study identified 1706 children who had febrile seizures and who were followed until age 7 years. Based on that study, one can conclude that febrile seizures do not increase the chance of mental retardation or serious neurological impairment. They are associated with an increased chance of recurrent febrile seizures and a slightly increased incidence of later epilepsy. Overall, the chance of later epilepsy after febrile seizures is 3%. In the presence of certain risk factors the risk increases (42,43) (Table 2).

The greatest risk of later epilepsy, 15.4%, occurs among those patients who are either neurologically or developmentally abnormal and who have focal seizures

TABLE 2. *Factors in febrile seizures associated with an increased risk of epilepsy at age 7 years[a]*

Family history of epilepsy
Preexisting neurological abnormality
Complex febrile seizure
   Greater than 15 minutes duration of seizure
   More than one febrile seizure in 24 hours
   Focal febrile seizure
Multiple (more than two) febrile seizures

[a]Modified from ref. 46.

(45,47). Among children with no risk factors, 2% subsequently develop epilepsy—approximately three to four times more than the children who do not have febrile seizures. Among those with one risk factor, 3% had epilepsy at age 7 years. When there are two or more risk factors, 13% have subsequent epilepsy. Among all patients with febrile seizures, the risk of epilepsy developing by age 7 years is 3%.

The risk of additional febrile seizures is related to the age at the time of the first febrile seizure. Overall, one-third of these patients have recurrent febrile seizures. However, the younger the patient at the time of the initial febrile seizure, the greater the chance of recurrence. When the first seizure occurs before the age of 12 months, the chance of a second is 50%. The rate of later epilepsy is twice as high among the children who have multiple febrile seizures.

The evaluation of children who convulse with fever is directed at excluding treatable causes of seizures, especially meningitis. The evaluation is also intended to identify the patients who have other forms of epilepsy, not febrile seizures. The latter problem is not so simple because the only sure test may be that of time. Patients who have partial or prolonged seizures with focal or diffusely paroxysmal EEG abnormalities are considered to have epilepsy. Neurologically abnormal patients and those who have prolonged, dangerous seizures are also treated as if they have epilepsy.

Effective treatment for preventing febrile seizures includes continuously administered phenobarbital and valproic acid (48–50) and intermittently administered diazepam (51). Because of the possibility of the rare, but potentially fatal, idiosyncratic hepatotoxicity, valproic acid is not recommended for febrile seizures. When phenobarbital is given, the doses must be sufficient to produce blood levels of 15 μg/ml or more; side effects are expected in 40% of patients. Reports from Europe indicate that diazepam solutions (0.5 mg/kg) given rectally when fever occurs will reduce the recurrence rate (51,52). In one study, diazepam (5–7.5 mg) administered rectally reduced the recurrence rate of febrile seizures from 39% in controls to 12% with 18 months follow-up. Mild side effects were seen in 64%. The most common were sedation (36%), euphoria (15%), and ataxia (8%) (53). Antipyretic therapy, although widely recommended, is not of proven benefit. Phenytoin and carbamazepine are ineffective.

It is unknown whether treatment with anticonvulsants deters the development of later epilepsy among patients with febrile seizures (47). Phenobarbital given continuously to prevent additional febrile seizures causes behavioral and possibly other side effects in a significant percentage of patients (54). Furthermore, patients who do develop serious complications of prolonged seizures associated with fever are more likely to do so during recurrent or complicated febrile seizures. Because of this, treatment has been recommended for children who are less than 18 months old or who have two or more risk factors (55).

DRUG THERAPY IN INFANTS AND YOUNG CHILDREN

Infants, children aged 1–12 months, usually require the largest relative doses of any age group because they have the highest relative capacities to eliminate most antiepileptics (17,20). The major exception to this is valproic acid, which is eliminated slowly unless it is given with other antiepileptic drugs that induce its metabolism (56,57).

Aside from valproate, infants eliminate most other antiepileptic drugs more rapidly than do any other age group. Phenobarbital half-lives decline from an average of 114.4 hours in the neonatal period to approximately 45 hours in infancy (58–61). Phenytoin is also rapidly eliminated by infants and has saturable, nonlinear kinetics (21,62). Because of both age-related effects and saturable elimination kinetics, the apparent half-lives of phenytoin are usually very short when phenytoin concentrations are low. Therefore, infants can require as much as 20 mg/kg/day phenytoin orally to produce levels in the therapeutic range. Phenobarbital maintenance doses usually range from 3 to 6 mg/kg/day as compared to adult doses, which range from 1 to 2 mg/kg/day.

After infancy, relative drug clearance progressively declines until adult values are achieved in early adolescence. For example, the relative clearance of carbamazepine is highest among infants and progressively declines during development. Carbamazepine half-lives as short as 4.6–12.6 hours have been reported in children aged 2–7 weeks (63). Children, especially those taking other drugs simultaneously, also accumulate higher concentrations of carbamazepine epoxide than do most adults.

EPILEPSIES ASSOCIATED WITH ABSENCE SEIZURES

Absence seizures cause paroxysmal, brief, nonconvulsive, staring behavior. The major differential diagnosis of ictal staring behavior is thus partial complex (psychomotor) versus absence seizures. Absence seizures occur in other epilepsies besides petit mal. They occur in myoclonic astatic epilepsy of childhood, in juvenile myoclonic epilepsy ("impulsiv petit mal" of Janz), in Lennox–Gastaut syndrome, and in other disorders (8,64). The distinction between the types of epilepsies with absence is important for prognostic and therapeutic reasons.

The clinical details of absence seizures have been quantified (65). The onset is abrupt (without warning), and the duration is usually less than 15 seconds. During the ictus, responsiveness is usually impaired, but not all EEG discharges are associated with behavioral seizures. Patients are variably amnesic and usually unaware of the absence. Recovery is prompt. If posture is altered, it does not cause the patient to fall down. Automatisms occur in more than half of absence seizures and most commonly involve the face, especially the eyelids. The occurrence of automatisms is directly related to the duration of the absence seizure. The longer the seizure, the more likely the patient will have automatisms.

Petit Mal Epilepsy (Pyknolepsy)

Petit mal epilepsy is characterized by absence seizures associated with a regular, monotonous 3-Hz spike-and-wave EEG pattern (5,65). Petit mal epilepsy is rare, probably accounting for less than half of the absence seizures in children.

The tendency to develop petit mal epilepsy is inherited, probably as an autosomal dominant trait with age-dependent expression (5). Not all studies of the genetics of this disorder agree, probably because of the difficulty of distinguishing the various epilepsies associated with absence seizures. Monozygotic twins are 85% concordant for the 3-Hz EEG trait and 75% concordant for the seizures in petit mal epilepsy.

Petit mal epilepsy (pyknolepsy) is benign, and it abates in adolescence (5,8,66). The patients are otherwise normal, have only absence seizures, and outgrow their epilepsy. Generalized tonic–clonic seizures thus do not seem to be a major problem here but are a regular feature of juvenile myoclonic epilepsy, which overlaps clinically with petit mal. As discussed below, when absences begin in later childhood or early adolescence, a diagnosis of juvenile myoclonic epilepsy is more likely.

Drugs that are effective in petit mal include ethosuximide, valproic acid, trimethadione, the ketogenic diet, a benzodiazepine such as clonazepam, or a carbonic anhydrase inhibitor such as acetazolamide. Because petit mal is benign, ethosuximide is recommended first; valproic acid is recommended when ethosuximide is insufficient or when the patient also has generalized tonic–clonic seizures.

Juvenile Myoclonic Epilepsy

This disorder was first described in 1956 by Janz, who labeled it "impulsiv petit mal" (8). Juvenile myoclonic epilepsy can be difficult to distinguish from classical petit mal epilepsy because absence seizures are common and may be the first sign. There are several differences between the two, but the most important difference between the two is the natural histories: Juvenile myoclonic epilepsy appears to be a lifelong form of epilepsy, whereas petit mal is transient (Table 3).

A diagnosis of juvenile myoclonic epilepsy should be suspected when absence seizures begin in the late childhood years or adolescence. Approximately one-third of patients with juvenile myoclonic epilepsy have myoclonic jerks involving the neck, usually in the morning after awakening. Patients do not often volunteer this

TABLE 3. *Differential features of petit mal epilepsy versus juvenile myoclonic epilepsy (JME)[a]*

Feature	Petit mal	JME
Age of onset	Midchildhood	Pubescence
Tonic–clonic seizure	Rare in 50%	Common; occurring early in the morning
Neck myoclonus	No	Common
Electroencephalogram	Spike-and-wave; 3 Hz	Polyspike-and-wave; 4–6 or 8–12 Hz
Genetics	? Age-dependent	? Polygenic
Treatment	Ethosuximide	Valproic acid
Prognosis	Remits in adolescence	Persists

[a]From ref. 8.

information and thus need to be questioned specifically about this symptom. In some cases the myoclonic jerks are repetitive and culminate in a clonic–tonic–clonic seizure. Generalized tonic–clonic seizures are also relatively common in juvenile myoclonic epilepsy and may be the chief complaint. These seizures can be refractory to the usual major anticonvulsant drugs but have a high probability of responding to valproic acid, which is the drug of choice in juvenile myoclonic epilepsy. The ictal EEG pattern also helps differentiate juvenile myoclonic epilepsy from petit mal. In juvenile myoclonic epilepsy the ictal discharge includes polyspikes and polyspike-and-wave patterns that usually occur at higher frequencies than the ictal discharges in petit mal.

BENIGN PARTIAL EPILEPSY OF CHILDHOOD (ROLANDIC EPILEPSY)

Although the principal seizure type in this disorder is partial, the natural history and familial nature of the benign partial epilepsies of childhood suggests that they are primary forms of epilepsy. Benign rolandic epilepsy, the most common type, usually appears in the middle to late childhood years (7,67–69). The predominantly nocturnal seizures have a simple partial onset, usually beginning in the face and infrequently generalizing to tonic–clonic convulsions. The family history is positive in 18% (70).

The electroencephalogram often shows focal spike activity, classically in the centrotemporal regions; in some patients, however, this activity occurs in the occipital, frontal, or temporal areas. The finding of rolandic spikes does not necessarily indicate that seizures will occur. In one large series of children with rolandic spikes, only 38% had seizures (71).

Rolandic epilepsy is usually controlled by a major antiepileptic drug such as phenytoin or carbamazepine. A majority of these patients are seizure-free 5 years after the onset. It has even been suggested that treatment may not be necessary (68). When antiepileptic therapy is warranted, it is important to recognize this diagnosis so that therapy is not unduly prolonged.

DRUG THERAPY OF EPILEPSY IN OLDER CHILDREN AND ADOLESCENTS

Children with epilepsy demonstrate the same pharmacokinetic complexities as adults; moreover, they have age-related kinetic issues and a high incidence of intercurrent illness. Thus in children the relationship between antiepileptic drug dose and actions is less predictable than in adults.

Pediatric patients require larger drug doses on a weight basis than do adults to achieve comparable blood levels and effects. They also have more variability in the relationship between drug dose and levels. Because this variability is so great, dosage based on weight is generally unreliable and should be used only as a starting point when initiating therapy. Thereafter, drug levels are helpful in individualizing each child's dose (Table 4). However, the end point of good therapy is clinical, not the production of a particular drug level. The goal of therapy is no seizures and no side effects.

During childhood, the relative clearance of antiepileptic drugs progressively declines until adult values are achieved at age 10–15 years (72). Because of the offsetting or contradictory effects of growth and reduced relative clearance, drug levels remain surprisingly constant in growing children even when doses are not increased (17). Young children require doses that are two to four times greater than adult doses on a weight basis. More importantly, children of any age have a greater within-group variability in dosage requirements. The situation is most unpredictable when children take antiepileptic drugs with short half-lives, when multiple drugs are given simultaneously, and when a drug with nonlinear kinetics is given.

Prescribing doses on a weight basis is helpful only when initiating therapy, and most children require one or two subsequent adjustments. Drug level measurements are important when children do not respond at low average doses or when they have symptoms suggestive of drug toxicity. When starting antiepileptic drug therapy,

TABLE 4. *Pharmacokinetics in children of frequently used antiepileptic drugs*

Drug	Initial dosage range (mg/kg/day)	$T_{1/2}$ range (hr)	Therapeutic range (µg/ml)
Phenobarbital	1–5	30–150	10–20
Primidone	10–20	6–8	8–?[a]
Carbamazepine	15–25	10–30	4–12
Phenytoin	4–12	3–60[b]	10–20
Methsuximide	10–20	18–30	10–20[c]
Ethosuximide	10–70	24–42	45–100
Valproic acid	10–70	4–15	50–100
Clonazepam	0.03–0.1	16–60	0.02–0.07

[a]Metabolized to phenobarbital.
[b]Effective half-life ($T_{1/2}$) varies with level.
[c]N-Desmethyl metabolite.

low average doses should be given initially unless there are frequent or severe seizures that necessitate higher doses acutely. Patients should be reevaluated clinically after an estimated five half-lives have transpired when drug levels have had time to stabilize.

Phenytoin dose–concentration relationships are precarious in many patients because of the nonlinearity of phenytoin elimination kinetics. When phenytoin elimination is nearly saturated, levels are highly vulnerable to (a) change resulting from intercurrent illness or (b) physiologic changes such as menses or drug interactions (73–76). Drug–protein binding is also an issue with phenytoin, which is approximately 90% bound. Phenytoin is thus highly vulnerable to interactions of several types, and it interacts with all of the major antiepileptic drugs (77,78). Unfortunately, the direction or extent of phenytoin interactions is often unpredictable, and one must reevaluate patients frequently when an interaction is anticipated.

Carbamazepine induces its own metabolism, a process termed *autoinduction* (79,80). This process is both time-dependent and concentration-dependent (81) but is usually complete 6 weeks after a change in dose (82,83). It is important to recognize autoinduction and not to misinterpret its consequences as patient noncompliance.

The range of drug doses required by children is wide. For example, valproate doses ranged from 26 to 154 mg/kg/day in one series (84). In addition, the clearance of most antiepileptic drugs varies between first and subsequent doses, with some patients having increasing while others have decreasing clearance (84,85). Levels of drugs with short half-lives (such as valproate) fluctuate more than levels of drugs with longer half-lives.

There is an inverse relation between age and clearance of all antiepileptic drugs (84–87). Multiple drug therapy (polytherapy) further increases antiepileptic drug clearance in children. For example, at equivalent doses the average valproate level is approximately 40% lower in children taking valproate plus other drugs than when valproate is taken alone (88). Conversely, when concomitant antiepileptic drugs are discontinued, the level of the remaining drug increases.

Polytherapy makes the regulation of most antiepileptic drugs more difficult. For example, in children on carbamazepine, monotherapy dosage increments of 2 mg/kg increase the carbamazepine level by 1 μg/ml. When other antiepileptic drugs are given simultaneously, a dosage of more than 3 mg/kg is required in order to increase the carbamazepine concentration by 1 μg/ml (89). All of the other antiepileptic drugs except valproic acid cause carbamazepine levels to decline (90). A similar situation is found for valproic acid. When other drugs are stopped, valproate levels increase 60–150% (88).

Dramatic changes in drug clearance are uncommon during adolescence. Most adolescents question the need for taking antiepileptic drugs; thus, some degree of noncompliance is to be expected. However, phenytoin levels can fluctuate during the menstrual cycle. Patients who have higher phenytoin levels (indicating a greater degree of saturation) have lower phenytoin levels at the time of menstruation than at midcycle (73).

PROBLEMS OF VARIABLE DRUG LEVELS
DURING CHRONIC THERAPY

Many factors contribute to the variability of drug levels during chronic therapy. Noncompliance is a foremost cause of unstable drug levels, but other factors also cause drug levels to fluctuate. These include intercurrent febrile illness, cyclical hormone levels, and drug interactions.

Intercurrent illness sometimes causes changes in both seizure threshold and drug levels. Relatively high phenytoin levels are most likely to be affected. Phenobarbital, which has a long half-life, is relatively resistant to short-term changes. The effect on carbamazepine is probably intermediate, but carbamazepine is more often affected by drug interactions.

Phenytoin biotransformation is modified by intercurrent illness and other factors. Infectious mononucleosis, flu immunization, streptococcal pharyngitis, and nonspecific viral illness causing fever have been implicated (74,75). During febrile illness, the phenytoin level can decrease by as much as 50%, allowing seizure recurrence.

Febrile illness is associated with other factors that cause drug levels to change. These include drug interactions and features of the illness (such as vomiting) that interrupt drug administration. Common problems include increased carbamazepine levels and toxicity due to co-medication with erythromycin (91–94). Carbamazepine toxicity appears 8–12 hours after erythromycin is added if the carbamazepine dose is not reduced. Patients usually recover 8–24 hours after the erythromycin treatment is stopped (94,95). Trimethoprim/sulfamethazole can increase the levels of unbound carbamazepine, and probably those of unbound phenytoin as well.

RECTAL ADMINISTRATION OF ANTIEPILEPTIC DRUGS

Rectal administration of certain antiepileptic drugs produces effective concentrations rapidly. Rectal administration is especially helpful in situations where children have severe seizures infrequently and in some cases of febrile seizures. Diazepam is absorbed rapidly and reliably after rectal administration of solutions; suppositories, however, do not produce the same effect (96–99). In fact, absorption is more rapid from the rectum than from muscle (100). After rectal administration of diazepam, peak concentrations are reached before 10 minutes in a majority of children (97,101). When diazepam cannot be given intravenously in status, rectal administration is next best. Pediatric doses range from 0.5 to 0.75 mg/kg to a maximum of 20 mg (102).

Other antiepileptic drugs, including paraldehyde, valproic acid, and lorazepam, have been administered rectally. Paraldehyde has been used the longest, accruing the most extensive experience (103–105). Although rectally administered valproic acid solutions have been used in refractory status epilepticus, seizures usually are not controlled for several hours. Absorption of valproic acid rectally is similar to

* no longer available

oral administration, producing peak levels in 2 hours (106–108). Thus far, experience with rectal lorazepam has been limited to volunteers, but lorazepam is absorbed more slowly from the rectum than diazepam (109). Carbamazepine is absorbed so slowly after rectal administration that retention of the dose until it can be absorbed is a problem (110).

REFERENCES

1. Mizrahi EM. Neonatal seizures: problems in diagnosis and classification. *Epilepsia* 1987:28(Suppl 1):S46–S55.
2. Moshe SL. Epileptogenesis and the immature brain. *Epilepsia* 1987;28(Suppl 1):S3–S15.
3. Commission on classification and terminology of the Internal League Against Epilepsy. Proposal for classification of epilepsies and epileptic syndromes. *Epilepsia* 1985;26:268–278.
4. Commission of classification and terminology of the International League Against Epilepsy. Proposal for revised clinical and electroencephalographic classification of epileptic seizures. *Epilepsia* 1981;22:489–501.
5. Gomez MR, Klass DW. Epilepsies of infancy and childhood. *Ann Neurol* 1983;13:113–124.
6. Duchowny MS. Complex partial seizures of infancy. *Arch Neurol* 1987;44:911–914.
7. Cavazutti GB. Epidemiology of different types of epilepsy in school age children of Modena, Italy. *Epilepsia* 1980;21:57–62.
8. Delgado-Escueta AV, Treiman DM, Walsh GO. The treatable epilepsies. *N Engl J Med* 1983;308:1508–1514.
9. Roger J, Dravet C, Bureau M, Dreifuss FE, Wolf P. *Epileptic syndromes in infancy, childhood, and adolescence*. London: John Libbey, 1985.
10. Volpe JJ. *Neonatal neurology*. Philadelphia: WB Saunders, 1986.
11. Poulin P. Benign neonatal convulsions (familial and nonfamilial). In: Roger J, Dravet C, Bureau M, Dreifuss FE, Wolff P, eds. *Epileptic syndromes in infancy, childhood and adolescence*. London: John Libbey, 1985;2–11.
12. Bankier A, Turner M, Hopkins IA. Pyridoxine dependent seizures—a wider clinical spectrum. *Arch Dis Child* 1983;58:415–418.
13. Goutieres F, Aicardi J. Atypical presentations of pyridoxine-dependent seizures: a treatable cause of intractable epilepsy in infants. *Ann Neurol* 1985;17:117–120.
14. Lacey DJ, Singer WD, Horwitz SJ, Goilmore H. Lorazepam therapy of status epilepticus in children and adolescents. *J Pediatr* 1986;108:771–774.
15. Gunawan S, Treiman DM. Pharmacokinetics of lorazepam in the treatment of status epilepticus. *Epilepsia* 1986;27:641.
16. Sorel L, Mechler L, Harmant J. Comparative trial of intravenous lorazepam and clonazepam in status epilepticus. *Clin Ther* 1981;4:326–336.
17. Dodson WE. Special pharmacokinetic considerations in children. *Epilepsia* 1987;28(Suppl 1):S56–S70.
18. Painter MJ, Pippenger C, Wasterlain C, Barmada M, Pitlick W, Carter G, Ahern S. Phenobarbital and phenytoin in neonatal seizures: metabolism and tissue distribution. *Neurology* 1981;31:1107–1112.
19. Fischer J, Lockman LA, Zaske D, Kreil R. Reply. *Neurology (NY)* 1982;32:789.
20. Dodson WE. Drug utilization in pediatric patients. *Epilepsia* 1984;25(Suppl 2):S132–S139.
21. Bourgeois BF, Dodson WE. Phenytoin elimination in newborns. *Neurology* 1983;23:173–178.
22. Lombroso CT, Fejerman N. Benign myoclonus of early infancy. *Ann Neurol* 1977;1:138–143.
23. Kellaway P, Frost JD, Hrachovy RA. Infantile spasms. In: Morselli PL, Pippenger CE, Penry JK, eds. *Antiepileptic drug therapy in pediatrics*. New York: Raven Press, 1983;115–136.
24. Jeavons PM, Harper JR, Bower BD. Long-term prognosis in infantile spasms: a follow-up report on 112 cases. *Dev Med Child Neurol* 1970;12:413–421.
25. Kurokawa T, Goya N, Fukuyama Y, et al. West syndrome and Lennox–Gastaut syndrome: a survey of natural history. *Pediatrics* 1980;65:81–88.
26. Matsumoto A, Wantanabe K, Negoro T, et al. Long-term prognosis after infantile spasms: a statistical study of prognostic factors in 200 cases. *Develop Med Child Neurol* 1981;23:51–65.

27. Lombroso CT. Differentiation of seizures in newborns and early infancy. In: Morselli PL, Pippenger CE, Penry JK, eds. *Antiepileptic drug therapy in pediatrics.* New York: Raven Press, 1983;85–102.
28. Singer WD, Haller JS, Sullivan LR, et al. The value of neuroradiology in infantile spasms. *J Pediatr* 1982;100:47–50.
29. Bertoni, JM, von Loh S, Allen RJ. The Aicardi syndrome: report of 4 cases and review of the literature. *Ann Neurol* 1979;5:475–482.
30. Willis J, Rosman NP. The Aicardi syndrome versus congenital infection: diagnostic considerations. *J Pediatr* 1980;96:235–239.
31. Singer WD, Rabe EF, Haller JS. The effect of ACTH therapy upon infantile spasms. *J Pediatr* 1980;96:485–489.
32. Chevrie JJ, Aicardi J. Convulsive disorders in the first year of life: neurological and mental outcome and mortality. *Epilepsia* 1978;19:678.
33. Riikonen R, Donner M. ACTH therapy in infantile spasms: side effects. *Arch Dis Child* 1980;55:664–672.
34. Aicardi J. The problem of the Lennox syndrome. *Dev Med Child Neurol* 1973;15:77–81.
35. Aicardi J. *Epilepsy in children.* New York: Raven Press, 1986.
36. Neidermeyer E. The Lennox–Gastaut syndrome: a severe type of childhood epilepsy. *Arch Z Nervenheilk* 1969;195:263–282.
37. Markand ON. Slow spike-wave activity in EEG and associated clinical features: often called Lennox or Lennox–Gestaut syndrome. *Neurology* 1977;27:746–757.
38. Gestaut H, Roger J, Soulayrol R, et al. Childhood epileptic encephalopathy with diffuse slow spike-waves (otherwise known as "petit mal variant"). *Epilepsia* 1966;7:139–179.
39. Blume WT, David RB, Gomez MR. Generalized sharp and slow wave complexes: associated clinical features and long-term follow-up. *Brain* 1973;96:289–306.
40. Yamatogi Y, Ohtsuka Y, Ishida T, et al. Treatment of the Lennox syndrome with ACTH: a clinical and electroencephalographic study. *Brain Dev* 1979;1:267–276.
41. Millichap JG. The definition of febrile seizures. In: Nelson KB, Ellenberg JH, eds. *Febrile seizures.* New York: Raven Press, 1981;1–3.
42. Nelson KB, Ellenberg JH. The role of recurrences in determining outcome in children with febrile seizures. In: Nelson KB, Ellenberg JH, eds. *Febrile seizures.* New York: Raven Press, 1981;19–26.
43. Nelson KB, Ellenberg JH. Predictors of epilepsy in children who have experienced febrile seizures. *N Eng J Med* 1976;295:1029–1033.
44. Levitan A, Cowan LD. Do febrile seizures increase the risk of complex partial seizures? An epidemiologic assessment. In: Morselli PL, Pippenger CE, Penry JK, eds. *Febrile seizures.* New York: Raven Press, 1981;65–74.
45. Falconer MA, Taylor DC. Surgical treatment of drug-resistant epilepsy due to mesial temporal sclerosis. Etiology and significance. *Arch Neurol* 1968;19:353–361.
46. Nelson KB, Ellenberg JH. Prognosis in children with febrile seizures. *Pediatrics* 1978;61:720–727.
47. Nelson KB. Can treatment of febrile seizures prevent subsequent epilepsy? In: Nelson KB, Ellenberg JH, eds. *Febrile seizures.* New York: Raven Press, 1981;143–146.
48. Minagawa K, Miura H. Phenobarbital, primidone, and sodium valproate in the prophylaxis of febrile convulsions. *Brain Dev* 1981;3:385–393.
49. Wolf SM, Carr A, Davis DC, et al. The value of phenobarbital in the child who has had a single febrile seizure: a controlled study. *Pediatrics* 1977;59:378–385.
50. Wallace SJ. Prevention of recurrent febrile seizures using continuous prophylaxis: sodium valproate compared to phenobarbital. In: Nelson KB, Ellenberg JH, eds. *Febrile seizures.* New York: Raven Press, 1981;135–142.
51. Thorn I. Prevention of recurrent febrile seizures: intermittent prophylaxis with diazepam compared with continuous treatment with phenobarbital. In: Nelson KB, Ellenberg JH, eds. *Febrile seizures.* New York: Raven Press, 1981; 119–126.
52. Milligan N, Shillon S, Richens A, Oxley J. Rectal diazepam in the treatment of absence status: a pharmacodynamic study. *J Neurol Neurosurg Psychiatry* 1981;44:914–917.
53. Knudsen FU. Effective short-term diazepam prophylaxis in febrile convulsions. *J Pediatr* 1985;106:487–490.
54. Stores G. Behavioral effects of antiepileptic drugs. In: Nelson KB, Ellenberg JH, eds. *Febrile seizures.* New York: Raven Press, 1981;185–192.

55. Fishman MA. An approach to the management of children with febrile seizures: a child neurologist's point of view. In: Nelson KB, Ellenberg JH, eds. *Febrile seizures.* New York: Raven Press, 1981;87–92.
56. Ishizaki T, Yokochi K, Chiba K, Tabuchi T, Wagatsuma T. Placental transfer of anticonvulsants (phenobarbital, phenytoin, valproic acid) and the elimination from neonates. *Pediatr Pharmacol* 1981;1:291–303.
57. Rating D, Koch S, Hauser I, Helge H. Valproic acid and its metabolites: placental transfer, neonatal pharmacokinetics, transfer via mother's milk and clinical status in neonates of epileptic mothers. *J Pharmacol Exp Ther* 1981;219:768–777.
58. Heinz E, Kampffmeyer HG. Biological half-life of phenobarbital in human babies. *Klin Wochenschr* 1975;53:445–446.
59. Painter MJ, Pippenger C, MacDonald H, Pitlick W. Phenobarbital and diphenylhydantoin levels in neonates with seizures. *J. Pediatr* 1978;92:315–319.
60. Painter MJ, Pippenger C, Wasterlain C, et al. Phenobarbital and phenytoin in neonatal seizures: metabolism and tissue distribution. *Neurology* 1981;31:1107–1112.
61. Fischer JH, Lockman LA, Zaske D, Kreil R. Phenobarbital maintenance dose requirements in treating neonatal seizures. *Neurology* 1981;31:1042–1044.
62. Chiba K, Ishizaki T, Miura H, Minagawa K. Michaelis–Menton pharmacokinetics of diphenylhydantoin and application in the pediatric age patient. *J Pediatr* 1980:96:479–484.
63. Morselli PL, Bossi L. Carbamazepine: absorption, distribution and excretion. In: Woodbury DM, Penry JK, Pippenger CE, eds. *Antiepileptic drugs.* New York: Raven Press, 1982;465–482.
64. Jeavons PM. Nosological problems of myoclonic epilepsies in childhood and adolescence. *Develop Med Child Neurol* 1977;19:3–8.
65. Penry JK, Porter RJ, Dreifuss FE. Simultaneous recording of absence seizures with video tape and electroencephalography. *Brain* 1975;98:427–440.
66. Gibberd FB. The prognosis of petit mal. *Brain* 1966;89:531–538.
67. Gastaut H, Gastaut JL, Goncalves e Silva GE, et al. Relative frequency of different types of epilepsy: a study employing the classification of the International League Against Epilepsy. *Epilepsia* 1975;16:457–461.
68. Beaussart M, Faou R. Evolution of epilepsy with rolandic paroxysmal foci: a study of 324 cases. *Epilepsia* 1978;19:337–342.
69. Loiseau P, Beaussart M. The benign seizures of childhood with rolandic paroxysmal discharges. *Epilepsia* 1973;14:381–389.
70. Blom S, Heijbel J, Bergfors PG. Benign epilepsy of children with centro-temporal EEG foci. Prevalence and follow-up study of 40 patients. *Epilepsia* 1972;13:609–619.
71. Lombroso CT. Sylvian spikes and midtemporal spike foci in children. *Arch Neurol* 1967;17:52–59.
72. Geulen PJM, Van der Kleijn E, Woudstra U. Statistical analysis of pharmacokinetic parameters in epileptic patients chronically treated with antiepileptic drugs. In: Schneider J, Janz D, Gardner-Thorpe C, Meinardi H, Sherwin AL, eds. *Clinical pharmacology of anti-epileptic drugs.* New York: Springer-Verlag, 1974;2–10.
73. Shavit G, Lerman P, Korczyn AD, Kivity S, Bechar M, Gitter S. Phenytoin pharmacokinetics in catamenial epilepsy. *Neurology* 1984;34:959–961.
74. Braun CW, Goldstone JM. Increased clearance of phenytoin as the presenting feature of infectious mononucleosis. *Ther Drug Monit* 1980;2:355–357.
75. Leppik IE, Fisher J, Kreil R, Sawchuck RJ. Altered phenytoin clearance with febrile illness. *Neurology* 1986;36:1367–1370.
76. Sawchuck RJ, Rector TS, Fordice JJ, Leppik IE. Effect of influenza vaccination on plasma phenytoin concentration. *Ther Drug Monit* 1979;1:285–288.
77. Kutt H. Interactions between anticonvulsants and other commonly prescribed drugs. *Epilepsia* 1984;25:S118–S131.
78. Mattson GF, Mattson RHK, Cramer JA. Interaction between valproic acid and carbamazepine: an *in vitro* study of protein binding. *Ther Drug Monit* 1982:4:181–184.
79. Levy RH, Pitlick WH, Troupin AS, Green JR, Neal JM. Pharmacokinetics of carbamazepine in normal man. *Clin Pharmacol Ther* 1975;17:657–668.
80. Dodson WE. Carbamazepine efficacy and utilization in children. *Epilepsia* 1987;28(Suppl 3):S17–S24.
81. Cloyd JC, Levy RH, Wedlund PH. Relationship between carbamazepine concentration and extent of enzyme autoinduction. *Epilepsia* 1986;27:592.

82. McNamara PJ, Colburn WA, Gibaldi M. Time course of carbamazepine self-induction. *J Pharmacokinet Biopharm* 1979;1:63–68.
83. Pitlick WH, Levy RH, Troupin AS, Green JR. Pharmacokinetic model to describe self-induced decreases in steady-state concentrations of carbamazepine. *J. Pharm Sci* 1976;65:462–463.
84. Cloyd JC, Kreil RL, Fischer JH, Sawchuck RJ, Eggerth RM. Valproic acid pharmacokinetics in children. I. Multiple antiepileptic drug therapy. *Neurology* 1983;33:185–191.
85. Dodson WE, Tasch V. Pharmacology of valproic acid in children with severe epilepsy: clearance and hepatotoxicity. *Neurology* 1981;31:1047–1069.
86. Chiba K, Suganuma T, Ishizaki T, et al. Comparison of steady-state pharmacokinetics of valproic acid in children between monotherapy and multiple antiepileptic drug treatment. *J Pediatr* 1985;106:653–658.
87. Fischer JH, Cloyd JC, Kreil RL, Kraus DM. Effects of age and concomitant antiepileptic drug (AED) therapy on valproic acid (VPA) protein binding and intrinsic clearance (Cl-int) in children. *Epilepsia* 1986;27:591.
88. Sackellares JC, Sato S, Dreifuss FE, Penry JK. Reduction of steady-state valproate levels by other antiepileptic drugs. *Epilepsia* 1981;22:437–441.
89. Rane A, Bengt H, Wilson JT. Kinetics of carbamazepine and its 10,11-epoxide metabolite in children. *Clin Pharmacol Ther* 1976;19:276–283.
90. Lander CM, Eadie MJ, Tyrer JH. Factors influencing plasma carbamazepine concentrations. *Proc Aust Assoc Neurol* 1977;14:184–193.
91. Mesdjian E, Dravert C, Cenraud B, Roger J. Carbamazepine intoxication due to triacetyloleandomycin administration in epileptic patients. *Epilepsia* 1980;21:489–496.
92. Hedrick R, Williams F, Morin R, Lamb WA, Cate JC. Carbamazepine–erythromycin interaction leading to carbamazepine toxicity in four epileptic children. *Ther Drug Monit* 1983;5:405–407.
93. Goulden KJ, Camfield PR, Camfield CS, et al. Changes in serum anticonvulsant levels with febrile illness in childhood epilepsy. *Ann Neurol* 1986;20:388.
94. Goulden KJ, Camfield PR, Dooely JM, et al. Severe carbamazepine intoxication after coadministration of erythromycin. *J Pediatr* 1986;109:135–138.
95. Wong YY, Ludden TM, Bell RD. Effects of erythromycin on carbamazepine kinetics. *Clin Pharmacol Ther* 1983;33:460–464.
96. Augrell S, Berlin A, Ferngren H, Hellstom B. Plasma levels of diazepam after parenteral and rectal administration in children. *Epilepsia* 1975;16:277–283.
97. Kanto J. Plasma concentrations of diazepam and its metabolites after peroral, intramuscular and rectal administration. *Int J Clin Pharmacol* 1975;12:427–432.
98. Franzoni E, Carboni C, Lambertini A. Rectal diazepam: a clinical and EEG study after a single dose in children. *Epilepsia* 1983;24:35–41.
99. Milligan N, Dhillon S, Oxley J, Richens A. Absorption of diazepam from the rectum and its effect on interictal spikes in the EEG. *Epilepsia* 1982;23:323–331.
100. Langslet A, Meberg A, Bresden JE, Lunde PKM. Plasma concentrations of diazepam and *n*-desmethlydiazepam in newborn infants after intravenous, intramuscular, rectal and oral administration. *Acta Paediatr Scand* 1978;67:699–702.
101. Dulac O, Aicardi J, Rey E, Olive G. Blood levels of diazepam after single rectal administration. *J Pediatr* 1978;93:1039–1041.
102. Farrell K. Benzodiazepines in the treatment of epilepsy. *Epilepsia* 1986;27:S45-S51.
103. Curless RG, Holzman BH, Ramsey RE. Paraldehyde therapy in childhood status epilepticus. *Arch Neurol* 1983;40:477–480.
104. Giacoia GP, Gessner PK, Zaleska MM, Boutwell WC. Pharmacokinetics of paraldehyde disposition in the neonate. *J Pediatr* 1984;104:291– 296.
105. Burstein CL. The hazard of paraldehyde administration. *JAMA* 1943;121:187–189.
106. Thorpy MJ. Rectal valproate syrup and status epilepticus. *Neurology* 1980;30:1113–1114.
107. Snead OC, Miles MV. Treatment of status epilepticus in children with rectal sodium valproate. *J Pediatr* 1985;106:323–325.
108. Cloyd JC, Kriel RL. Bioavailability of rectally administered valproic acid syrup. *Neurology* 1981;31:1348–1352.
109. Graves NM, Kriel RL, Jones-Saete C. Rectal administration of lorazepam. *Ann Neurol* 1986;20:429.
110. Graves NM, Kriel RL, Jones-Saete C, Cloyd JC. Relative bioavailability of rectally administered carbamazepine suspension in humans. *Epilepsia* 1985;26:429–433.

Epilepsy: Current Approaches to Diagnosis and Treatment,
edited by Dennis B. Smith,
Raven Press, Ltd., New York © 1990.

6

Antiepileptic Drug Selection in Adults

Dennis B. Smith

Oregon Comprehensive Epilepsy Program,
Good Samaritan Hospital & Medical Center,
Portland, Oregon 92710; and
Department of Neurology, Oregon Health Sciences University,
Portland, Oregon 92710

Currently available antiepileptic drugs have some selective efficacy for different seizure types. Appropriately classifying a patient's major seizure type narrows the choice of antiepileptic drug, but consideration of toxicity, cost, ease of administration, and the urgency of the clinical situation may also influence the choice. Balancing the efficacy of an antiepileptic drug against its toxicity is not always straightforward, and it requires (a) a basic understanding of the differences in the spectrum of activities of different antiepileptic drugs and (b) an appreciation of the impact that different toxicities may have on individual patients and patient populations. For example, drug-induced toxicity, particularly changes in cognition or mood, may develop so insidiously that the behavioral change may go undetected by both the patient and the treating physician. This subtle toxicity may significantly affect the patient's quality of life, and it is important to know which drugs are more likely to produce long-term cognitive effects. When choosing an antiepileptic drug for a woman of childbearing potential, however, mild cognitive side effects may be less important than considerations of teratogenicity.

In this chapter, some basic pharmacological principles for the management of seizures will be reviewed which increase the likelihood of achieving maximum seizure control while minimizing the likelihood of producing significant drug toxicity. Compelling evidence from a number of recently completed controlled clinical trials will be presented and used as a basis for recommending specific antiepileptic drugs for specific epileptic syndromes and seizure types in teen-age and adult patients.

BASIC PRINCIPLES

The most important principle in the pharmacological management of epilepsy is that initiation of therapy *should always begin with a single antiepileptic drug*. Not only should therapy always begin with a single drug, but if the initial drug is not successful, it should be replaced by a second single antiepileptic agent. Of course, more than one drug may be necessary to control seizures in some patients, and if a patient is already being treated with two or more drugs, it may be difficult to change to single-drug therapy. Nonetheless, the vast majority of patients can be successfully managed on one antiepileptic drug, and seizure control as well as toxicity may actually improve in some patients as their drug regimen is simplified.

This recommendation for using a single antiepileptic drug whenever possible is based on multiple sound pharmacological principles, personal experience, and data from recent clinical studies (1–3). Whenever two or more drugs are used at the same time, therapeutic decisions become much more complex—particularly when trying to interpret and manage adverse events and subtle toxicity (4).

Advantages of Monotherapy

1. *Management of Toxicity*. Many dose-dependent side effects of different antiepileptic drugs are similar, and when two or more drugs are used concurrently, it may not be possible to discern which drug is responsible for the symptoms of toxicity, even when the serum levels of both drugs are known. For example, the combination of phenytoin and carbamazepine frequently results in clinical symptoms of toxicity, even when serum levels of both drugs are well within established therapeutic range. In contrast, if side effects occur when a single antiepileptic drug is used, appropriate modification of the therapeutic regimen can be made with relative ease.

2. *Compliance*. Probably the most common reason for antiepileptic drug failure or lack of efficacy is lack of compliance (5). When a single drug fails, evidence for noncompliance should be sought before another drug is substituted for the first. When seizure frequency has not been effectively reduced despite apparently adequate dosage of the anticonvulsant, it is a mistake to assume that the drug is not effective until serum anticonvulsant blood levels (both free and total) are documented and compliance is assessed.

It is axiomatic that the more simple and easy to remember the drug regimen is, the more likely the patient is to be compliant. Patients tend to rebel or deny their illness when they have to take *any* medication chronically. The more medication they have to take and the more complex the regimen, the more likely it is that the rebellion and/or denial will affect compliance. Rebellion and/or denial of illness, of course, are not the only reason for noncompliance: It is simply easier to remember and understand a single-drug schedule than to remember a dosing schedule involving multiple drugs taken at different times during the day.

3. *Drug Interaction*. One of the consequences of using more than one drug at a time is the occasional unpredictable effect one drug may have on the other. Although some interactions may be of little consequence, some can precipitate undesirable toxicity. Other interactions (e.g., between valproate and clonazepam) may even result in loss of seizure control. Dose-related side effects become compounded when two drugs are used simultaneously, even when neither drug is present in the

blood in what is usually considered an unacceptable range (6). The combination of carbamazepine and phenytoin is a good example of this kind of interaction. The toxicities of these two antiepileptic drugs add more quickly than their combined therapeutic efficacy.

The addition of a second drug to a therapeutic regimen may induce hepatic enzyme systems and speed the metabolism of the first drug, leading to decreases in serum concentration of the first drug. Alternatively, the first drug may speed up the anticipated metabolism of the added drug. This kind of interaction may make it difficult to achieve adequate serum levels of *either* drug (5). Not only is this kind of interaction not completely predictable, but the difficulty is compounded by the fact that some drugs may inhibit the metabolism of others. Monitoring serum levels of both drugs is helpful to avoid these complications, but the interactions may take weeks or months to become apparent, and it is often impractical to monitor serum levels with sufficient frequency to avoid clinically significant changes in serum drug levels.

Perhaps the most common example of one antiepileptic drug inducing a more rapid metabolism of another is the effect of phenobarbital on phenytoin. When phenobarbital is added to the regimen of a patient on monotherapy with phenytoin, the serum phenytoin levels tends to fall toward "subtherapeutic" ranges, resulting in an increased likelihood of a breakthrough in seizure control. In response to loss of seizure control, it is a common mistake for the treating physician to raise the phenobarbital dose. This, however, may further increase the metabolism of phenytoin and may exacerbate an already iatrogenic worsening of the patient's condition.

Induction is not the only problematic drug interaction. Valproate, for example, may displace phenytoin from protein-binding sites, and even though total serum phenytoin levels fall or remain constant, clinical toxicity may result because of an increase in free or "active" unbound phenytoin (7). Some drugs may even *inhibit* the metabolism of others, leading to an unexpected accumulation of one or both drugs—a situation seen, for example, when methsuximide is added to phenytoin therapy (8). A more commonly encountered and troublesome interaction is the inhibiting effect valproate has on the metabolism of phenobarbital. When valproate is added to phenobarbital therapy, phenobarbital levels may quickly rise to toxic levels. If this interaction is not recognized, the toxicity may be wrongly attributed to the valproate.

4. *Synergism.* Unfortunately, there is no evidence that the anticonvulsant properties of different anticonvulsant compounds are additive. Adequate blood levels of each anticonvulsant drug must be achieved to effect a good therapeutic result regardless of the presence of other drugs.

5. *Idiosyncratic Side Effects.* Idiosyncratic side effects are, by definition, unpredictable and may occur at the initiation of therapy with any drug, or they may take some months or (rarely) years to develop (9). If two drugs are given simultaneously and an idiosyncratic allergic reaction is seen, it is virtually impossible to tell which drug is responsible. Of equal importance is the fact that cross-hypersensitivity reactions have been reported, particularly with drugs that have similar chem-

ical configuration (such as phenobarbital or phenytoin). Both drugs may then have to be discontinued, and a potentially safe and effective anticonvulsant agent may thereby be removed from the therapeutic armamentarium for that patient.

6. *Chronic Toxicity.* There is growing evidence that polypharmacy increases the development of frequently unrecognized chronic toxicity (4). Reduction to monotherapy may reduce undesirable metabolic or cognitive effects of polytherapy. Several studies have documented an improvement in neuropsychological test scores when therapy with two or more anticonvulsants was reduced to therapy with a single agent (1,10–12).

7. *Seizure Control.* In at least one study (1), it has been shown that simply by reducing polytherapy to monotherapy, seizure control was improved in greater than 36% of patients. Whether this was simply because of increased compliance, however, is not known.

Treatment with a single anticonvulsant drug may not always be possible. Monotherapy is less likely to succeed in severe prolonged epilepsy and in patients with brain damage or progressive structural lesions. However, even in these circumstances, there is no good evidence that therapy with multiple drugs is any more effective than therapy with a single agent.

Finally, and perhaps most importantly, there is now compelling objective clinical evidence that polypharmacy has no advantage in terms of seizure control over monotherapy in the majority of patients (1,3,4,13,14). Schmidt (1), in an evaluation of 36 patients, showed that simplifying their regimen from two anticonvulsants to monotherapy was accomplished with no increase in seizures in 83% of these patients, while 36% actually showed some decrease in seizure frequency. Reynolds and Shorvon (4) similarly found that 70–75% of their patients could be controlled completely with one drug.

A nationwide multicenter Veterans Administration (VA) Cooperative Study (3) designed to prospectively compare the efficacy and toxicity of four major anticonvulsant drugs (carbamazepine, phenytoin, primidone, and phenobarbital) has provided significant additional scientific evidence for the effectiveness of monotherapy. In this study, 622 carefully screened adults (15) with partial or secondarily generalized tonic–clonic seizures were randomized to carbamazepine, phenobarbital, phenytoin, or primidone and followed for at least 2 years or until the drug they were placed on failed to control their seizures and/or caused unacceptable side effects. Sixty percent of the patients were adequately managed [meaning that their seizure frequency or manifestation (and/or toxic side effects) did not significantly interfere with their overall quality of life] (16) on the first sole drug they were placed on (Fig. 1). The failures were randomized to one of the three remaining anticonvulsant drugs. Of the 40% who failed on the first drug, more than half responded to monotherapy with the second drug.

One hundred twelve patients of the original 622 required two-drug therapy; of these, 54 (48%) had better seizure control on the two drugs. More than half of those patients who failed on monotherapy also failed to be significantly improved on two-

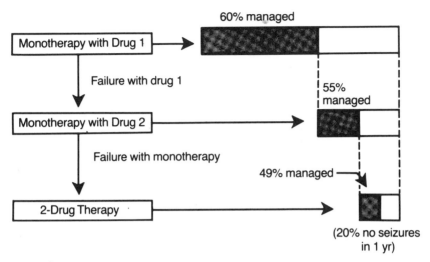

FIG. 1. Percent of patients successfully managed on monotherapy, with first or second drug randomly assigned (combined data for all drug groups).

drug therapy (3). What these statistics do not reveal is the fact that side effects—not loss of seizure control—resulted in most drug failures whether on monotherapy or two-drug therapy. In addition, the side-effect scores on two-drug therapy were consistently higher than the scores on monotherapy throughout the study.

PRIMARY DRUG SELECTION

While the advantages of treating a patient with a single anticonvulsant agent are clear, the principles for guiding the selection of the best anticonvulsant for any given patient are less clear. With the exception of generalized absence seizures, until recently there had been no convincing clinical or scientific evidence that can justify the recommendation of any single anticonvulsant drug for any specific seizure type in adults (17,18). Phenobarbital, phenytoin, primidone, and carbamazepine are still the most commonly used anticonvulsant drugs in the treatment of epilepsy in adults. Each of these drugs possesses considerable efficacy in the treatment of partial seizures, although each has undesirable side effects. Sodium valproate is clearly an effective anticonvulsant in the treatment of absence, myoclonic seizures, and generalized tonic–clonic seizures, but its effectiveness in the treatment of partial seizures has not been as well documented (19). Ongoing prospective studies, including another nationwide VA study, are currently evaluating the efficacy of sodium valproate in the treatment of complex partial seizures. While the results are not yet in, preliminary indications from the VA study suggest that valproic acid may have a broader spectrum of clinical activity than is now widely accepted.

Recommendations for choosing one drug over another as the initial therapy for any individual patient is still frequently influenced by personal biases, based on perception of toxicity and anecdotal experience rather than on well-controlled and well-documented studies. Fragmentary and sometimes conflicting information from published clinical trials of the relative efficacy and toxicity of different anticonvulsant drugs (18) add to the confusion. However, there is now some sound statistical evidence from the VA Cooperative Study (3) upon which to base recommendations for primary drug selection. Of the several measures employed in that study for assessment of the comparative efficacy of the study drugs in seizure control, the most straightforward and simple analysis was examination of the percentage of patients seizure-free after 1 year. Complete control of tonic–clonic seizures for 12 months was not significantly different among the study drugs: 55% of patients were seizure-free in the carbamazepine group, 58% in the phenobarbital group, 48% in the phenytoin group, and 63% in the primidone group. Control of partial seizures was significantly better with carbamazepine than with the other three study drugs after 18 months of follow-up ($p < 0.05$) (Table 1). Partial seizures were controlled in 65% of the patients receiving carbamazepine as opposed to 33% taking phenobarbital, 34% taking phenytoin, and 26% taking primidone.

Another method of comparing the efficacy of these four drugs was to examine the number of patients on each drug remaining active in the study over time. A decreasing retention of patients over time represents an inability of the drug to manage seizures, whether because of poor seizure control, unacceptable toxicity, or both. Figure 2 shows the number of patients successfully managed with each drug during 36 months of follow-up. This analysis combines data for all seizure types (53% of all the patients had more than one seizure type). Retention rates were significantly better among patients receiving carbamazepine or phenytoin than among those receiving primidone ($p < 0.001$). Phenobarbital also had a better retention rate than primidone ($p < 0.05$). Retention rates were better for carbamazepine or phenytoin than for phenobarbital, but this difference did not reach statistical significance.

Very few patients failed to remain on their original antiepileptic drug because of a lack of seizure control alone; most failures occurred because of both toxicity and lack of seizure control (Table 2).

TABLE 1. *Percent of patients free of all seizures*

Drug group	Generalized tonic–clonic (12 months)	Partial complex (18 months)
Phenobarbital	58	33
Phenytoin	48	34
Primidone	63	26
Carbamazepine	55	65[a]
All	55	42

[a] $p < 0.05$.

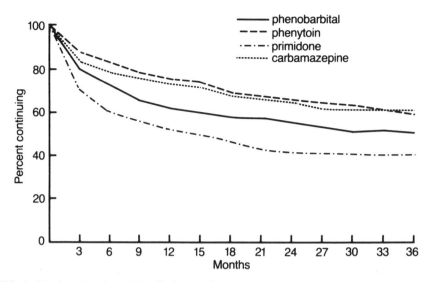

FIG. 2. Number of patients (classified according to treatment group) remaining active in the study for 36 months.

Patients receiving primidone experienced the highest incidence of toxicity. Most of these patients experienced unacceptable toxicity within the first 1–3 months of therapy. The side effects included nausea, vomiting, dizziness, ataxia, and somnolence, resulting in early discontinuation of the drug. Patients tolerating the initiation of therapy with primidone, however, experienced no more toxicity with chronic therapy than did patients taking any of the other three antiepileptic drugs.

A total behavioral toxicity score was derived by combining the scores of the individual subtests transformed into weighted ordinal units of change based upon published norms. The higher the score on the behavioral toxicity battery, the more the deterioration from baseline performance is indicated.

When the effect of each antiepileptic drug on the total behavioral toxicity battery was examined at both 1 and 3 months, significant differences between the drugs were apparent (Table 3). None of the groups showed an improvement in performance at either 1 or 3 months when comparisons were made with their predrug test

TABLE 2. *Reasons for drug failure in the four treatment groups*

Reason	Treatment group			
	Carbamazepine	Phenobarbital	Phenytoin	Primidone
Toxicity alone	12%	19%	18%	36%
Toxicity plus seizures	30%	33%	29%	35%
Seizures alone	3%	4%	1%	3%
Total failures	45%	56%	48%	74%

TABLE 3. *Total behavioral toxicity score for each drug at 1, 3, 6, and 12 months*

Months: p value: Drug	1 <0.001	3 <0.002	6 NS[a]	12 <0.01
Carbamazepine	15.5	14.9	14.8	16.1
Phenytoin	17.3	20.1	15.9	20.1
Phenobarbital	21.3	17.2	15.8	18.5
Primidone	17.5	18.5	16.1	18.3

[a]NS, not significant.

scores. Carbamazepine patients showed the least deterioration, achieving a total battery score of 15.5 at 1 month and 14.9 at 3 months. Patients with primidone also showed relatively little deterioration at 1 and 3 months, having a total score of 17.5 at 1 month and 18.5 at 3 months. In contrast, patients taking phenobarbital or phenytoin showed significant deterioration in the total behavioral toxicity score at both 1 and 3 months ($p<0.001$ at 1 month); scores for the phenobarbital, phenytoin, and primidone groups all showed deterioration in total scores at 3 months, whereas patients taking carbamazepine showed no such deterioration at 3 months ($p<0.002$ at 3 months). Drug levels for all groups were within the well-accepted therapeutic range. The total behavioral toxicity score for phenobarbital was 21.3 and 17.2 at 1 and 3 months, respectively, whereas for phenytoin the scores were 17.3 and 20.1.

On the basis of the results of this long-term prospective comparison of phenobarbital, primidone, carbamazepine, and phenytoin, the most successful drugs when used as initial antiepileptic treatment in adults appear to be carbamazepine and phenytoin. Because of the relative lack of adverse behavioral effects of carbamazepine, carbamazepine may be the preferred drug for initiation of therapy in some adults with generalized tonic–clonic seizures, partial seizures, or both.

In addition to consideration of the efficacy/toxicity ratio of a given drug, factors such as the ease of administration, cost, and urgency of achieving therapeutically acceptable levels also play a role in the selection of the most appropriate drug for an individual patient. A brief overview of some of the advantages and disadvantages of the major antiepileptic drugs will be provided in the following section.

ADVANTAGES AND DISADVANTAGES OF THE MOST COMMONLY USED ANTIEPILEPTIC DRUGS

Carbamazepine

Advantages

1. *Particularly Effective Against Partial Seizures and Symptomatic Epilepsy.*
Carbamazepine has been shown to be effective against partial seizures with both
simple and complex symptomatology and against generalized tonic–clonic seizures.
Experimentally, it is extremely potent against maximal electroshock (MES) seizures—a seizure model that is felt to be a good representation of the localization-
related epilepsies in humans. Carbamazepine is only weakly effective against
Metrazol (MTZ)-induced seizures in animals. MTZ-induced seizures are felt to be a
model for cortical reticular epilepsy, manifested by primary generalized seizures in
humans. Clinically, carbamazepine appears somewhat less effective than phenobarbital or valproate in the treatment of primary generalized tonic–clonic seizures, and
it is ineffective against generalized absence seizures. Dodson (19) and others have
reported worsening of absence, myoclonic, and atonic seizures with the use of carbamazepine. In another recent study (20), carbamazepine provided significantly
better total control of partial seizures than phenobarbital, phenytoin, or primidone.

2. *Lack of Adverse Cognitive Effects.* The major advantage of carbamazepine, in
addition to its efficacy in the treatment of partial seizures, is its relative lack of long-
term adverse effects on cognitive function. Its lack of sedation, particularly compared with phenobarbital or primidone, is also a major advantage. In some patients,
carbamazepine has positive psychotropic effects (21).

Disadvantages

1. *Initiation of Therapy.* Side effects are particularly pronounced at the onset of
therapy, and they make the initiation of therapy complex but certainly manageable.
Complaints of nausea as well as dizziness, sedation, and lightheadedness are common during initiation of therapy, but they rarely persist after the first few days or
weeks. Idiosyncratic reactions (such as rashes) are not common, and they can be
observed with most antiepileptic drugs.

2. *Rare Bone Marrow Suppression.* The initial fears of bone marrow suppression
associated with carbamazepine treatment have been overemphasized. Although it is
important to monitor platelet count and white blood cell count, both before initiation
of therapy and at 3-month intervals for at least 1 year thereafter, fear of bone marrow suppression should not be a major consideration if carbamazepine is otherwise
indicated. Some leukopenia is common in patients treated with carbamazepine, but
in the VA Cooperative Study, some leukopenia was found in association with all of
the major antiepileptic drugs. In that study, no clinically significant leukopenia
occurred during treatment with any of the antiepileptic drugs.

As a general rule, if the white blood cell count falls to less than 3000 during
carbamazepine therapy, the granulocyte count should be used as the guide for determining when to switch to another antiepileptic drug. When the granulocyte count
falls to less than 1000, carbamazepine should be discontinued and another antiepileptic drug substituted. Unfortunately, the very rare idiosyncratic agranulocytosis cannot be satisfactorily predicted regardless of the frequency of laboratory
testing. Warning patients of signs and symptoms of bone marrow suppression such

as bleeding, easy bruisability, and sore throat remains the best preventative approach.

3. *Dose-Related Toxicity.* Dose-related side effects include diplopia, blurred vision, dizziness, and even sedation. Even though carbamazepine is used in the treatment of some affective disorders, worsening of depression and the appearance of frank psychosis appear to be related to carbamazepine therapy in some patients. Hyponatremia and a syndrome of inappropriate antidiuretic hormone secretion are infrequently encountered. Both seem to be related to plasma serum concentration of carbamazepine, but they can occur with therapeutic serum levels. It has been suggested that water retention with carbamazepine is secondary to increased renal sensitivity to serum vasopressin.

Other Considerations

Carbamazepine is moderately expensive, and because of a relatively short half-life averaging less than 12–14 hours, it must be given in divided doses. Generic forms of carbamazepine are available, but they are unsatisfactory. Differences in absorption between different products cause wide fluctuations in blood levels which can result in unexpected loss of seizure control or toxicity on the same dose. The difficulty with generic substitution is serious enough that the Epilepsy Foundation of America cautions against the use of generic carbamazepine, and the Food and Drug Administration (FDA) has recently recalled several carbamazepine generics because of difficulty with absorption. It is not available in parenteral form, limiting its usefulness in urgent situations and when patients are unable to take their medicines orally.

The advantages and disadvantages of carbamazepine are summarized as follows:

Advantages	Disadvantages
1. Broad spectrum of activity	1. Lack of parenteral formulation
2. Superior efficacy in the control of partial seizures	2. Short half-life, necessitating multiple daily dosing
3. Lack of cognitive side effects	
4. Absence of sedation	
5. Absence of dysmorphic side effects	

Phenytoin

Advantages

1. *Broad Spectrum of Clinical Effectiveness.* Phenytoin has a spectrum of anti-epileptic activity similar to that of carbamazepine, and it has clinically been demonstrated to be equally as effective as carbamazepine, phenobarbital, or primidone in the treatment of secondarily generalized tonic–clonic seizures (3,20). The data shown in Tables 1 and 2 suggest that phenytoin is somewhat less effective than carbamazepine in achieving complete control of partial seizures. In experimental models of epilepsy, phenytoin is very potent against MES seizures but is completely ineffective against MTZ seizures. Clinically, phenytoin is ineffective against generalized absence seizures and may, in fact, make absence seizures worse.

2. *Ease of Administration.* Phenytoin has a variable half-life but can usually be given in a twice-daily dosing schedule; in some patients it can be administered in a single bedtime dose. Before prescribing a single bedtime dose, it is advisable to obtain blood levels in the early morning (10–12 hours post-dose) and to repeat the determination in the late afternoon (18–20 hours post-dose). If there is too great a morning peak or too low a near-trough level, b.i.d. dosing will be necessary.

Intravenous phenytoin is available for emergency administration (*note*: it will precipitate in a glucose solution), though oral "loading" doses are usually effective and well tolerated in "urgent," but not "emergent," situations.

Oral suspension of phenytoin has greater bioavailability than capsules and may be useful for patients with irradic absorption of the drug. A problem occasionally encountered with the oral suspension is the failure to properly mix the drug in the bottle. Patients may then be undermedicated with initial doses and overmedicated with the final dose from the bottle. Because of its very alkaline pH, phenytoin is poorly absorbed when given rectally and should not be given intramuscularly because it may precipitate in muscle. Concomitant ingesting with meals or antacids decreases its absorption.

Disadvantages

1. *Dose-Related Adverse Effects.* Phenytoin probably has less sedative effects than the barbiturates, but some sedation, dizziness, and difficulty in coordination are frequently seen with initiation of therapy, particularly after loading doses. The dose-related effects include nystagmus, ataxia, sedation, incoordination, and even an exacerbation of seizures. Cerebellar degeneration has been reported with chronic use, particularly when toxic levels have been sustained for some period of time. The effects of chronic phenytoin administration on cognition are controversial. Difficulty with concentration and perceptual tasks has been well documented, but Dodrill and Temkin (22) have recently provided some evidence that previous interpretation of the effects of phenytoin on cognition has been confounded by its effect on motor speed and dexterity.

When administered intravenously at a high rate, phenytoin may cause hypotension and cardiac arrhythmias. This cardiac toxicity occurs more frequently in older patients. Finally, at high serum levels (>30–35 µg/ml) a paradoxical increase in seizure frequency can occur. If this is not recognized, the treating physician may inadvertently aggravate the situation by further increasing the dose as the seizure frequency increases!

2. *Dysmorphic Effects.* The chronic dysmorphic side effects are particularly disturbing and limit the usefulness of this drug, particularly in young adults and women. Coarsening of features, acne, and hirsuitism (particularly of the face) seem inevitable with chronic administration. In addition, the gingival hyperplasia and gingivitis, which are exacerbated by poor oral hygiene, can also be troublesome.

3. *Idiosyncratic Reactions.* Bone marrow suppression is rare. In the VA Cooperative Study a benign leukopenia with white blood cell count less than 3000/mm^2 occurred with equal frequency to that associated with carbamazepine monotherapy. Idiosyncratic side effects such as rash, lupus-like syndromes, and Stevens–Johnson syndrome appear with somewhat greater frequency than is seen with the barbiturates or carbamazepine. Long-term treatment can lead to lymphadenopathy that is nonprogressive and does not evolve to a lymphoproliferative disorder.

Folic-acid-dependent megaloblastic anemia is encountered in up to one-third of patients on chronic phenytoin therapy. It is a self-limited disturbance and does not evolve into aplastic marrow disorders. It is managed by supplementing the diet with folic acid. The chronic use of phenytoin has been associated with osteomalacia manifested by hypocalcemia, elevated alkaline phosphatase, and radiologically demonstrable bone demineralization. It has no clinical significance in a great majority of cases, but decreased exposure to sunlight and the presence of other concurrent diseases such as seen in the elderly and institutionalized patients may increase the risk of pathologic bone fractures. When there is radiologic evidence of osteoporosis, administration of vitamin D is indicated. Phenytoin compares with thyroxine (T4) for binding sites on the thyroxine-binding globulin and may spuriously lower the levels of T4 and protein-bound iodine. Long-term follow-up, however, indicates that these patients remain euthyroid. Hyperglycemia and glycosuria are occasionally seen and have been attributed to inhibition of insulin secretion.

Other Considerations

Phenytoin demonstrates nonlinear kinetics, which makes the dosage adjustment particularly difficult. A small adjustment in dose may cause dramatic changes in blood levels with resultant toxicity on the one hand, or loss of seizure control on the other. Patients are sometimes wrongly accused of poor compliance because of widely fluctuating serum levels of phenytoin, when in fact the fluctuations are secondary to minor dosage adjustments made by the physician, or secondary to the substitution of a generic product.

There is a mild teratogenetic risk for women of childbearing potential. The most common birth defects associated with phenytoin therapy are relatively minor and include cleft palate and cleft lip. Cardiac defects are extremely rare. This teratogenicity, coupled with the dysmorphic side effects, limits the use of this drug in women and children.

The advantages and disadvantages of phenytoin are summarized as follows:

Advantages	Disadvantages
1. Well-documented efficacy in tonic–clonic and partial seizures 2. Lack of sedative side effects at usual dose 3. Reasonable cost 4. Parenteral form available	1. Dysmorphic side effects 2. Teratogenicity 3. Unpredictable metabolism 4. Possible cumulative effects on cerebellar/motor functions

Phenobarbital

Advantages

1. *Broad Spectrum of Clinical Efficacy*. Phenobarbital has a wide spectrum of anticonvulsant properties in experimental models of the epilepsies (20) and is extremely effective in the treatment of both generalized tonic–clonic and complex or simple partial seizures. The VA Cooperative Study showed no significant difference in efficacy between phenobarbital, carbamazepine, phenytoin, and primidone except in the complete control of partial seizures, where carbamazepine proved superior. Because phenobarbital is very effective against MTZ-induced seizures in animals, it would be predicted that phenobarbital would be very effective against generalized absence seizures in humans. In fact, phenobarbital is probably only minimally effective against generalized absence seizures, and it may even exacerbate absence seizures in some patients. Phenobarbital is probably ineffective against myoclonic seizures.

2. *Long Half-Life*. While the long half-life allowing a long dosage interval is a major advantage, it can be a double-edged sword. Longer dosing intervals and a simplified regimen can help achieve compliance, but the long half-life means that weeks can elapse before a steady state is achieved during initiation of therapy. In addition, the long half-life makes withdrawal of the drug a prolonged and difficult procedure: Because withdrawal seizures are common as the dose is reduced, dosage reduction must be done slowly and over several months. In my experience, the greatest danger of withdrawal seizures occurs in the final phases of withdrawal

when levels of phenobarbital are less than 5–10 µg/ml, having fallen from levels in the mid-20s.

Disadvantages

Adverse Effects on Cognition; Sedation. The major disadvantage of using phenobarbital is that it is sedating. Pharmacological tolerance develops fairly rapidly to the more serious sedative effect, and patients frequently do not complain of sedation on chronic therapy. When a nonsedating drug such as carbamazepine is substituted for phenobarbital, however, many patients report that they feel significantly more alert. Gastrointestinal side effects are rare, as are side effects such as dizziness, diplopia, and difficulty with coordination (ataxia). The chronic effects of phenobarbital on higher cognitive function have been well documented (10) and, in some patients, have been shown to cause depression. There is also some evidence that phenobarbital interferes with concentration and learning.

Other Considerations

The major disadvantage of phenobarbital is its sedative side effects along with its effects on cognition and learning. Phenobarbital may therefore not be a wise initial choice for a patient in whom even a subtle deterioration in cognitive abilities would interfere with his or her vocation or schooling (12). Connective tissue changes such as Dupuytren's contracture are not uncommon with chronic therapy, and the frequent occurrence of impotence may also limit its usefulness.

Phenobarbital is generally a safe drug with rare idiosyncratic reactions. It can cause depression, and it should be avoided in anyone with a history of depression or suicidal ideation. Although the incidence of birth malformations is rare in infants exposed to phenobarbital *in utero*, developmental delay, low APGAR scores, and respiratory distress can be problems. Phenobarbital is transmitted readily in breast milk, and it may cause undesirable general neurological suppression of the infant.

The advantages and disadvantges of phenobarbital are summarized as follows:

Advantages	Disadvantages
1. Long half-life, making single daily dosing practical	1. Sedation
2. Parenteral formulation is available	2. Chronic effects on learning and cognition
3. Broad spectrum of efficacy	3. Impotence
4. Cost	4. Affective disturbances
5. Lack of teratogenicity	5. Developmental delay in infants exposed *in utero*

Primidone

Advantages

Broad Spectrum of Clinical Efficacy. Since the demonstration in 1956 (23) that primidone is prominently converted to phenobarbital, there has been controversy over whether primidone is simply a prodrug for phenobarbital. Animal studies clearly demonstrate that primidone has antiepileptic properties independent of its derived phenobarbital, and they also show that its spectrum of antiepileptic activity is similar to that of phenytoin and carbamazepine and is distinct from that of phenobarbital. It has also been demonstrated that the combination of primidone and derived phenobarbital produces superior antiepileptic efficacy than either drug used alone without expected additive toxicity. Primidone alone has less hypnotic effects than phenobarbital. Human studies have confirmed that primidone is an effective antiepileptic drug in its own right, particularly against generalized tonic–clonic seizures. In the VA Cooperative Study, it was found that there was no significant difference in the control of tonic–clonic seizures between carbamazepine, phenobarbital, phenytoin, and primidone. However, 63% of the patients taking primidone remained seizure-free after 1 year, contrasting with 58%, 55%, and 48% of patients being seizure-free while taking phenobarbital, carbamazepine, and phenytoin monotherapy, respectively (see Table 1).

In the VA study, it was shown that the mean derived phenobarbital level during the first 12 months of the study was 13.4 µg/ml, well below the accepted therapeutic range for phenobarbital. In contrast, the mean phenobarbital level for patients on phenobarbital monotherapy for 12 months was 24.4 µg/ml. Despite these differences in phenobarbital level, seizure control was actually somewhat better in the patients taking primidone compared with patients taking phenobarbital. Furthermore, patients taking phenobarbital as monotherapy showed some deterioration in seizure control when levels fell into the mid-teens.

The half-life of primidone varies considerably between patients, ranging from 3.3 to over 20 hours but averaging well over 8 hours. This relatively short half-life of primidone necessitates b.i.d. or t.i.d. dosing schedules. With frequent dosing schedules, however, little fluctuation in plasma levels of primidone can be expected in most patients. Plasma binding of primidone is negligible, and there is a good correlation between plasma levels of primidone and the level of primidone found in cerebrospinal fluid and brain. PEMA, the other major metabolite of primidone, probably does not contribute significantly to the antiepileptic properties of primidone. Primidone has antiepileptic properties independent of phenobarbital, and its spectrum of activity in both animals and humans is different than that of phenobarbital.

On the basis of both animal and clinical studies, primidone should be considered as primary therapy in the treatment of patients with both partial and secondarily generalized seizures. If therapy with phenobarbital has failed to achieve adequate seizure control, it should not be assumed that primidone will also fail because primidone is also a barbiturate.

Disadvantages

1. *Toxicity with Initiation of Therapy.* Most toxicity occurs during initiation of therapy and includes nausea, vomiting, dizziness, lightheadedness, blurred vision, and sedation. Evidence from both animal and human studies indicates that this early toxicity is a result of the rapid buildup of primidone concentration in brain. In order to avoid these troublesome side effects, it is advisable to initiate treatment slowly by giving 125 mg (1.8 mg/kg) only at bedtime for 3 days and then increasing the dose by 125 mg increments every 3 days.

2. *Dose-Related Toxicity.* Chronic toxicity with primidone seems to be somewhat less than that associated with phenobarbital. Behavioral toxicity data derived from the VA study (Table 3) indicate that primidone has a different behavioral profile than phenobarbital and that it has less adverse effects on mood scales than does phenobarbital. Complaints during long-term therapy are minimal on primidone. The effects of primidone on concentration and learning have not been adequately assessed. Similarly, there is insufficient evidence to assess the specific teratogenicity of primidone independent of its derived phenobarbital.

In summary, it is clear that if the side effects associated with initiation of therapy are tolerated, patients do well with minimal long-term side effects on primidone monotherapy. Controlled studies such as the VA study support the fact that patients on primidone monotherapy do as well as patients on carbamazepine, phenytoin, or phenobarbital, discounting the adverse events associated with the initiation of therapy.

Other Considerations

No parenteral formulation is available, so that the drug cannot be given in acute situations or when patients cannot take medicines orally. Long-term behavioral effects are not well documented, but they appear to be somewhat fewer than those associated with phenobarbital. Connective tissue changes similar to those produced by phenobarbital also occur during primidone therapy, and the incidence of impotence tends to parallel that of phenobarbital.

The advantages and disadvantages of primidone are summarized as follows:

Advantages	Disadvantages
1. Spectrum of antiepileptic activities similar to carbamazepine and phenytoin 2. Relative lack of sedation and behavioral effects compared with phenobarbital	1. Short half-life, making multiple dosing necessary 2. High cost 3. Difficulty in initiation of therapy 4. No parenteral form available

Valproate

$$CH_3-CH_2-CH_2 \diagdown \quad \diagup O \\ C \\ CH_3-CH_2-CH_2 \diagup \quad \diagdown OH$$

Advantages

1. *Efficacy in Idiopathic Generalized Epilepsies.* Valproate, while clearly effective against generalized tonic–clonic seizures, has less well documented efficacy against complex or simple partial seizures (24). Because valproate is effective against generalized tonic–clonic seizures as well as against nonconvulsive generalized seizures such as absence, myoclonic, and akinetic (or drop) attacks, this drug is the drug of choice for patients having seizures of both types. There is no evidence to suggest that valproate is superior to carbamazepine, phenytoin, primidone, or phenobarbital in the control of partial seizures, but there is evidence to support the assertion that valproate is equally effective. Valproate is also equally as effective as ethosuximide in the control of generalized absence seizures, and it has a distinct advantage when the patient has both generalized absence and generalized tonic–clonic seizures.

2. *Lack of Sedation.* Valproate appears to have fewer cognitive and behavioral effects than phenytoin or the barbiturates. Sedation reported with valproate is almost always due to its effect on co-medication; for example, valproate blocks the metabolism of phenobarbital and may cause acutely high barbiturate levels when the drug is used as co-medication.

Disadvantages

1. *Dose-Related Side Effects.* Cognitive side effects appear to be minimal (25), but there has been a suggestion that valproate may have some effect on memory.

Reports of sedation, ataxia, and lightheadedness are in large part due to the use of valproate in combination with phenobarbital, phenytoin, or carbamazepine. Because valproate inhibits the metabolism of phenobarbital and tends to displace phenobarbital, phenytoin, and carbamazepine from protein-binding sites, the toxicity of the concurrent medication is exaggerated and frequently becomes intolerable to the patient. In this circumstance, both the patient and the prescribing physician may misinterpret the effects as being due to valproate resulting in the premature discontinuation of valproate, which is then regarded as a failure. Obtaining free levels of the antiepileptic drugs and decreasing the dose of the other antiepileptic drugs may solve the problem and allow a therapeutic trial on valproate.

Nausea and vomiting may be seen with the initiation of therapy and may persist in some patients. These symptoms usually occur 1–2 hours after oral intake, but they may also be seen after rectal administration. Nausea is probably secondary to both the gastric irritation and the central effects of the drug. Administration of valproate with or after meals can be helpful. In our hands, ranitidine has not been successful in controlling the symptoms of nausea, but some patients have responded well to prochlorperazine.

Dose-related intention tremor can be quite disabling in some individuals. Equally troublesome is weight gain apparently related to central stimulation of appetite. Asterixis may be seen at high doses, and it bears an inconsistent relationship to blood ammonia levels. Nausea and vomiting are not infrequent during the initiation of therapy, but they have been minimized with the use of the divalproic sodium formulation and do not usually necessitate discontinuation of the medication.

2. *Idiosyncratic Side Effects.* Thrombocytopenia and platelet dysfunction can occur in patients taking valproate. This is probably infrequent but should be taken into consideration when such patients are about to undergo surgery. An IgM platelet autoantibody directed against a free fatty acid present in the platelet wall that has a configuration similar to valproate has been postulated as the possible mechanism (26).

3. *Hepatic Toxicity.* The hepatic toxicity of valproate has been overstated. Transient abnormalities of liver function are not unusual, but idiosyncratic hepatotoxicity requiring discontinuation of the drug is extremely rare. In infants under the age of 2, there has been some concern about a fatal hepatotoxicity, but this has been shown to occur especially when other antiepileptic drugs are used concomitantly. The risk is much lower during monotherapy, and it decreases dramatically later in childhood. No fatal cases have been reported above the age of 2. The incidence of rash and other dermatologic problems on valproate is very low. Hair loss may occur at higher doses, but it is a rare complication.

Reversible and irreversible hepatitis-like syndrome, Reyes-like syndrome, and hyperammonemia have been reported. Transient elevation of serum aminotransferase between two and three times the upper limit of normal is seen in approximately 10% of patients. The majority of these patients are asymptomatic and have normal serum bilirubin and alkaline phosphatase. Less than 1% of patients develop malaise, lethargy, and anorexia, all of which rapidly resolve on reducing the dose or stopping the drug (27). Symptomatic valproate-induced hyperammonemia can occur in the absence of overt liver disease and can be confused with fulminant hepatic failure. Higher ammonia levels are more commonly seen when valproate is associated with other antiepileptic drugs, notably phenobarbital (28). Return to baseline ammonia levels is usually seen within 2–5 days of stopping the drug. Concomitant administration of L-carnitine may be of benefit in these patients. Cases of Reyes-like syndrome have been reported in children receiving aspirin while on valproate therapy. The mechanisms mediating this reaction are not known. The drugs may have additive hepatotoxicity in susceptible individuals, and for this reason this combination should be avoided.

4. *Teratogenicity*. Neural tube defects and spinal bifida have been reported in children of women taking valproate. The incidence is extremely low, and it is similar to the incidence of cleft lip and palate seen in association with phenytoin therapy. Nonetheless, until the incidence and nature of the teratogenicity of valproate are clarified in further clinical studies, the potential teratogenicity may limit its usefulness in women of childbearing potential.

Other Considerations

The drug is quite expensive, but with the divalproic sodium formulation the drug can now be given in a simplified twice daily regimen. Hepatotoxicity is rare (29), but nonetheless any evidence for preexisting hepatic dysfunction is probably a contraindication for the use of this drug. The drug has very complex interactions with other antiepileptic drugs, making it particularly difficult to use in combination with other drugs. For example, when used in combination with phenytoin, it may be necessary to administer as much as 3 or 4 g of valproate to achieve antiepileptic drug blood levels (ABLs) in an acceptable range, whereas 1–1.5 g is usually sufficient when valproate is used alone. In addition, the percentage of unbound phenytoin may increase dramatically, resulting in toxicity despite total phenytoin levels in the low therapeutic range (Table 4).

Advantages	Disadvantages
1. Superior efficacy against primary generalized seizures, including absence seizures, myoclonic seizures, akinetic seizures, and primary generalized tonic–clonic seizures	1. Complex interaction with other antiepileptic drugs
	2. Absence of a parenteral formulation
	3. Cost
2. Broad spectrum of effectiveness against partial and secondarily generalized seizures	4. An incidence of teratogenicity similar to that of phenytoin
3. Relative lack of cognitive side effects	
4. Rare idiosyncratic side effects	

TABLE 4. *Change in original AED blood level produced by adding a second AED[a]*

Added AED	Original AED				
	CBZ	PHT	VPA	PRM	Pb
CBZ	↓ auto-induct	↓	↓	↓ PRM ↑ Pb	↓
PHT	↓		↓	↓	↓
VPA	↑ (↓)	↑ Free ↓ Total		↑ Pb	↑
PRM	↓ (↑)	↑ ↓	↑ ↓		↑
Pb	↓	↓	↓	↓	

[a]AED, antiepileptic drug; CBZ, carbamazepine; PHT, phenytoin; VPA, valproic acid; PRM, primidone; Pb, phenobarbital. An arrow pointing upward denotes an increase, whereas one pointing downward denotes a decrease.

OTHER FACTORS INFLUENCING THE SELECTION OF A PRIMARY ANTIEPILEPTIC DRUG

The urgency of the clinical situation and need for achieving a rapid and stable protective serum anticonvulsant level may influence the choice of the primary anticonvulsant agent. If a patient is having frequently recurring seizures that significantly interfere with his or her functioning, it may be necessary to select a drug that may be given in a loading dose parenterally or orally in order to rapidly achieve stable therapeutic effect. This kind of urgent clinical situation virtually limits the selection to either phenytoin or phenobarbital. Of the two, loading with phenytoin is associated with far fewer side effects and, in this circumstance, is probably the drug of choice.

Dysmorphic and idiosyncratic side effects such as gum hypertrophy, hirsuitism, acne, and rash have been documented to be higher for phenytoin than for carbamazepine, phenobarbital, or primidone (3). This fact, coupled with the worrisome teratogenetic risk, should alert clinicians not only to consider carbamazepine as the drug of choice in women and young adults, but to switch patients in this population group from phenytoin to either phenobarbital, primidone, or carbamazepine. Because of the high protein binding of both valproate and phenytoin, their use in uremia or hepatic disease may be limited.

Chronic toxicity may be difficult to recognize, and careful monitoring on the part of the physician is necessary. Dysmorphic side effects of phenytoin increase over time, and gradual changes in endocrine function, immunosuppression, folic acid deficiency, osteomalacia, subtle cognitive changes, and cerebellar dysfunction may occur. While these chronic side effects are all associated with phenytoin therapy, carbamazepine and the barbiturates may produce similar effects, with the probable exception of dysmorphic changes. Dupuytren's contracture occurs with increasing frequency over time during monotherapy with the barbiturates, occurring to a lesser extent with phenytoin. Bone marrow suppression and hepatic toxicity associated with carbamazepine are uncommon, but liver function tests and blood counts should be monitored at least three to four times per year.

Phenobarbital and primidone are most likely to cause sexual dysfunction, and the changes in cognitive and motor functions associated with these drugs have already been discussed. Long-term effects of sodium valproate therapy are less well documented, but they include weight gain, alopecia, edema, and behavioral change. Hepatic toxicity is rare in adults; if it does occur, it usually occurs within the first 6 months of therapy and is reversible with discontinuation of the drug.

SELECTION OF ALTERNATE DRUG THERAPY

The first alternative, if more than one trial of monotherapy for two or more of the five major anticonvulsant drugs has failed, is the use of a combination of two of these same drugs. If an intelligently chosen combination of two of these drugs is ineffective, the substitution of a second-line anticonvulsant for one of the first two drugs may then be necessary. It is rarely necessary to add a third drug to any regimen. If seizure frequency is not affected by a combination (or combinations) of two drugs, it is likely that the patient will be found to be refractory to medical therapy. The addition of more anticonvulsants serves only to compound dose-related side effects and increase the risks of serious (perhaps fatal) idiosyncratic side effects.

Guidelines for Combination Therapy

Avoid a combination of two drugs that have similar or additive side effects. Primidone and phenobarbital, both barbiturates, should *never* be used in combination. Mephenytoin in combination with phenytoin may increase the likelihood of development of toxic parenchymal systemic side effects.

Be aware of pharmacokinetic interactions. Whenever two drugs are used in combination, compulsive monitoring of the anticonvulsant blood levels of each compound is essential. When phenytoin and carbamazepine are used in combination, mutual induction tends to decrease the blood level of each agent. With this combination, it is frequently difficult to achieve "adequate" blood levels of either compound without experiencing exaggerated and unexpected side effects. Valproate displaces phenytoin from protein-binding sites, resulting in increased free phenytoin and therefore an increased rate of excretion and a tendency toward lower serum phenytoin levels. The increased "free" or unbound fraction, however, results also in an increased "active" fraction. Hence, a lower total phenytoin level may not be representative of lower available or "unbound" phenytoin. In fact, without access to both free and total phenytoin levels, pushing phenytoin dosage on the basis of decreasing total phenytoin levels in this situation can result in unexpected toxicity and a paradoxical deterioration in seizure control. The multiplicity of drug interaction with valproate makes polypharmacy using this drug particularly difficult.

Avoid combining drugs from the same chemical family. The disadvantages of combining primidone and phenobarbital, and mephenytoin and phenytoin, have been discussed. The same disadvantages of additive toxicity with little, if any, increased efficacy apply to any barbiturate combination or any combination of hydantoins (mesantoin, phenytoin, ethotoin) or succinimides (ethosuximide, methsuximide, or phensuximide).

Try two drugs with differing spectra of activity. Phenobarbital has an entirely different spectrum of anticonvulsant activity than does phenytoin in experimental models. (This may be the reason for the success of this combination in some selected patients.) Similarly, valproate, a gamma-aminobutyric acid agonist, acts in very different ways than phenobarbital, phenytoin, carbamazepine, or ethosuximide, and it is a good choice for combination therapy with any of those agents if it has been found that monotherapy has failed.

Try a combination of the least toxic first-line anticonvulsants before using second-line (more toxic) agents. The major feature discriminating the "first-line" anticonvulsants from the "second-line" anticonvulsants is their side effects. The second-line anticonvulsants are not commonly used because for the most part they are highly toxic (e.g., methsuximide and mephenytoin) or have questionable long-term efficacy (e.g., acetazolamide and the currently available benzodiazepines).

Interactions of Antiepileptic Drugs

Inhibition of Metabolism

Inhibition of metabolism of antiepileptic drugs can be competitive or noncompetitive. Noncompetitive inhibition leads to increasing antiepileptic-drug serum levels that are proportional to the doses of both the antiepileptic drug and the inhibiting drug. The metabolism of hydantoin, for example, is noncompetitively inhibited by concomitant administration of disulfiram and isoniazide (30). Competitive inhibitors raise serum levels of antiepileptic drugs to a variable higher plateau and then stabilize. Clinically, this is most commonly seen with a combination therapy of phenobarbital and hydantoin. Phenobarbital is a competitive inhibitor of hydantoin and tends to increase serum levels of the latter. This effect, however, is partially canceled by a different mechanism—namely, the faster hepatic metabolism of phenytoin, determined by phenobarbital enzymatic induction.

Enzymatic Induction. Carbamazepine, phenobarbital, phenytoin, and primidone are potent enzyme inducers. When used in combination, reciprocal stimulation of metabolism of these drugs may occur. The clinical consequences of enzyme induction can be seen at three different levels:

1. *Autoinduction.* This is most clearly observed with carbamazepine: An initially effective dosage may lose its efficacy and require increasingly higher doses to

achieve the same serum concentration. This, however, is a self-limited process that plateaus within 3–6 weeks. No significant further increase in carbamazepine clearance rates occurs thereafter.

2. *Stimulation of metabolism of a concurrently administered drug.* The effect of adding a second drug on serum concentration of the original drug can be seen in Table 4.

Other well-documented examples of clinically important interactions include: decreased serum warfarin and dicoumarol concentration with decreased anticoagulant response; increased metabolism of estrogens and progestagens with decreased efficacy of birth control pills; increased elimination and decreased clinical efficacy of prednisone, cortisol, dexamethasone, and metyrapone when used for therapeutic or diagnostic purposes; and increased metabolism of quinidine with decreased antiarrhythmic efficacy (31). Acetaminophen metabolism is induced by phenobarbital and may lead to accumulation of toxic metabolites in children.

3. Stimulation of metabolism of endogenous substances may account for increased inactivation of vitamin D (rickets and osteomalacia), increased metabolism of sex hormones (acne, hirsutism, menstrual irregularities, and decreased libido), and (a) altered metabolism of triglycerides and cholesterol, (b) folate deficiency, and (c) precipitation of attacks of acute porphyrias.

USE OF ANTIEPILEPTIC BLOOD LEVELS

Regardless of which antiepileptic drug is selected for an individual patient, periodic determination of serum or plasma antiepileptic drug level is critical for guiding not only the total dose of the drug but also the dosing interval. Although the initial dosing schedule can be based on knowledge of the drug's average half-life, wide interindividual variations in half-life and in dosage requirements occur. Dosing recommendations such as those given in Table 4 are based on the average dose needed to achieve antiepileptic blood levels in the intermediate to high "therapeutic" range. These figures are derived from large population statistics and are meant to serve as a guide to dose and dosing interval in individual patients.

To use antiepileptic drug levels effectively, it is important to realize that published accepted therapeutic ranges are based on "trough" levels. A trough level is defined as the lowest concentration of drug present during a dosing interval. It is important to prescribe a dose and dosing schedule such that the trough level does not fall below the minimal effective concentration for that drug. If the drug concentration does fall below that level at any time between doses, the patient is at risk for an exacerbation of seizures. If blood levels are used for dosing adjustment, it is crucial that the blood levels be obtained just prior to the next scheduled dosing. The drug level obtained at that time should be well within the published therapeutic range for that drug. A drug level obtained at any other time can give very misleading information and can lead to a false sense of security or, worse, may lead to the conclusion that the drug had been given an adequate trial without achieving seizure control, when in fact a trough level would have revealed a low or even subtherapeutic con-

TABLE 5. *Summary of dosing data in adults*

Drug	Initial dose[a]	Average maintenance dose range	Average half-life in adults (hours)	Time to reach steady state[b] (days)	Recommended "therapeutic" blood level range	Percent protein bound
Carbamazepine	100 mg hs	600–1800 mg (15 mg/kg)	12–20	3–4	8–12 µg/ml	60–90
Phenobarbital	100 mg hs	100–160 mg (1.5 mg/kg)	72–168	14–21	15–30 µg/ml	40–60
Phenytoin	300 mg hs	300–500 mg (5 mg/kg)	10–30	3–7	12–20 µg/ml	80–95
Primidone	125 mg hs	750–1500 mg (18 mg/kg)	6–22	3–4	8–14 µg/ml	0
Divalproex sodium	250 mg hs	1–3 g (30 mg/kg)	15–20	2–4[c]	50–150 µg/ml	80–95

[a]To reach average maintenance dose, increase by increments of the initial dose no more frequently than the average number of days to reach "steady state."
[b]After any dosage adjustment.
[c]Clinical response may lag by 2–3 weeks.

centration. The timing of drug-level determination is particularly crucial for drugs with a relatively short half-life such as carbamazepine, primidone, or even phenytoin. The timing is perhaps less crucial for a drug such as phenobarbital, the levels of which fluctuate very little over a 24-hr period (Table 5).

A Note on the Use of Generic Antiepileptic Drugs

Attempts to lower the cost of medical care are laudable. The push by the federal government and by some Health Maintenance Organizations (HMOs) to use generic products is based on just such a goal. Unfortunately, the use of generic antiepileptic drugs is fraught with danger and compromises the clinical care of patients with epilepsy. The reason why generic products cause a particular problem in the treatment of the epilepsies is very straightforward: It is not possible to maintain consistent antiepileptic blood levels with generic products.

In the treatment of some disorders, consistent blood levels of the appropriate medicine are not crucial for effective treatment. The therapeutic range for most antiepileptic drugs is so narrow, however, that stability of ABLs is essential for an effective therapeutic response. FDA regulations require that for a generic drug to be licensed, an equivalent dose of the generic product must result in a blood level within 20% of the brand name product—"proving" equivalent absorption. This would be an adequate safeguard *if* the prescribing physician could be assured that the patient always received the same generic product. Blood levels could be followed during the switch from brand name to generic, and the dose could be adjusted to maintain a constant blood level. In reality, the pharmacist buys from a distributor, who, in turn, buys from a number of different manufacturers. The result is that the physician cannot be assured of a constant product, and the patient may experience fluctuations in ABLs up to 40%! The clinical implications of that kind of fluctuation is clear. Secondly, quality control is not consistent among the generics, as demonstrated by the recent FDA recall of several generic carbamazepine products.

The problem with the use of generic compounds in the treatment of epilepsy is serious enough that the Epilepsy Foundation of America has issued a position statement:

> The Epilepsy Foundation of America is seriously concerned about mandatory substitution of generic anticonvulsants without prior approval of the patient and treating physician. Generic formulations of a number of widely used anticonvulsants (carbamazepine, phenytoin, primidone and valproic acid) have recently become available and present the opportunity to reduce costs. Some states and some institutions (including prepaid health plans) have mandated that the pharmacist fill a prescription with the least expensive available drug. There may be significant differences between the characteristics of brand name and generic anticonvulsants, as well as among generic anticonvulsant drugs. The fact that these differences may exist could result in adverse effects, including loss of seizure control and the development of toxic side effects. Change from one formulation of the drug to another can usually be accomplished, and risks minimized, if physicians and patients monitor blood levels, seizures and toxicity.
>
> The Epilepsy Foundation of America therefore strongly advises that all rule making bodies—including those at the federal and state levels, as well as prepaid medical plans, institutions such as hospitals, correctional facilities, residential facilities, and others who make decisions about the availability of certain medications—be made aware of the potential adverse effects of changing from one formulation of an anticonvulsant to another without the prior expressed permission of the treating physician and the agreement of the patient.

Use of Antiepileptic Drug During Pregnancy

Many pregnant women with epilepsy will experience an increase in seizure frequency during gestation. In most cases, it is not possible to predict which patients will lose seizure control. Occurrence or absence of seizures during previous pregnancies is not a reliable indicator. There is some evidence that patients with frequent seizures, catamenial seizures, or excessive weight gain may be at increased risk for breakthrough seizures. While partial seizures seem to have little impact on the fetus, generalized seizures may pose a risk to the patient and the fetus.

Several factors seem to contribute to the increased susceptibility to seizures during pregnancy. In most cases there is a decline in serum levels of anticonvulsant drugs despite steady doses of these drugs. Decreased intestinal absorption, decreased serum albumin associated with an increased body weight, increased volume of distribution due to hemodilution, and increased renal and hepatic clearances are the likely causes. Noncompliance should also be considered.

While the incidence of prematurity, low birth weight, and congenital malformations is increased in infants of women with epilepsy independent of drugs, hemorrhage and microcephaly seem to be directly related to the use of antiepileptic drugs. A vitamin-K-responsive hemorrhagic disorder can occur with the use of all major antiepileptic drugs except valproate and occurs within the first 24–48 hours of life.

The hemorrhage is the result of a deficiency of clotting factors II, VII, IX, and X and is secondary to a competitive inhibition of prothrombin precursors. Prophylactic administration of vitamin K during the last 4 weeks of pregnancy is usually sufficient to prevent it. Bleeding in infants of epileptic mothers taking antiepileptic drugs should be treated with fresh-frozen plasma.

For a more detailed discussion, see Chapter 8.

Principles of Management

All nonsterilized women of childbearing age should be alerted to the fact that oral contraceptives may lose their therapeutic efficacy when taken with enzyme-inducing antiepileptic drugs, as a result of increased hormonal metabolism. The occurrence of breakthrough bleeding in such patients should alert the physician to this possibility. The use of barrier methods of contraception should be encouraged.

In an already pregnant woman, changing or discontinuing medication serves little purpose, because most congenital malformations occur within the first 6 weeks of gestation. Nonetheless, attempts should be made to simplify the therapeutic regimen to monotherapy, and the lowest effective dose should be given. Frequent verifications of serum levels to adjust dose are often necessary. While carbamazepine appears to be less teratogenetic than other currently available antiepileptic drugs, all the evidence is not yet in. The fetal hydantoin syndrome is probably unique to phenytoin. Spinal bifida is a worrisome risk associated with valproate, occurring in up to 1% of infants born to women taking valproate.

Breastfeeding

The concentration of an antiepileptic drug in the maternal milk is similar to the concentration of the unbound drug in the plasma. For this reason, sedation, poor feeding, irritability, and idiosyncratic side effects can be seen in the infant. Withdrawal symptoms can also occur if the mother has been on phenobarbital or primidone.

Long-Term Management

It is clear not only from anecdotal experience but also from the results of long-term follow-up studies such as the VA Cooperative Study that the number of patients who remain seizure-free on any single drug or drug combination decreases over time (3). This increased failure rate over time is particularly prominent during the first 2–3 years of treatment. The implications in terms of discontinuing treatment with antiepileptic drugs are discussed in Chapter 7.

Partial seizures are particularly difficult to control completely, and in some patients it may be necessary to settle for elimination of secondary generalization. In other cases it may be possible to limit the anatomic spread of the seizure so that it remains a simple partial seizure and so that the clinical manifestation of the seizure interferes only minimally with the patient's conscious awareness and interaction with the environment.

In the long-term management of adult epilepsy patients, anticonvulsant therapy alone is not likely to succeed unless there is considerable attention given to the psychosocial, educational, and vocational problems these patients experience. It is the responsibility of the treating physician not only to prescribe the most appropriate anticonvulsant therapy but also to consider and manage the behavioral and physiological effects of long-term toxicity, the behavioral effects caused by living with a chronic disorder, and the psychosocial effects of stressful and often inappropriate environmental interactions. These considerations are discussed in detail in Chapter 10.

CONCLUSIONS AND RECOMMENDATIONS

From all of these considerations and from weighing the advantages and disadvantages of different antiepileptic drugs, some specific recommendations for the first choice of antiepileptic drugs can be made:

1. For children with uncomplicated generalized absence seizures, the drug of choice is *ethosuximide*.

2. For children with atypical absence seizures, particularly when associated with myoclonic, tonic, or tonic–clonic seizures, *valproate* is the drug of first choice. (Any evidence of preexisting hepatic dysfunction is a contraindication for the use of this drug.)

3. For adults and children with complex partial seizures, *carbamazepine* is probably the best initial choice. Although phenytoin is probably nearly as effective (as judged by the results of the VA study using predominantly males), its dysmorphic side effects and the emerging documented effects on behavior, concentration, and motor skills make this drug less attractive as a choice, particularly for children and young women.

4. For adults and children with primary generalized seizures or tonic–clonic seizures, as well as when secondarily generalized tonic–clonic seizures are the demonstrated seizure type, *valproate* is a good first choice drug. Carbamazepine and phenytoin may be equally effective (except for myoclonic seizures), but the side effects of phenytoin make it somewhat less satisfactory.

5. *Valproate* is also the drug of choice for atonic, akinetic, tonic, and myoclonic seizures.

The absence of barbiturates from this list of recommendations is not intended to impugn the effectiveness of either phenobarbital or primidone. Both are excellent anticonvulsants and continue to have an important role in the treatment of the epilepsies, particularly in adults. The sedative and behavioral effects of phenobarbital, however, limit its usefulness as a first choice anticonvulsant when initiating therapy. Behavioral studies of patients on primidone indicate that if the initial systemic side effects are tolerated, this drug has substantially fewer behavioral side effects than phenobarbital or even phenytoin. Nonetheless, the significant incidence of intolerable side effects of the start-up period militate against using this drug as a *first choice* when initiating therapy for complex partial or generalized tonic–clonic seizures in adults. It is an extremely effective antiepileptic drug, and it is also an excellent alternative should therapy with carbamazepine, phenytoin, or valproic acid fail.

Regardless of which drug is chosen as the initial therapy for an individual patient, therapy should always begin with a single drug, and dose should be guided by antiepileptic-drug blood levels measured just before the patient's next dose.

ACKNOWLEDGMENT

The author wishes to acknowledge the contribution of Dr. John DeToledo, particularly in the section on drug interactions and pregnancy.

REFERENCES

1. Schmidt D. Reduction of two-drug therapy in intractable epilepsy. *Epilepsia* 1983;24:368–376.
2. Shorvon SD, Reynolds EH. Reduction in polypharmacy for epilepsy. In: Johannessen SI, Morselli PL, Pippenger CE, Richers A, Schmidt D, Memardi H, eds. *Antiepileptic therapy: advances in drug monitoring*. New York: Raven Press, 1980;203–209.
3. Mattson RH, Cramer JA, Collins JF, et al. Comparison of carbamazepine, phenobarbital, phenytoin and primidone in partial and secondarily generalized tonic–clonic seizures. *N Engl J Med* 1985;313:145–151.
4. Reynolds EH, Shorvon SD. Monotherapy or polytherapy for epilepsy? *Epilepsia* 1981;22:1–10.
5. Pippenger CE, Lesser RP. An overview of therapeutic drug monitoring principles. *Cleve Clin Q* 1984;51:241– 254.
6. Kutt H, Penry JK. Usefulness of blood levels of antiepileptic drugs. *Arch Neurol* 1974;31:283–288.
7. Mattson RH. Valproate: interaction with other drugs. In: Woodbury DM, Penry JK, Pippenger CE, eds. *Antiepileptic drugs*. New York: Raven Press, 1982;579–589.
8. Browne TR, Feldman RG, Buchanan RA, et al. Methsuximide for complex partial seizures: efficacy, toxicity, clinical pharmacology, and drug interactions. *Neurology* 1983;33:414– 418.
9. Sparberg M. Diagnostically confusing complications of diphenylhydantoin therapy: a review. *Ann Intern Med* 1963;59:914–930.
10. Trimble MR, Thompson PJ. Anticonvulsant drugs, cognitive function and behavior. *Epilepsia* 1983;24:S55– S63.
11. Shorvon SD, Reynolds EH. Reduction of polypharmacy for epilepsy. *Br Med J* 1979;2:1023.
12. Theodore WH, Porter RJ. Removal of sedative–hypnotic antiepileptic drugs from the regimens of patients with intractable epilepsy. *Ann Neurol* 1983;13:320–324.
13. Lesser RP, Pippenger CE, Luders H, Dinner DS. High-dose monotherapy in treatment of intractable seizures. *Neurology* 1984;34:707–711.
14. Morris HH, Lesser RP, Luders H, Dinner DS. Medical therapy for intractable complex partial seizures. *Cleve Clin Q* 1984;51:255– 260.
15. Mattson RH, Cramer JA, Delgado-Escueta AV, et al. A design for the prospective evaluation of the efficacy and toxicity of antiepileptic drugs in adults. *Neurology* 1983;33(Suppl 1):14–25.
16. Cramer JA, Smith DB, Mattson RH, et al. A method of quantification for the evaluation of antiepileptic drug therapy. *Neurology* 1983;33(Suppl 1):26–37.

17. Gram L, Bentsen KD, Parnas J, Flachs H. Controlled trials in epilepsy: a review. *Epilepsia* 1982;23:491–519.
18. Smith DB, Delgado-Escueta AV, Cramer JA, Mattson RH. Historical perspective on the choice of antiepileptic drugs for the treatment of seizures in adults. *Neurology* 1983;33(Suppl 1):2–7.
19. Dodson WE. Carbamazepine efficacy and utilization in children. *Epilepsia* 1987;28(Suppl 3):S17–S24.
20. Smith DB, Mattson RH, Cramer JA, et al. Results of a nationwide veterans administration cooperative study comparing the efficacy and toxicity of carbamazepine, phenobarbital, phenytoin, and primidone. *Epilepsia* 1987;28(Suppl 3):S50–S58.
21. Post RM, Uhde TW, Roy-Byrne PP, Joffe RT. Antidepressant effects of carbamazepine. *Am J Psychiatry* 1986;143:29–34.
22. Dodrill CB, Temkin NR. Motor speed is a contaminating variable in the measurement of the "cognitive" effects of phenytoin. *Epilepsia* 1987;28:587.
23. Butler TC, Waddell WJ. Metabolic conversion of primidone (mysoline) to phenobarbital. *Proc Soc Exp Biol Med* 1956;93:544–546.
24. Bruni J, Albright F. Valproic acid therapy for complex partial seizures. *Arch Neurol* 1983;40:135–137.
25. Thompson PJ, Trimble MR. Sodium valproate and cognitive function in normal volunteers. *Br J Clin Psychol* 1981;12:819–824.
26. Sandler WP, Emberson C, Robert GE, Vaak A, Darnborough J, Heeley AF. IGM platelet antibody due to sodium valproate. *Br Med J* 1978;2:1683.
27. Powell-Jackson PR, Tredger JM, Williams R. Hepatotoxicity to sodium valproate: a review. *Gut* 1984;25:673–681.
28. Warter JM, Marescaux C, Brandt C, et al. Sodium valproate associated with phenobarbital: effects on ammonia metabolism in humans. *Epilepsia* 1983;24:628–633.
29. Pinder RM, Brogden RN, Speight JM, Avery GS. Sodium valproate: a review of its pharmacological properties and therapeutic efficacy in epilepsy. *Drugs* 1977;13:81–123.
30. Kutt M. Phenytoin: interactions with other drugs. In: Levy R, Mattson R, Meldrum B, et al., eds. *Antiepileptic Drugs*. New York: Raven Press, 1989;215–232.
31. Perucca E, Richens A. General principles: biotransformation. In: Woodbury DM, Penry JK, Pippenger CE, eds. *Antiepileptic drugs*. New York: Raven Press, 1982;31–55.

Epilepsy: Current Approaches to Diagnosis and Treatment,
edited by Dennis B. Smith,
Raven Press, Ltd., New York © 1990.

7

Epilepsy in the Elderly

A Pharmacologic Perspective

Alan S. Troupin* and Svein I. Johannessen**

*Department of Neurology, Louisiana State University Medical Center,
New Orleans, Louisiana 70112
Neurology & Epilepsy Program, Fairview Training Center,
Salem, Oregon 97310; and
Department of Neurology, Oregon Health Sciences University,
Portland, Oregon 97210; and
**Department of Research, The National Center for Epilepsy,
Sandvika, Norway 1301*

Epilepsy generally affects young people, with the peak incidences occurring in childhood and adolescence. For most patients, the seizures are well controlled while they are young; and for many, the medication can be withdrawn by early to middle adulthood. Some patients, however, will continue to need medication for many years and will reach a time when pharmacologic changes due to advancing age will influence the management of their drug program. Furthermore, there is an increase in the incidence of onset of new epilepsy past age 50 (1), so there will be an additional population of patients needing new therapy with anticonvulsant drugs. However, since not all seizures in the elderly herald the onset of epilepsy, not all seizures will require treatment with antiepileptic drugs.

SEIZURES IN THE ELDERLY

In addition to the fact that there is an increase in the incidence of epilepsy past age 50, there is also an increase in the incidence of sporadic seizures occurring in this same population. Single seizures can be precipitated in patients of any age as a result of certain physiologic or pharmacologic stresses. Epilepsy, on the other hand, is the presence of recurrent spontaneous seizures unassociated with such stresses. Since the events and situations that produce seizures are often the result of pathophysiology in other organ systems, and since the incidence of disease generally increases with age, it is not surprising that elderly people have sporadic seizures arising from other illnesses or their treatments. Since sporadic seizures resulting from other illnesses do not require specific antiepileptic therapy, management of these seizures first requires adequate diagnosis followed by a decision whether treatment is appropriate at all. Roughly half of the seizures in the elderly are directly identifiable as being caused by external events (2). The largest category of sporadic seizures in this age group is the result of some impairment of delivery of blood, oxygen, or glucose to the brain (3). Most commonly, this is the result of cardiac arrhythmia or major cardiac output failure, with hypotension, diabetes, and major respiratory embarrassment also being significant events leading to seizures. Such patients will not get protection from subsequent seizures due to the same cause by the use of anticonvulsants but will respond to an attack on the disease which provoked the seizure in the first place. Similarly, other systemic illnesses that alter the milieu of the brain can lead to seizures. Uremia, hyponatremia, and other metabolic encephalopathies will generate seizures that will not recur following the restoration of homeostasis by appropriate therapeutic intervention.

Another prominent cause of seizures that do not represent epilepsy is the use of medication that lowers the seizure threshold. Since many elderly people have illnesses for which various medications are prescribed, the problem is more common in this age group than in younger individuals. Although this effect is commonly recognized for some drugs, such as the phenothiazines, tricyclic antidepressants, and xanthines (e.g., theophylline and aminophylline), certain other drugs that lower the seizure threshold are often overlooked as causes of seizures. The non-narcotic analgesics propoxyphene and pentazocine are common offenders in this category. All the antihistamines lower the seizure threshold, although seizures are not common. Usually, this problem can be handled by removing the drug that lowers the seizure threshold, but occasionally that is not possible. Under such circumstances, treatment with an anticonvulsant will provide protection against seizures stimulated in this fashion.

A more common pharmacologic event producing seizures is the withdrawal of sedative and anxiolytic drugs. The overuse of these agents in the population is a noteworthy public health problem, and the elderly are very much at risk. It is not uncommon to find elderly patients taking several sedative and anxiolytic agents, the need for which is currently questionable. When a different physician diligently removes the inappropriate drugs, their discontinuation may produce withdrawal seizures. All of the barbiturates and all of the benzodiazepines present a risk of withdrawal seizures. Another common scenario involves the elderly patient who is admitted to the hospital or chronic care facility where the new physician is unaware of some of the patient's prior medications and writes appropriate orders for a new drug program for this patient. The prior drugs are thus circumstantially discontinued, and seizures may again supervene. This situation does not require particular treatment after the fact, but these seizures may be avoided by being aware of the problem, realizing nevertheless that the relevant information is sometimes not forthcoming.

The onset of frank epilepsy (repeated, spontaneously occurring seizures), however, will require ongoing drug management. The list of etiologies of new epilepsy in the elderly does not differ strikingly from the list for the younger age group, with the exception of the absence of hereditary or birth injury causes. Occlusive cerebral vascular disease represents the most frequent identified cause and is responsible for about one-third of cases (4,5). There are both (a) acute seizures at the time of the vascular event, which may not forecast the appearance of chronic epilepsy, and (b) the evolution of subsequent recurrent seizures developing from the region of cortical damage (6). In the latter category, about half the patients develop obviously focal seizures, while the remainder appear clinically generalized. Many of the focal seizures will generalize secondarily as well (7). Seizures may also, of course, follow cerebral hemorrhages in patients.

The incidence of tumors—both primary and metastatic—is also higher in the elderly. Tumor accounts for a modest number of patients with the onset of epilepsy in the age group 40–70 (4), but the concern that any seizure onset after age 40 might represent tumor plays a large part in directing the evaluation of older adults with the onset of epilepsy. The neurologic degenerative diseases more common in the elderly are only occasionally associated with seizures.

The evaluation of the elderly patient with the new onset of seizures must concentrate first on the identification of any external or pathophysiologic event that may have produced the seizure, and then it must distinguish these symptomatic seizures from the onset of epilepsy. The most effective therapy for the symptomatic seizures is management of the precipitating event without the use of anticonvulsants. Patients with the actual onset of epilepsy also need an evaluation to identify whether additional remediable illnesses are present. In addition to the group of patients with a new onset of epilepsy, there will be a modest number of chronic epilepsy patients who will have survived to the point where the pharmacologic changes related to aging will have some bearing on the continued therapy of their seizures.

PHARMACODYNAMIC DIFFERENCES

Once it has been determined that treatment with antiepileptic drugs is indicated, the pharmacodynamic differences between the elderly and younger people need to be considered. It has been a frequent observation that the elderly are more "sensitive" to the effects of any drugs producing sedation and alteration of mental functioning (8). This certainly applies to the anticonvulsants as well as to the sedative–hypnotic drugs, although relatively little documentation of this fact exists. Studies of the benzodiazepine anticonvulsants have shown, however, that with careful neuropsychological testing, a difference in motor performance at equal serum levels can be demonstrated between the elderly and the young adult population (9). A decrease in cognition was seen to run parallel to the motor performance decrement. Equal end-points in terms of sedative and depressant effects were reached at considerably lower serum levels in the elderly as opposed to younger adults (10). A confusional syndrome has been demonstrated in the elderly who take nitrazepam (11) and has been identified with other benzodiazepines and the barbiturates as well. It is considered that these problems are due to increased receptor sensitivity on a physiologic basis (8,12) or to a diminished number of receptors (13). This heightened sensitivity to the side effects of sedating drugs is unrelated to the anticonvulsant effect of these drugs, which means that the therapeutic index of sedating drugs essentially decreases with age.

A paradoxical excitement in response to sedating agents occurs in the elderly much as it does in the younger child. The barbiturates particularly, and the benzodiazepines as well, have been seen to produce a syndrome of restlessness, inattention, manic behavior, and sleeplessness. This syndrome also is unrelated to therapeutic effectiveness but generally results in the need to withdraw that particular drug from that patient.

PHARMACOKINETIC MECHANISMS

There are age-related changes in several of the pharmacokinetic parameters that influence steady-state serum levels. Actually, some of these changes are in opposite directions and may vary in relative significance from patient to patient and drug to drug. Most of the changes are those that progress slowly with aging, but there are also problems that vary acutely with other disease states. Renal clearance of drugs, for instance, tends to decrease gradually with age (14); however, with the exception of phenobarbital, most of the anticonvulsants are extensively metabolized prior to actual renal excretion. These hydroxylated and conjugated metabolites are not biologically active and have little bearing on accumulation of the active substances in healthy individuals. Acutely, however, there can be a major diminution of renal clearance with renal failure; furthermore, the metabolites can accumulate to high levels, forcing a reduction in the speed of metabolism of the parent drug along with symptomatically elevated levels.

In general, absorption of drugs is not altered with age (14,15), unless antacids or kaolin products are taken with the drugs, usually as over-the-counter remedies. The changes in volume of distribution are more problematic, however, since there is a tendency for lean body mass to decrease with age with a relative increase in body fat. This means that the volume of distribution for lipid-soluble drugs, including most anticonvulsants, may very well increase (16). It has been shown, for instance, that the volume of distribution of nitrazepam (lipid soluble) increases prominently with age (17), whereas the volume of distribution of lorazepam, which is considerably more polar, decreases with age (18). The relatively large lipid distribution volume can delay reaching useful serum levels initially and can also delay the fading of side effects with dose reduction for the highly lipid-soluble drugs.

Changes in binding to serum albumin with advancing age have a notable bearing on overall drug clearance for those drugs that are extensively bound. Actually, binding affinity per se does not change with age, but the binding percentage changes with serum albumin content, which is, in turn, age-related (19,20). With drugs that are highly bound, the changes in binding must be taken into account before changes in clearance and speed of hepatic metabolism can be clearly identified. These factors have led to confusion about phenytoin metabolism and levels, for instance.

When binding decreases, clearance increases because more free drug is presented to hepatic metabolizing enzymes (15), yet there is a modest increase in serum levels as a result of decreased hepatic metabolism in those patients whose binding has not been altered (21). Therefore, prediction of the influence that binding will have on the speed of metabolism of a given individual can be estimated only roughly from serum albumin levels.

Overall, there is a general trend toward diminished metabolism of drugs with age (20,22). The above paragraphs describe various factors that may interfere with the identification of this reduction in speed of metabolism and diminished total body clearance, but the overall trend toward slower metabolism is a background reality with advancing age. There is both a diminution of enzyme mass and a reduction in hepatic blood flow (23). There is specifically a reduction in the number of liver cells as well as a reduction in the number of mitochondria per cell (24). Consequently, the hepatic mixed function oxidative system (P450) is reduced in mass and capability (25). The Stage I (microsomal) drug-metabolizing processes of hydroxylation, *N*-dealkylation, and so on, are thereby reduced, whereas the Stage II process of conjugation, which takes place in intracellular "water," is unaffected. With less enzyme mass available, induction of metabolism is reduced with age (25), whereas inhibition, which presumably represents totally different mechanisms, is unchanged (23). Hepatic blood flow does tend to diminish with age chronically, but it also will diminish acutely with decreases in cardiac output in disease states (16). Bedridden patients, therefore, tend to have longer half-lives and decreased total body clearance because of decreased hepatic blood flow (17).

DRUG INTERACTIONS

Drug interactions represent a major problem in the therapy of epilepsy. In most patients, every effort is made to treat with a single agent in order to avoid both (a) the alterations in metabolism which each drug may produce in the other and (b) the addition of side effects. It is the latter (which usually involves the summation of alterations in mental functioning produced by the various agents) that can be subtle and quite perturbing. In older patients, many of whom have diseases other than their seizures, the use of various other medications can have a bearing on the metabolism of an anticonvulsant, and vice versa. The specific drug interaction pairs that have been evaluated are numerous, and yet only a small proportion of the potential interactions have been evaluated. Several publications deal specifically with this subject (26,27).

The interactions between anticonvulsants shall not be considered specifically here. In elderly patients it is of greater importance to examine some of the interactions in which anticonvulsants alter the serum levels of other therapeutic agents (Table 1). The induction of hepatic metabolizing enzymes by phenytoin provides a good example of these problems. Similar but less extensively documented information is available for phenobarbital and carbamazepine. The potential problems are

TABLE 1. *Some interactions between anticonvulsants and other drugs*

I. Anticonvulsants induce the metabolism of:	
Quinidine	Warfarin
Digitalis glycosides	Steroids
Disopyramide	Metyrapone
Lidocaine	Theophylline
Furosemide	Doxycycline
Propranolol	Acetaminophen
Tricycline antidepressants	Haloperidol
Phenothiazines	Meperidine
II. Anticonvulsant metabolism is inhibited by:	
Isoniazid	Dextropropoxyphene
Para-aminosalicylic acid	Allopurinol
Chloramphenicol	Phenylbutazone
Sulfonamides	Disulfiram
Trimethoprim	Propranolol
Trioleandomycin[a]	Warfarin
Erythromycin[a]	Cimetidine
III. Anticonvulsant metabolism is induced by:	
Phenothiazines	Tetracyclines
Benzodiazepines	Rifampin

[a]Affects carbamazepine only.

greatest for cardioactive drugs, since the induction of metabolism produced by the anticonvulsants will lower serum levels of quinidine and the digitalis glycosides, leading to diminished therapeutic effects. Furosemide levels will also fall. These combined effects can strikingly decrease the efficacy of the therapy of cardiac failure.

Phenytoin or phenobarbital will induce the metabolism of the warfarin anticoagulants, which could lead to inadequate anticoagulation. More subtle is the clinical situation in which the anticoagulant dose is raised to compensate for the accelerated metabolism. The danger exists that when the phenytoin is removed, the metabolism of the warfarin will gradually return to its previous lower rate with an increased bleeding tendency and potentially disastrous consequences. The metabolism of the tricyclic antidepressants and haloperidol is also accelerated with reduced therapeutic effect. The metabolism of both endogenous and exogenous steroids is likewise induced by the anticonvulsants. This is usually of little consequence where an intact pituitary–end-organ relationship exists; but when steroid hormones are used for therapeutic purposes, the reduced serum level can lead to diminished therapeutic effect. The acceleration of metabolism of thyroid hormones by anticonvulsants will only rarely lead to clinical hypothyroidism, however.

Another significant hormonal effect is the stimulation of antidiuretic hormone (ADH) release from the brain by carbamazepine both in normal individuals and in those with diabetes insipidus (28). There is a decrease in serum sodium and in serum osmolalities in some patients. This antidiuretic effect can lead to water intoxication and is more prominent with increasing serum carbamazepine levels (29).

Symptomatically, these patients can experience weight gain, peripheral edema, irritability, and other mental changes. Somewhat more worrisome is the presence of dyspnea, pulmonary edema, and frank cardiac failure—especially in elderly patients (30,31).

Another cardiovascular event is the addition of slowing of cardiac conduction produced by phenytoin to that same pharmacologic effect of the digitalis glycosides. This can lead to increased bradycardia and frank heart block at levels and doses lower than would be expected for each agent given individually. A similar pharmacodynamic interaction exists between phenytoin and disopyramide and between phenytoin and lidocaine (32).

Agents provided for other illnesses can alter the metabolism or protein binding of anticonvulsants, usually involving acceleration of metabolism of the anticonvulsant with a resulting drop in its serum level. With careful monitoring, this can be identified before the return of seizures. Somewhat less common is inhibition of metabolism of the anticonvulsant by the other drugs in question, leading to an initially subtle evolution of drug side effects. The most common reaction leading to the displacement of phenytoin from serum albumin is the one caused by acetylsalicylic acid in modest doses over a period of 1–2 days. Less commonly, the same reaction occurs with the use of phenylbutazone or sulfasoxazole. This displacement of bound phenytoin will lead to high free levels and a consequent increase in drug effect and dose-related side effects. While for most people there can eventually be some compensation for this as a result of an increase in speed of metabolism, acute symptoms may appear before metabolic changes evolve. Less commonly, if phenytoin levels are high, an increase in unbound drug will not be compensated for by increased clearance resulting from the saturable nature of hydantoin metabolism.

SPECIFIC DRUG CLEARANCES IN THE ELDERLY

We report data from 467 inpatients and outpatients seen at The National Center for Epilepsy at Sandvika, Norway, and 87 inpatients from the Fairview Training Center, Salem, Oregon. These were all patients from whom accurately measured anticonvulsant levels of phenytoin, phenobarbital, and carbamazepine were available. Ages, weight, sex, and drug dose were also available and tabulated. All serum levels were drawn at the morning trough. Compliance was checked against hospital records. This study was performed retrospectively. The patient data were separated into groups of patients taking either (a) phenytoin alone or with phenobarbital or carbamazepine, (b) phenobarbital alone or with phenytoin or carbamazepine, or (c) carbamazepine alone or with phenytoin or phenobarbital.

The total body clearance, a measure of drug metabolism at steady state (33), is felt to represent a more meaningful measure of drug turnover than half-life for long-term evaluation (20). Clearance is the ratio between total daily dose in mg/kg/day and the steady-state serum level measured at the lowest daily trough, usually just prior to the first morning dose. This is expressed here in liters/kg/day but has also been expressed in other works in ml/kg/hr. For each drug or combination the data were grouped according to age, and the mean drug clearances were calculated for each decade group. Comparison between regression lines evaluated slopes and intercepts separately by *t*-test.

The mean clearance for each decade for each drug or combination was plotted. There was excessive scatter for these data in younger patients for all drugs or combinations. Past age 40 (age 30 for carbamazepine) there was a log-linear decrement in clearance. Regression analysis for the data above ages 30 for carbamazepine and 40 for phenytoin and phenobarbital yielded regression lines with meaningful correlation coefficients (Table 2).

Examination of the regression analyses for the three groups shows that there is a consistent decrement in clearance with age for all groups and combinations (Figs. 1–3). It is also obvious that the presence or absence of co-medication makes no difference in the rate of decrease in clearance of carbamazepine or phenobarbital. The rate of decrease seems modest and may be of less clinical importance for some patients than the enhanced sensitivity to side effects in this age group. The speed of decrease in clearance is observably greater for phenytoin, however. Although there is no significant difference in phenytoin clearance changes over time for co-medication with carbamazepine or phenobarbital (Fig. 2), the clearance of phenytoin used alone falls less rapidly with age ($p = 0.06$ for the slope and $p < 0.05$ for the intercept). The more abrupt fall with co-medication is related to the diminished capacity of the liver for induction of microsomal metabolism with advancing age (25). Presumably, the presence of a saturable kinetic mechanism makes this difference apparent for phenytoin but not for carbamazepine or phenobarbital. Since the populations studied were basically free of major systemic illnesses and were not over age 75, the possibility that a similar separation of clearance rates for these agents would be seen later in life remains unexplored. The consistent fall in anticonvulsant clearance with age shown here does extend previously theoretical considerations to the realm of practical clinical pharmacology. The data suggest, therefore, that goal dose estimates for older patients should be revised downwards from those used for younger adults, who comprised the original populations for the drug studies from which the therapeutic recommendations were drawn.

TABLE 2. *Total body clearances—older patients*

Treatment	Correlation coefficient	Slope	N
Phenytoin alone	− 0.86	− 0.38	50
with phenobarbital	− 0.91	− 1.20	50
with carbamazepine	− 0.65	− 1.15	20
Phenobarbital alone	− 0.90	− 0.10	47
with phenytoin	− 0.99	− 0.10	50
with carbamazepine	− 0.94	− 0.09	49
Carbamazepine alone	− 0.78	− 0.01	87
with phenytoin	− 0.84	− 0.02	19
with phenobarbital	− 0.74	− 0.01	49

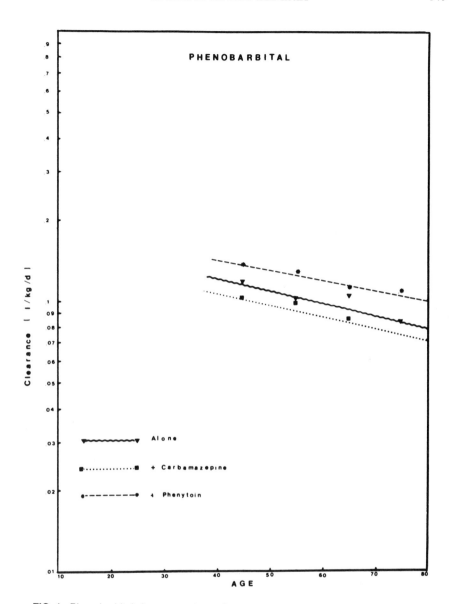

FIG. 1. Phenobarbital clearances at steady state: means for age groups, by decades.

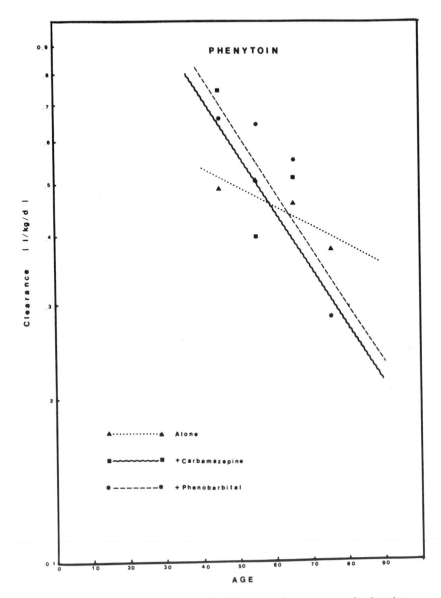

FIG. 2. Phenytoin clearances at steady state: means for age groups, by decades.

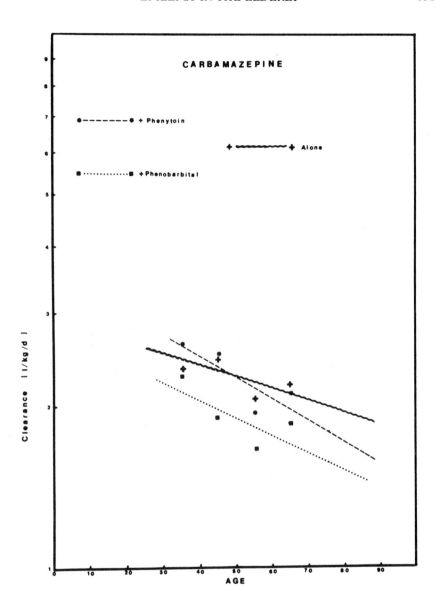

FIG. 3. Carbamazepine clearances at steady state: means for age groups, by decades.

SUMMARY AND GUIDELINES

In the elderly, there is a large incidence of single seizures or short runs of single seizures that are the direct result of pathophysiology in some other organ system only distantly producing symptomatic seizures. These seizures should not be treated as epilepsy, but the underlying disease should be managed vigorously. Monotherapy, the use of single agents for the therapy of epilepsy, is even more important in the elderly because of the addition of side effects and the increased sensitivity to these side effects in these patients. For this reason, nonsedating agents are even more valuable for the elderly patient. One should particularly avoid the barbiturates.

The kinetics of the anticonvulsants are different in the elderly than in the younger population, the latter of whom have a higher incidence of epilepsy. The speed of metabolism is generally slowed—progressively more with advancing age, as shown herein. However, for particular drugs and particular individuals, changes in the volume of distribution may exacerbate or diminish this influence. Overall, however, lower goal doses of anticonvulsants are beneficial in the elderly. Furthermore, reduction in serum albumin and the consequent diminution of drug binding will likewise have a bearing on drug effect and drug side effects. In this age group, not only are serum levels vital for monitoring therapy, but levels of unbound drug will be valuable in assessing complex symptomatic problems. Prominent side effects at "average" serum levels, for instance, may represent reduced binding. Useful and comfortable therapy with that agent might still be possible if the unbound drug level is used as the guide value.

One needs also to keep in mind the multiple problems of drug interactions. There are interactions between anticonvulsants if more than one are used, but the anticonvulsants can also have effects on other drugs that the patient is taking; furthermore, these effects may alter both the therapeutic benefit and the side-effect picture of those other agents. There are also pharmacodynamic interactions between cardioactive drugs and some of the anticonvulsants. Adequate appreciation of the influence of the anticonvulsants (as well as of the drugs with which they interact) upon the heart is of prime importance in managing epilepsy in older patients. The above cautions are meant to cast some light on the potential problems that can arise in the treatment of epilepsy in senior citizens but should by no means be taken as an excuse for compromising on control of seizures in this group.

REFERENCES

1. Hauser WA, Kurland LT. The epidemiology of epilepsy in Rochester, Minnesota, 1935–1967. *Epilepsia* 1975;16:1–66.
2. Schold C, Yarnell PR, Earnest MP. Origins of seizures in elderly patients. *JAMA* 1977;238:1177–1178.
3. Carney LR. Seizures after the age of sixty. *Practitioner* 1976;217:74–81.
4. Luhdorf K, Jensen LK, Plesner AM. Etiology of seizures in the elderly. *Epilepsia* 1986;27:258–263.
5. Oles KS, Gal P, Penry JK, Tapscott WH. Use of antiepileptic drugs in the elderly population. *Public Health Rep* 1987;120:335–337.

6. Lesser RP, Luders H, Dinner DS, Morris HH. Epileptic seizures due to thrombotic and embolic cerebrovascular disease in older patients. *Epilepsia* 1985;26:622–630.

7. Luhdorf K, Jensen LK, Plesner AM. Epilepsy in the elderly: incidence, social function, and disability. *Epilepsia* 1986;27:135–141.

8. Gordon M, Preksaitis HG. Drugs and the aging brain. *Geriatrics* 1988;43:69–78.

9. Castelden CM, George CF, Marcer D, Hallett C. Increased sensitivity to nitrazepam in old age. *Br Med J* 1977;1:10–12.

10. Reidenberg MM, Levy M, Warner H, et al. Relationship between diazepam dose, plasma level, age, and central nervous system depression. *Clin Pharmacol Ther* 1978;23:371–374.

11. Evans JG, Jarvis EH. Nitrazepam and the elderly. *Br Med J* 1972;4487.

12. Everitt DE, Avorn J. Drug prescribing for the elderly. *Arch Intern Med* 1986;146:2393–2396.

13. Wang F, Wagner HN, Dannals RF, et al. Effects of age on dopamine and serotonin receptors measured by positron emission tomography in the living human brain. *Science* 1984;226:1393–1396.

14. Crooks J, O'Malley K, Stevensen IH. Pharmacokinetics in the elderly. *Clin Pharmacokinet* 1976;1:280–296.

15. Hayes MJ, Langman MJS, Short AH. Changes in drug metabolism with increasing age. 2. Phenytoin clearance and protein binding. *Br J Clin Pharmacol* 1975;2:73–79.

16. Triggs EJ, Nation RL. Pharmocokinetics in the aged: a review. *J Pharmacokinet Biopharm* 1975;3:357–418.

17. Kangas L, Iisalo E, Konto J, et al. Human pharmacokinetics of nitrazepam: effect of age and diseases. *Eur J Clin Pharmacol* 1979;15:163–170.

18. Greenblatt DJ, Allen MD, Locniskar A, et al. Lorazepam kinetics in the elderly. *Clin Pharmacol Ther* 1979;26:103–113.

19. Bender AD, Post A, Meier JP, et al. Plasma protein binding of drugs as a function of age in adult human subjects. *J Pharm Sci* 1975;64:1711–1713.

20. Greenblatt DJ, Sellers EM, Shader RI. Drug therapy: drug therapy in old age. *N Engl J Med* 1982;306:1081–1088.

21. Houghton GW, Richens A, Leighton M. Effect of age, height, weight, and sex on serum phenytoin concentration in epileptic patients. *Br J Clin Pharmacol* 1975;2:251–256.

22. Klotz U, Muller-Seydlitz P. Altered elimination of desmethyldiazepam in the elderly. *Br J Clin Pharmacol* 1979;7:119–120.

23. Loi CM, Vestal RE. Drug metabolism in the elderly. *Pharmacol Ther* 1988;36:131–149.

24. Tauchi H, Sato T. Effect of environmental conditions upon age changes in the human liver. *Mech Ageing Dev* 1975;4:41–80.

25. Schmucker DL. Subcellular and molecular mechanisms underlying the age-related decline in liver drug metabolism. In: Butler RN, Bearn AG, eds. *The aging process: therapeutic implications.* New York: Raven Press, 1984;117–131.

26. Hansten PD. *Drug interactions,* 5th ed. Philadelphia: Lea & Febiger, 1985.

27. Woodbury DM, Penry JK, Pippenger CE, eds. *Antiepileptic drugs,* 2nd ed. New York: Raven Press, 1982.

28. Leiba A, Rusecki Y, Ber A, et al. The antidiuretic effect of carbamazepine (Tegretol) in diabetes insipidus. *Harefuah* 1976;89:1–4.

29. Henry DA, Lawson DH, Reavey P, Renfrew S. Hyponatremia during carbamazepine treatment. *Br Med J* 1977;6053:83–84.

30. Stephens WP, Espir ML, Tattersall RB, et al. Water intoxication due to carbamazepine. *Br Med J* 1977;6063:754–755.

31. Flegel KM, Cole CH. Inappropriate antidiuresis during carbamazepine treatment. *Ann Intern Med* 1977;87:722–723.

32. Wood RA. Sinoatrial arrest on interaction between phenytoin and lignocaine. *Br Med J* 1971;1:645.

33. Guelen PJM, van der Kleijn E. *Rational anti-epileptic drug therapy.* Amsterdam: Elsevier/North-Holland, 1978.

Epilepsy: Current Approaches to Diagnosis and Treatment,
edited by Dennis B. Smith,
Raven Press, Ltd., New York © 1990.

8

Special Treatment Problems in Adults

David M. Treiman

Neurology and Research Services,
West Los Angeles VA Medical Center, and
Department of Neurology, UCLA School of Medicine,
Los Angeles, California 90073

There are a number of issues in the management of adults with epilepsy which cause special concerns for medical practitioners. This chapter will address some of these special treatment problems and attempt to provide guidelines for rational decision-making in clinical practice. The following questions will be considered: (a) When should the first seizure be treated? (b) Should antiepileptic drugs be given prophylactically to prevent the development of epilepsy after head trauma or surgery? (c) How should the pregnant patient with epilepsy be managed? (d) When should antiepileptic drug therapy be discontinued? (e) What is the best approach to the management of status epilepticus?

TREATMENT OF THE SINGLE SEIZURE

Perhaps one of the more perplexing decisions that the practitioner must face is what to do about a single seizure in an adult. Any cerebral seizure, but especially a generalized tonic–clonic seizure, is a frightening event to patient, family, and even the physician. There is concern that the seizure may be indicative of some other underlying and more serious condition such as a brain tumor. There is also concern that, should another seizure occur, it could seriously jeopardize the well-being of the patient and his employability and could pose a significant risk to him and others should he continue to drive. On the other hand, there are serious social and medical consequences associated with making the diagnosis of epilepsy and prescribing anti-epileptic drugs. Thus the physician is faced with a dilemma: how best to ensure that another seizure will not occur while at the same time avoiding inappropriate or unnecessary prescription of antiepileptic drugs, which may themselves produce serious consequences.

The evaluation of an adult who presents with a single seizure is as follows: (a) to decide whether the seizure was the first of a series of epileptic seizures or whether it was nonepileptic and caused by some other disorder such as alcohol withdrawal, cardiac arrhythmia, acute central nervous system (CNS) infection, or acute metabolic encephalopathy; (b) to look for a treatable cause of the seizure; and (c) if the diagnosis of epilepsy is made, to determine the seizure type, so that the appropriate medication can be selected.

Epilepsy is a disorder characterized by recurrent nonprovoked cerebral seizures. Thus the diagnosis of epilepsy may be made only if the patient has had two or more nonprovoked seizures. There is considerable controversy regarding the frequency of recurrence of spontaneous nonprovoked seizures in the adult after a first seizure. Reynolds and colleagues (1) have suggested that at least 80% of patients will have a recurrence of a seizure within 2 ¹/₂ years after the first seizure, whereas Hauser et al. (2) have recently suggested that the true recurrence rate following a single nonprovoked seizure in an adult with a normal neurological exam and normal electroencephalogram (EEG) is less than 20% (2,3) and perhaps less than 10% in children (4). Seven other studies have found recurrence rates between 27% and 71% (5–11). The discrepancies in reported recurrence rates after a single seizure will have to be resolved by a consideration of methodological differences between these various studies. Nonetheless, the problem facing the physician is how best to predict whether or not a patient will have a second seizure after experiencing one single seizure. Data from Hauser et al. (3) and from Annegers et al. (10) suggest that the risk of recurrence after a single seizure is approximately double in patients with a history of prior neurological insult compared with patients with no history of neurological insult. Hauser's data also show that a positive family history for seizures increases the risk of recurrence. Electroencephalographic patterns of generalized spike and wave, focal spikes and slowing, and nonspecific slowing are also associated with a high risk of recurrence (7,10). On the other hand, in the 1982 Hauser study (2), only generalized spike-and-wave discharges were associated with a higher rate of recurrence (approximately four times greater than in patients with normal EEGs). Johnson et al. (6) also observed an increased rate of recurrence in Navy personnel who exhibited a spike-and-wave pattern at the time of evaluation for an initial seizure.

Two studies have evaluated the role of the computed tomography (CT) scan as a predictor of recurrence risk. Russo and Goldstein (12) found abnormal CT scans in about half of a group of 62 patients, many of whom (69%) also had abnormal neurological examinations. They therefore concluded that the CT scan is only useful in patients who have neurological deficits and not in patients with normal neurological examinations. On the other hand, Ramirez–Lessepas et al. (13) found 14 patients with structural lesions out of a total of 148 patients being evaluated for their first seizure who had no abnormality on neurological examination. A more recent study using magnetic resonance imaging was able to identify lesions in the majority of patients undergoing temporal lobectomy (14).

The fundamental question with regard to management of a single seizure is whether to initiate antiepileptic drug therapy. Clearly, if a single seizure is the result of alcohol withdrawal, other metabolic insult, or other acute cerebral insult, then antiepileptic drug therapy should not be started. However, if the seizure is the first of what will be a group of spontaneous recurrent epileptic seizures, then antiepileptic drug therapy should be started. Thus the answer to the question "When should antiepileptic drug therapy be started?" is "When the diagnosis of epilepsy is made." Ordinarily, a diagnosis of epilepsy is dependent on the recurrence of two or more spontaneous cerebral seizures. However, when one seizure presents with a clear focal onset or is accompanied by signs of a focal lesion on the neurological examination, EEG, or cerebral image study which suggest a significant increase in the risk of recurrence of subsequent spontaneous nonprovoked seizures, antiepileptic drug therapy should be initiated.

PROPHYLAXIS

There continues to be considerable debate regarding whether a patient who has experienced serious head trauma or a craniotomy should be treated prophylactically with antiepileptic drugs to prevent the development of chronic epilepsy. In the largest study of the incidence of epilepsy after intercranial surgery for nontraumatic conditions, Foy et al. (15) reported that 20% of their patients developed epilepsy within 5 years of a craniotomy, regardless of the reason for which it was done. Even after placement of a burr hole for biopsy or for an interventricular catheter, 13% of the patients developed seizures. Dan and Wade (16) reported a 9% incidence of epilepsy after the placement of an intercranial catheter; the incidence was 55% when the catheter was inserted frontally.

Post-traumatic epilepsy is generally divided into early and late epilepsy. Early traumatic epilepsy refers to the occurrence of seizures within the first week after head injury. Jennett (17) has suggested that the risk of recurrence of seizures is 25% in patients who suffer early traumatic epilepsy and is 75% in those who have late traumatic epilepsy. The incidence of traumatic epilepsy is quite variable, depending on the severity of the head injury. About one third of the patients with missile injuries to the head develop late epilepsy, compared with only 5% of patients with non-missile injuries severe enough to require hospitalization (17). The incidence of post-traumatic epilepsy—28% within 5 years following 130 war injuries (18) and 29% following 1425 civilian head injuries (19)—is thus similar to the incidence reported following craniotomy for nontraumatic conditions (15). Data such as these have been cited as the justification for antiepileptic drugs in the prophylactic treatment of patients after severe head injury and after intracranial surgical procedures, even when no seizure has been observed. However, there are as yet no data which provide convincing evidence that prophylactic use of antiepileptic drugs prevents the development of post-traumatic or post-surgical epilepsy. Studies by Young et al. (20,21) provided some indication that phenytoin given within hours after injury and maintained for at least 3 months may provide long-lasting protection against the development of seizures. However, there were methodological flaws with these studies. More recently published studies of the prophylactic value of phenytoin in preventing the development of post-traumatic epilepsy after severe injury have been disappointing (22–24). Large studies of the prophylaxis of post-traumatic epilepsy are now being carried out in Seattle, Los Angeles, and San Diego which are intended to provide definitive information regarding the potential prophylactic role of antiepileptic drugs. However, data currently available provide no convincing evidence that antiepileptic drug prophylactic therapy prevents the later development of epilepsy.

MANAGEMENT OF THE PREGNANT PATIENT

Three questions must be addressed when considering the management of a pregnant woman who has epilepsy: (a) What is the effect of the pregnancy on the patient's epilepsy? (b) What is the effect of the patient's epilepsy on the developing fetus? (c) What is the effect of antiepileptic drugs on the developing fetus?

The effect of pregnancy on seizure frequency in epileptic women has been evaluated in a number of studies with variable results. Schmidt (25) compiled the results of 27 studies published between 1884 and 1980. Of the 2165 patients included in these 27 studies, 24% experienced an increase in seizure frequency, 22% experienced a decrease in seizure frequency, and 53% experienced no change in seizure frequency. Knight and Rhind (26) studied 153 pregnancies in 59 patients. They found that patients with intractable epilepsy (one or more seizures per month) were four times more likely to have an increase in seizure frequency during pregnancy than patients who had seizures less than once every 3 months. In another study of 52 patients, Remillard et al. (27) observed that an increase in seizure frequency during pregnancy was three times more likely in patients who had complex partial and secondarily generalized tonic–clonic seizures than in patients with primary generalized epilepsy. Although seizure frequency may increase in some epileptic women during pregnancy, there is no evidence for an increase in the incidence of epilepsy during pregnancy and no evidence that status epilepticus occurs more frequently during pregnancy (25). The main causes for an increase in the frequency of seizures during pregnancy are poor compliance and altered absorption of antiepileptic drugs (28). With an increasing awareness of potential teratogenic effects of antiepileptic drugs, compliance problems are likely to increase. This emphasizes the need for vigorous educational efforts to ensure that a woman with epilepsy who desires to have children is aware of the potential risks to both herself and her fetus should she become pregnant.

There is a general assumption on the part of neurologists and obstetricians that seizures are bad for a fetus, but evidence to support this hypothesis has been difficult to obtain. Yerby (28) has suggested that partial seizures do not appear to pose a significant risk to the fetus but that generalized convulsive seizures can be extremely hazardous to the mother and fetus. He was able to record the fetal heart rate of a fetus whose mother experienced a generalized seizure during labor. Although the seizure lasted less than 1 minute, the fetal heart rate was significantly depressed for over 20 minutes after the episode (Fig. 1). Furthermore, Yerby (28) has pointed out that while stillbirths are rare in pregnant women with epilepsy they have been reported following a single generalized convulsion or following a series of convul-

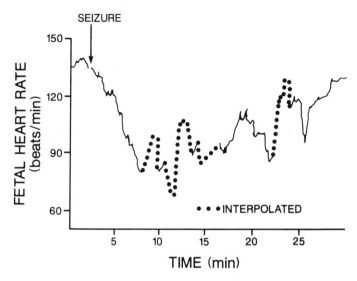

FIG. 1. Fetal heart rate as monitored during maternal seizure. (From ref. 28.)

sions (29–31). When status epilepticus does occur during pregnancy, it has poten-tially devastating effects on both the mother and child. Teramo and Hiilesmaa (32) reported that in 29 cases of status epilepticus that occurred during pregnancy, nine of the mothers and 14 of the infants died during the episode of status, or shortly thereafter.

There is general recognition of an increase in the incidence of congenital malfor-mations in infants born to epileptic mothers when compared with control popula-tions. The malformation rate in the general population is 29.6 per 1000 live births (28). The malformation rate in infants born to epileptic mothers is 70 per 1000, which represents a 2.4-fold increase in risk (33–36). Most of the increase in risk of malformations has been attributed to the use of antiepileptic drugs, particularly in the first trimester. Yerby (28) has suggested four lines of evidence that support the concept that the increase in fetal malformation rate is due to the use of antiepileptic drugs: (a) Higher malformation rates are seen in children born to mothers with epilepsy who are treated during pregnancy than in children born to mothers who are not treated with antiepileptic drugs during pregnancy (34,36–40). (b) Antiepileptic drug concentrations are higher in mothers with malformed children compared with the levels found in the mothers of healthy children (41). (c) Malformation rates are higher in children born to women being treated with polytherapy than in children born to women being treated with only one drug (38,42). (d) There is no increase in malformation rates in infants born to mothers who have seizures during pregnancy when compared with infants born to mothers who have no seizures during preg-nancy (33,34).

Trimethadione has been associated with very high rates of stillbirth and fetal malformation (43). A characteristic syndrome consisting of cleft lip and palate, congenital cardiac malformations, and minor skeletal abnormalities which produce an unusual facial appearance because of a short neck with a low posterior hairline, broadly rooted nose, wide-spaced prominent eyes, and deformity of the pinna was first reported by Meadow (44) in 1968. An expanded series that included an additional 40 cases was described by him in 1970 (45). Although it was initially attributed to the use of phenytoin by the mothers during the first trimester of pregnancy, similar malformations have been observed with other antiepileptic drugs such as phenobarbital (46), diazepam (46), and valproic acid (47). Valproic acid has also been reported to have a specific risk of neural tube defects approximately twice that of the normal population. The risk of spina bifida in infants born to mothers taking valproic acid during pregnancy is approximately 1.2% compared with 0.6% in infants whose mothers are neither taking antiepileptic drugs nor have epilepsy (48).

The goal of management of the pregnant epileptic is to reduce the risk to the fetus from teratogenic effects as much as possible while at the same time not exposing the mother and the fetus to complications from an increased frequency of seizures. With these goals in mind, it becomes apparent that the best way to manage a pregnant woman with epilepsy is to treat her with the lowest dose of the least teratogenic antiepileptic drug consistent with the prevention of generalized tonic–clonic seizures during the pregnancy. Ideally, it would be desirable to prevent any exposure of the fetus to an antiepileptic drug during the first trimester. However, realistically, for most women with epilepsy, withdrawal of antiepileptic medication presents an unacceptable risk of exacerbation of seizures. However, the goal of minimal antiepileptic drug exposure for the fetus suggests several principles of management: A plan for antiepileptic drug management should be developed before a woman with epilepsy becomes pregnant. The neurologist is frequently the only physician a young woman with epilepsy may see prior to the onset of pregnancy. Thus the neurologist (or other primary-care physician) treating the patient's epilepsy has a special responsibility regarding education of the female patient at risk for pregnancy as to the potential risks to her and her fetus, should she become pregnant. Such patient education efforts should be carried out early in the relationship between the physician and a female of childbearing potential, ideally long before the patient contemplates pregnancy. It is, however, important that the relative risk of pregnancy to the mother and fetus be presented in an objective and dispassionate fashion so that the patient will have a realistic understanding of the issues involved. It is equally tragic for a 14-year-old girl with epilepsy to request a tubal ligation because of fear caused by an overstated risk of pregnancy in epilepsy as it is for that same 14-year-old to become pregnant with no knowledge of the potential risks involved.

Part of the development of a management plan before a pregnancy occurs must involve a reassessment of the evidence that the patient has epilepsy. Because there is a clear increase in the risk of teratogenicity from antiepileptic drugs, these drugs should only be prescribed when they are essential to prevent epileptic seizures that will cause risk to the fetus or the pregnant patient. When the decision is made by the patient to become pregnant after consideration of the risk of teratogenic effects and possible complications of the patient's epilepsy, efforts should be made to select the drug with the least risk to the fetus. Such a drug should be prescribed at the minimal doses necessary to maintain control over generalized tonic–clonic seizures. When selecting the best drug, a consideration should be given to the patient's family history because congenital abnormalities tend to be familial. Clearly, if there is a history of spina bifida within a family, valproic acid is not an appropriate drug.

With regard to the selection of drugs, all of the antiepileptic drugs appear to be associated with an increased risk of fetal malformation somewhere in excess of two times that of the normal population. Midline facial defects and other stigmata of the fetal anticonvulsant syndrome have been reported for both phenytoin and phenobarbital, and neural tube closure defects have been reported for valproic acid. Although much still remains to be learned, current knowledge suggests that carbamazepine has the lowest risk of producing fetal malformations (46). Thus carbamazepine is the drug of choice for women with epilepsy whose seizures can be controlled adequately with this drug. If another drug must be used, then the lowest possible dose should be prescribed.

DISCONTINUATION OF THERAPY

When patients become seizure-free for 2 or more years, many physicians consider discontinuing antiepileptic therapy. The reasons given in support of such discontinuation are the chronic toxic effects (49) and the adverse effects on the CNS function (50). Rates of remission of 2 or more years have been reported to range between 10% and 70%, depending on the population in which the study was done (50,51). In general, remission rates have been higher in community-based studies than in hospital-based studies (52,53). The probability of remission is greatest when epilepsy starts after the age of 1 but before the age of 20 (52,54), when seizures are controlled early in the course of treatment (50), and when the patient experiences only generalized tonic–clonic seizures (55–57). Patients who have partial-onset seizures with secondary generalization have a low probability of remission (51,54).

When the decision is made to discontinue antiepileptic drug medication, a number of factors influence the probability of relapse of seizures during or after antiepileptic drug withdrawal. These have been summarized by Schmidt (58), who compiled the results from 17 studies that included a total of 2909 patients. Overall, the relapse rate in adults was about 50% for patients who had been completely seizure-free for 1–3 years, but it dropped to 33% when patients had been seizure-free for 4 or more years before medication was discontinued. Eighty-five percent of the patients who relapsed did so in the first 6 months, and virtually all relapses occurred within the first 4 years after discontinuation of medication.

In general, the same factors that predict a high probability of remission from seizures while being treated with antiepileptic drugs predict a lower probability of relapse after drug withdrawal. Relapse rates are lowest in patients with petit mal epilepsy manifested as absence seizures without generalized tonic–clonic seizures, and they are highest in patients who have complex partial seizures. Among the

TABLE 1. *Assessment of risk for relapse following the discontinuation of antiepileptic drugs[a]*

| | Risk of relapse | | |
Clinical characteristics	High	Intermediate	Low
Seizure control (years)	1–2	2–3	4 or more
Therapy prior to control (years)	More than 5	2–5	1–2
Duration of epilepsy (years)	More than 5	2–5	1–2
Type of seizure	Complex partial absence and GTC[b]	GTC only	Absence only
	GTC on awakening	GTC during sleep	
Multiple type of seizures	Yes		
High previous seizure frequency	Yes		
Lack of sleep	Yes		
Intake of alcoholic beverages following discontinuation	Yes		
Mental retardation	Yes		
Increase in generalized or focal paroxysmal discharges during reduction or following discontinuation	Yes		
Patient is not convinced to discontinue treatment	Yes		
Duration of discontinuation of treatment (months)	1–6	6–12	More than 12

[a]Modified from ref. 58.
[b]GTC, generalized tonic–clonic seizure.

generalized epilepsies, the rate of relapse is highest in patients with juvenile myoclonic epilepsy (59). The rate of relapse increases with the duration between the onset of the seizure disorder and the time required to obtain complete control.

Predictors of the risk for relapse following discontinuation of antiepileptic drugs are provided in Table 1, taken from Schmidt (58). From the data presented above and in the table, a set of clinical guidelines can be developed for the discontinuation of antiepileptic drugs in the adult. *In general, in an adult in whom the diagnosis of epilepsy has been properly made, the probability of successful discontinuation of antiepileptic medication is quite low.* Schmidt (58) has suggested that only about 14% of patients will continue to remain seizure-free after withdrawal of antiepileptic medication. However, if a neurologically normal adult whose seizures have been controlled completely within 1 or 2 years after onset is sufficiently desirous of discontinuing antiepileptic medication to accept the risk of having another seizure, then consideration can be given to medication withdrawal. Because the rate of relapse decreases from 50% to 33% when patients are completely seizure-free for 4 or more years, discontinuation should not be considered until the patient is seizure-free for at least 4 years.

There is no general agreement as to how quickly antiepileptic drugs should be withdrawn. Schmidt (58) suggests that the dose be decreased by 25% every 6 months or even longer. Such a slow withdrawal regimen is designed to avoid the risk of withdrawal seizures. Unfortunately, there are no data regarding the risk of withdrawal seizures in patients who have been previously well-controlled. A few studies of withdrawal seizures have been carried out on patients with medically intractable epilepsy on polypharmacy undergoing changes in treatment regimens (60) or who had a transient reduction in medication while on an epilepsy monitoring unit (61,62). These studies do not provide data regarding the rate of drug withdrawal.

For most adult patients with well-controlled epilepsy, maintenance of driving privileges is of paramount importance. Clearly, withdrawal of medication from a well-controlled patient increases that patient's risk of having a seizure and thus decreases the safety with which such an individual can operate a motor vehicle. Therefore, a rational approach to the establishment of any procedure for antiepileptic drug discontinuation in an adult is to withhold driving privileges during the period of discontinuation and for some arbitrary period after discontinuation has been completed. Because most relapse seizures occur within the first 6 months after completion of drug withdrawal, withholding of driving privileges for 6 months after antiepileptic drugs have been stopped would seem appropriate. Therefore, in order to reduce the duration of the loss of driving privileges to as short a period as possible, drug withdrawal should be carried out in the shortest period of time consistent with the avoidance of withdrawal seizures. No clear and generally accepted guidelines have been established. However, one common approach to switching patients from polypharmacy to monotherapy is to taper each drug at a rate no faster than 25% of the initial dose every five half-lives. Although such a reduction schedule may avoid the precipitation of withdrawal seizures, perhaps a more prudent and conservative regimen would involve a 25% reduction of dose every 2–4 weeks. Because the patient should be instructed not to drive during the period of drug withdrawal and for 6 months thereafter, such a schedule would still involve an 8- to 10-month period during which the patient would be unable to drive. The necessity to restrict driving privileges should be presented to the patient in any discussion of possible discontinuation of antiepileptic drugs and should enter into the patient's decision as to whether or not he or she wishes to consider discontinuation of antiepileptic drug therapy.

STATUS EPILEPTICUS

Status epilepticus is a medical emergency that requires vigorous and effective treatment in order to prevent the occurrence of significant neurological morbidity and even mortality. In the past, only generalized tonic–clonic status epilepticus has been thought to present a serious threat to the individual because of systemic complications of hypoxia, acidosis, and hyperpyrexia. However, there is abundant evidence from experimental and clinical studies that sustained ictal electrical discharges in the brain, even in the absence of motor convulsive activity, can produce profound neuronal damage (63). Thus the current view among a number of epileptologists is that all forms of status epilepticus should be treated as an emergency and that the ictal discharges should be stopped as soon as possible.

Status epilepticus is defined in the International Classification of Epileptic Seizures as "whenever a seizure persists for a sufficient length of time or is repeated frequently enough that recovery between attacks does not occur" (64). Operationally, the term "status epilepticus" is now applied to any situation in which there are two or more seizures without full recovery of consciousness between seizures. In the case of simple partial status epilepticus (where there is no loss of consciousness), continuous or repetitive seizure activity for a period lasting longer than 30 minutes is usually thought to represent status epilepticus (65). From these operational definitions, it is apparent that status epilepticus may occur in many forms and that recurrent uncontrolled seizures of any of the varieties listed in the International Classification of Epileptic Seizures can represent status epilepticus. Although there is as yet no international classification of status epilepticus, Table 2 presents a classification of status epilepticus which we have found useful. In general, status epilepticus can be divided into convulsive status epilepticus and nonconvulsive status epilepticus (66). Convulsive status epilepticus includes both primarily and secondarily generalized tonic–clonic status, myoclonic status, and simple partial motor status. Nonconvulsive status epilepticus includes petit mal status (sometimes known as spike-and-wave stupor or absence status), complex partial status, and simple partial sensory status.

The most common form of status epilepticus seen in the adult is generalized convulsive status epilepticus. In most cases, adults present with secondarily generalized tonic–clonic seizures. This form of status epilepticus refers to a situation where there is (a) bilateral ictal activity on the EEG associated with a profound alteration of consciousness and (b) bilateral convulsive activity on clinical examina-

TABLE 2. *Classification of status epilepticus*[a]

I. Convulsive status epilepticus
  Primarily generalized convulsive status epilepticus
    Tonic–clonic status epilepticus
    Myoclonic status epilepticus
    Clonic–tonic–clonic status epilepticus
    Tonic status epilepticus
  Partial or focal status epilepticus
    Focal motor status epilepticus (jacksonian status epilepticus)
    Epilepsia partialis continuans
  Generalized convulsive status epilepticus with partial onset
II. Nonconvulsive status epilepticus or prolonged epileptic fugue states
  Spike-and-wave stupor
  Complex partial status epilepticus

[a]Modified from ref. 66.

tion. However, the clinical presentation of this form of status may be markedly asymmetrical, and thus cases of generalized convulsive status epilepticus sometimes are mistakenly described as focal motor status. Even though the motor activity may be largely unilateral, the presence of a profound alteration of consciousness implies bilateral ictal discharges on the EEG. The term "simple partial motor status epilepticus" should be applied only to situations where the patient is fully conscious but exhibits continuous or intermittent focal convulsive activity limited to one side of the body.

Generalized convulsive status epilepticus usually starts out with the patient exhibiting discrete generalized tonic–clonic seizures separated by quiet periods during which the patient has a significant attentuation of consciousness. These discrete seizures are associated with typical ictal discharges on the EEG and are separated by interictal slowing during the quiescent period. However, if the patient is allowed to continue in status epilepticus long enough before treatment is effective, there is a merging of the discrete seizures into a waxing-and-waning pattern on the EEG (67). The patient may undergo an electromechanical disassociation where the ictal discharges continue on the EEG, but the patient's clinical presentation becomes subtle and is manifested only by intermittent twitching of the eyes, face, trunk, or extremities (68). Ultimately, the electromechanical disassociation may become complete, at which time the patient may have no motor convulsive activity but may continue to exhibit ictal discharges on the EEG. The ictal discharges may consist of continuous rapid rhythmical spikes or, after prolonged episodes of status epilepticus, may consist of only periodic epileptiform discharges on a relatively flat background (67). Because of the electromechanical disassociation and the possibility that a patient may exhibit little or no clinical seizure activity at a time when electrical seizure activity is continuing unabated, it is important to monitor success of treatment with the EEG. Although treatment should never be withheld while awaiting an EEG, if the patient does not rapidly respond to treatment with cessation of clinical seizure activity and rapid recovery of consciousness, an EEG is essential to verify that all ictal activity has stopped.

The treatment of status epilepticus can be divided into a consideration of general principles and a consideration of specific details of management. Treiman (63) has suggested the following goals for the management of status epilepticus: (a) Terminate electrical and clinical seizure activity as soon as possible, preferably within 30 minutes. (b) Prevent recurrences of seizures. (c) Ensure adequate cardiorespiratory function and brain oxygenation. (d) Correct any precipitating factors such as hypoglycemia and electrolyte imbalance or fever. (e) Stabilize metabolic balance by prevention or correction of lactic acidosis, electrolyte imbalance, and dehydration. (f) Prevent or correct any other systemic complications. (g) Evaluate and treat possible causes of status epilepticus.

Rapid termination of the seizure activity of status epilepticus requires detailed knowledge of the pharmacokinetics of the antiepileptic drugs to be used. Ideally, the most potent drugs should be used. It should be administered intravenously to ensure effective serum and brain tissue concentrations to stop the seizures. The drug

TABLE 3. Properties of drugs of importance in treating status epilepticus[a]

Property	Diazepam	Phenytoin	Phenobarbital	Paraldehyde	Lorazepam
Route of administration	Intravenous	Intravenous	Intravenous	Intravenous	Intravenous
Time to enter brain	10 sec	1 min	20 min	<2 min	1–3 min
Time to peak brain concentration	8 min	15–30 min	30 min	20 min	23 min
Effective serum concentration in status epilepticus (μg/ml)	0.2–0.8	35	45	120–150	0.1–0.2
Time to stop status epilepticus	1 min	5–30 min	20 min	?	<5 min
Effective half-life (hr)	0.25	22+	50–120 min	6	14
Brain/plasma ratio	?	0.6–1.4	0.6–0.9	0.61	3.3
pK_a	3.4	8.3	7.41	?	1.3
Partition coefficient	309	295.1	26.3	32.6	240
Protein binding	97–99%	87–93%	45–50%	90%	85–93%
Volume of distribution	1–2 liters/kg	0.5–0.8 liter/kg	0.7 liter/kg	0.9 liter/kg	0.7–1.0 liters/kg

[a]Modified from ref. 63.

must be able to cross the blood–brain barrier rapidly. Treatment should not be started with intramuscular or oral administration because absorption by these routes is too slow and too variable. Furthermore, because of the rapid redistribution from the circulation that occurs with some drugs, serum concentrations adequate to stop ongoing seizures may never be achieved by these routes. Caution should be used in selecting the rate of intravenous infusion in order to avoid hypotension, cardiac arrhythmias, and respiratory depression. When therapy is started, sufficiently high doses should be used and adequate time allowed for the drug to enter the brain before changing to a second drug. After status epilepticus is controlled, an adequate loading dose of a long-acting maintenance antiepileptic drug should be given intravenously (or orally if the patient is awake) to prevent recurrence of seizures. The patient should then be continued on maintenance therapy.

A variety of drugs have been used successfully in the management of status epilepticus. Tables 3 and 4 summarize the pharmacological properties of anticonvulsant drugs important in the management of status epilepticus. Because any one of these drugs may be effective, the choice of drugs is not nearly as important as the skill with which they are used. Having a preestablished protocol for the management of status epilepticus results in far more successful treatment than when status epilepticus is treated in a haphazard and nonsystematic way, as is frequently the case in the hospital and emergency room—where the quality of treatment of status epilepticus is dependent on the knowledge and competence of the house officer who is on call. Table 5 presents our current approach to the management of status epilepticus. The protocol represents a modification of several previously published protocols as the result of observations we have made during the course of our studies of status epilepticus.

TABLE 4. *Drugs of importance in treating status epilepticus: clinical parameters*

Parameter	Diazepam	Phenytoin	Phenobarbital	Lorazepam
Indications	Most forms of status epilepticus	Phenytoin withdrawal intracranial bleed	Phenobarbital withdrawal	Most forms of status epilepticus
Loading dose	0.15–0.25 mg/kg up to 20 mg	20 mg/kg	20 mg/kg	0.1 mg/kg
Maximum rate of administration	2 mg/min	50 mg/min	100 mg/min	2 mg/kg
Potential side effects				
Depression of consciousness	10–30 min	None	>0.5 g	Several hours
Respiration	0.5–1 min	None	>0.5 g	Occasional
Hypotension	Occasional	50% of patients	Occasional	Occasional
Atrial fibrillation	None	Rare	None	None

[a]Modified from ref. 63.

TABLE 5. *Treatment protocol for generalized convulsive status epilepticus*

Make diagnosis by observing one additional seizure in patient with history of recent seizures or impaired consciousness, or by observing continuous seizure activity for more than 30 minutes.

Call EEG technician and start EEG as soon as possible, but do not delay treatment while waiting for the EEG unless necessary to verify diagnosis.

Establish intravenous catheter with normal saline.

Draw blood for serum chemistries, hematology studies, and antiepileptic drug concentrations.

Administer 100 mg thiamine followed by 50 ml of 50% glucose by direct push into the intravenous line.

Administer lorazepam (0.1 mg/kg) by intravenous push (<2 mg/min).

If status epilepticus does not stop, start phenytoin (20 mg/kg) by slow intravenous push (<50 mg/min) directly into port closest to patient. Monitor blood pressure and EEG closely during infusion.

If status epilepticus does not stop after 20 mg/kg phenytoin, give an additional 5 mg/kg; if necessary, give another 5 mg/kg, to a maximum dose of 30 mg/kg.

If status epilepticus persists, intubate patient and give phenobarbital (20 mg/kg) by intravenous push (<100 mg/min).

If status persists, start barbiturate coma. Give pentobarbital (5 mg/kg) slowly as initial intravenous dose to induce an EEG burst–suppression pattern. Continue 0.5–2 mg/kg/hr to maintain burst–suppression pattern. Slow rate of infusion every 2–4 hours to see if seizures have stopped. Monitor blood pressure, electrocardiogram, and respiratory function closely.

We now initiate therapy with intravenous lorazepam. This drug enters the brain nearly as rapidly as diazepam, but, because of a significantly smaller volume of distribution, it does not rapidly redistribute to body fat with a resultant precipitous drop in brain concentrations, as has been described for diazepam (69,70). The incidence of breakthrough seizures is small, even when no other drug is given within the first 24 hours (71). Therefore, a loading dose of phenytoin can be given in a careful and controlled manner either intravenously or even orally, should the patient rapidly recover from the episode of status epilepticus. If lorazepam fails to stop the episode of status epilepticus, we then give phenytoin at a loading dose of 20 mg/kg as quickly as possible. However, we never administer phenytoin faster than 50 mg/min in order to avoid precipitating cardiac arrhythmias or hypotension. Because of our recent observation that a postinfusion phenytoin level of 35 µg/ml is necessary to stop status epilepticus (72), if status epilepticus persists we now follow the initial 20-mg/kg loading dose of phenytoin with an additional 5 or 10 mg/kg before we consider switching to a third drug.

If a third drug is necessary we now use phenobarbital at a loading dose of 15 or 20 mg/kg intravenously. Although there are no data regarding the appropriate dose of phenobarbital for the treatment of status epilepticus in the adult, several studies of neonatal status epilepticus have suggested a dose of 20 mg/kg (73,74). Data from treatment of experimental status epilepticus in the rat, if extrapolated to humans, suggest that a loading dose of 15 mg/kg may be effective in the initial treatment of status epilepticus (75). When phenobarbital is used as a third drug in the management of medically intractable status epilepticus, high loading doses may be necessary. Before phenobarbital is used as a third drug, the patient should be intubated.

We have used paraldehyde successfully in a 4% saline solution administered intravenously to stop intractable generalized convulsive status epilepticus. We start the infusion at a rate of 50 ml/hr and increase the rate at increments of 50 ml/hr every 5 minutes until all clinical and electrical signs of status epilepticus stop or hypotension necessitates slowing the rate of infusion. Unfortunately, sterile paraldehyde was withdrawn from the American market in October 1986, and its future status is uncertain.

Eighty-five percent of patients in generalized convulsive status epilepticus can be treated successfully with lorazepam and/or phenytoin (71). Most of the remaining 15% can be treated successfully with the addition of phenobarbital as described in the protocol. In the few cases that remain resistant to treatment, barbiturate coma can be used, following procedures similar to those described in the protocol (76).

SUMMARY AND CONCLUSIONS

In this chapter we have discussed a number of the special problems facing the clinician in the management of the adult patient with epilepsy. A solution to these problems is best found by a critical consideration of the available data and by an intelligent application of these data to clinical management. Antiepileptic drug therapy should be initiated when the diagnosis of epilepsy is made. This may be after a single seizure if there is a sufficient probability (from the presence of focal findings on the examination or image studies, or epileptiform discharges on the EEG) that a second seizure will occur if treatment is not initiated. There is as yet no good evidence that prophylactic use of antiepileptic drugs prevents the development of post-traumatic epilepsy after head injury or intracranial surgery. Management of the pregnant epileptic requires adequate dialogue between the patient and physician before conception, so that a rational plan can be developed which minimizes the risk to the patient and to the fetus. There does appear to be a twofold increase in the risk of congenital malformations in fetuses born to epileptic mothers taking antiepileptic drugs. Although the data are not yet adequate, carbamazepine appears to be the antiepileptic drug associated with the least risk to the fetus at this time. Discontinuation of antiepileptic drugs is unlikely to be successful in most adults with well-documented epilepsy. If drug discontinuation is considered, it should not be initiated until the patient has been seizure-free for at least 4 years; moreover, the patient should not drive during the period of drug withdrawal and for at least 6 months after antiepileptic drugs have been stopped. Status epilepticus needs to be stopped as rapidly as possible, ideally within 30 minutes. Success is most likely when a fixed protocol is used, such as the one presented in this chapter.

REFERENCES

1. Elwes RDC, Chesterman P, Reynolds EH. Prognosis after a first untreated tonic–clonic seizure. *Lancet* 1985;ii:752–753.
2. Hauser WA, Anderson VE, Loewenson RB, McRoberts SM. Seizure recurrence after a first unprovoked seizure. *N Engl J Med* 1982;307:522–528.
3. Hauser WA, Rich S, Anderson VT. Seizure recurrence after a first unprovoked seizure: an extended follow-up. *Epilepsia* 1986;27:617.
4. Shinnar S, Zeitlin-Gross L, Moshe SL, Berg AT, Goldensohn A, Hauser WA. Risk of seizure recurrence in untreated children following a first unprovoked idiopathic seizure. *Epilepsia* 1986;27:615.
5. Thomas MH. The single seizure: its study and management. *JAMA* 1959;169:457–459.
6. Johnson LC, De Bolt WL, Long MT. Diagnostic factors in adult males following initial seizures. A three year follow up. *Arch Neurol* 1972;27:193–197.
7. Saunders M, Marshall C. Isolated seizures: an EEG and clinical assessment. *Epilepsia* 1975;16:731–733.
8. Blom S, Heijbel J, Bergfors PG. Incidence of epilepsy in children: a follow-up study three years after the first seizure. *Epilepsia* 1978;19:343–350.
9. Cleland PG, Mosquera I, Steward WP, Foster JB. Prognosis of isolated seizures in adult life. *Br Med J* 1981;283:1364.
10. Annegers JF, Shirts SB, Hauser WA, Kurland LT. Risk of recurrence after an initial unprovoked seizure. *Epilepsia* 1986;27:43–50.
11. Luhdorf K, Jensen LK, Plesner AM. Epilepsy in the elderly: prognosis. *Acta Neurol Scand* 1986;74:409–415.
12. Russo LS, Goldstein KH. The diagnostic assessment of single seizures. Is cranial computed tomography necessary? *Arch Neurol* 1983;40:744–746.
13. Ramirez-Lessepas M, Golla RJ, Morilo LR, Gumnit RJ. Value of computed tomographic score in the evaluation of adult patients after their first seizure. *Ann Neurol* 1983;15:536–543.
14. Kuzniecky R, de la Sayette V, Ethier R, et al. Magnetic resonance imaging in temporal lobe epilepsy: pathological correlations. *Ann Neurol* 1987;22:341–347.

15. Foy PM, Copeland GP, Shaw MDM. The incidence of post-operative seizures. *Acta Neurochirurg* 1981;55:253–264.
16. Dan NQ, Wade MJ. The incidence of epilepsy after ventricular shunting procedures. *J Neurosurg* 1986;65:19–21.
17. Jennett B. Epilepsy after head injury and intracranial surgery. In: Hopkins A, ed. *Epilepsy*. New York: Demos, 1987;401–412.
18. Caveness WF, Meirowsky AM, Risk BL, et al. The nature of post-traumatic epilepsy. *J Neurosurg* 1979;50:545–553.
19. Jennett B. *Epilepsy after non-missile head injuries*, 2nd ed. London: Heinemann, 1975.
20. Young B, Rapp R, Perrier D, Kostenbauder H, Hackman J, Blacker M. Early post-traumatic epilepsy prophylaxis. *Surg Neurol* 1975;4:339.
21. Young B, Rapp R, Brooks WH, Madauss W. Post-traumatic epilepsy prophylaxis. *Epilepsia* 1979;20:671.
22. Serist Z, Musil F. Prophylactic treatment of post-traumatic epilepsy: results of long term follow-up in Czechoslovakia. *Epilepsia* 1981;23:315–320.
23. North JB, Penhall RK, Haneich A, et al. Phenytoin and post-operative epilepsy. *J Neurosurg* 1983;58:672–677.
24. Young B, Kapp RP, Norton JA, et al. Failure of prophylactically administered phenytoin to prevent post-traumatic seizures. *J Neurosurg* 1983;58:236–241.
25. Schmidt D. The effect of pregnancy on the natural history of epilepsy: review of the literature. In: Janz D, Dam M, Richens A, Bossi L, Helge H, Schmidt D, eds. *Epilepsy, pregnancy and the child*. New York: Raven Press, 1982;3–14.
26. Knight AH, Rhind EG. Epilepsy and pregnancy: a study of 153 pregnancies in 59 patients. *Epilepsia* 1975;16:99–110.
27. Remillard G, Dansky L, Andermann E, Andermann F. Seizure frequency during pregnancy and the puerperium. In: Janz D, Dam M, Richens A, Bossi L, Helge H, Schmidt D, eds. *Epilepsy, pregnancy and the child*. New York: Raven Press, 1982;15–26.
28. Yerby MS. Problems and management of the pregnant woman with epilepsy. *Epilepsia* 1987;28:S29–S36.
29. Burnett CWF. A survey of the relationship between epilepsy and pregnancy. *J Obstet Gynecol* 1946;53:539–556.
30. Suter C, Klingman WO. Seizure states and pregnancy. *Neurology* 1957;7:105–118.
31. Higgins TA, Comerford JB. Epilepsy in pregnancy. *J Irish Med Assoc* 1974;67:317–329.
32. Teramo K, Hiilesmaa VK. Pregnancy and fetal complications in epileptic pregnancies: a review of the literature. In: Janz D, Dam M, Richens A, Bossi L, Helge H, Schmidt D, eds. *Epilepsy, pregnancy and the child*. New York: Raven Press, 1982;53–59.
33. Nakane Y, Oltuma T, Takahashi T, et al. Multiinstitutional study of teratogenicity and fetal toxicity of anticonvulsants: a report of a collaborative study group in Japan. *Epilepsia* 1980;221:663–680.
34. Fedrick J. Epilepsy and pregnancy: a report from the Oxford Record Linkage Study. *Br J Med* 1983;2:442–448.
35. Kelly TE. Teratogenicity of anticonvulsant drugs. I. Review of the literature. *Am J Med Genet* 1984;19:413–434.
36. Lander CM, Smith MT, Chalk JB, et al. Bioavailability and pharmacokinetics of phenytoin during pregnancy. *Eur J Clin Pharmacol* 1984;27:105–110.
37. South J. Teratogenic effects of anticonvulsants. *Lancet* 1972;2:1154.
38. Lowe CR. Congenital malformations among infants born to epileptic women. *Lancet* 1973;1:9–10.
39. Monson RR, Rosenberg L, Hartz SC. Diphenylhydantoin and selected congenital malformations. *N Engl J Med* 1973;289:1049–1052.
40. Nakane Y. Congenital malformations among infants of epileptic mothers treated during pregnancy. *Folia Psychiatr Neurol Jpn* 1979;33:363–369.
41. Dansky L, Andermann E, Sherwin AI, et al. Maternal epilepsy and congenital malformations: a prospective study with monitoring of plasma anticonvulsant levels during pregnancy. *Neurology* 1980;3:15.
42. Lindhout D, Hoppener RJ, Meinardi H. Teratogenicity of antiepileptic drug combinations with special emphasis on epoxidation of carbamazepine. *Epilepsia* 1984;25:77–83.
43. Feldman GL, Weaver DD, Lovrien EW. The fetal trimethadione syndrome. *Am J Dis Child* 1977;131:1389–1392.
44. Meadow SR. Anticonvulsant drugs and congenital abnormalities. *Lancet* 1968; ii:1296.

45. Meadow SR. Congenital abnormalities and anticonvulsant drugs. *Proc R Soc Med* 1970;63:48–49.
46. Schardein JL. Drugs affecting the central nervous system: psychotropic agents. In: *Chemically induced birth defects*. New York: Marcel Dekker, 1985;191–196.
47. Tein I, MacGregor DL. Possible valproate teratogenicity. *Arch Neurol* 1985;42:291–293.
48. Lindhout D, Schmidt D. *In-utero* exposure to valproate and neural tube defects. *Lancet* 1986;1:1392–1393.
49. Schmidt D. *Adverse effects of antiepileptic drugs*. New York: Raven Press, 1982.
50. Chadwick D. The discontinuation of antiepileptic therapy. In: Pedley TA, Meldrum BS, eds. *Recent advances in epilepsy 2*. Edinburgh: Churchill Livingstone, 1985;111–124.
51. Rodin EA. *The prognosis of patients with epilepsy*. Springfield, IL: Charles C Thomas, 1968.
52. Annegers JF, Hauser WA, Elverback LR. Remission of seizures and relapse in patients with epilepsy. *Epilepsia* 1979;20:729–737.
53. Goodridge DMG, Shorvon SD. Epileptic seizures in a population of 6000. I. Treatment and prognosis. *Br Med J* 1983;287:645–647.
54. Group for the Study of the Prognosis of Epilepsy in Japan. Natural history and prognosis of epilepsy: report of a multi-institutional study in Japan. *Epilepsia* 1981;22:35–53.
55. Juul-Jensen P. *Epilepsy, a clinical and social analysis of 1020 adult patients with epileptic seizures*. Copenhagen: Munksgaard, 1963.
56. Reynolds EH, Shorvon SD, Galbraith AW, Chadwick D, Dellaportas CI, Vydelingum L. Phenytoin monotherapy for epilepsy: a long-term prospective study, assisted by serum level monitoring, in previously untreated patients. *Epilepsia* 1981;22:475–488.
57. Turnbull DM, Rawlins MD, Weightman D, Chadwick DW. A comparison of phenytoin and valproate in previously untreated epileptic patients. *J Neurol Neurosurg Psychiatry* 1982;45:55–59.
58. Schmidt D. Discontinuation of antiepileptic drugs. In: Porter RJ, Morselli PL, eds. *The epilepsies*. London: Butterworth, 1985;227–241.
59. Janz D, Kern A, Mossinger HJ, Puhlmann U. Ruckfall-prognose nach reduktion der medikamente bei epilepsiebehandlung. *Nervenarzt* 1983;54:525–529.
60. Spencer SS, Spencer DD, Williamson PD, Mattson RH. Ictal effects of anticonvulsant medication withdrawal in epileptic patients. *Epilepsia* 1981;22:297–307.
61. Theodore WH, Porter RJ. Removal of sedative–hypnotic antiepileptic drugs from the regimens of patients with intractable epilepsy. *Ann Neurol* 1983;13:320–324.
62. Marciani MG, Gotman J, Andermann F, Olivier A. Patterns of seizure activation after withdrawal of antiepileptic medication. *Neurology* 1985;35:1537–1543.
63. Treiman DM. General principles of treatment: responsive and intractable status epilepticus in adults. In: Delgado-Escueta AV, Wasterlain CG, Treiman DM, eds. *Advances in neurology, vol 34: status epilepticus: mechanisms of brain damage and treatment*. New York: Raven Press, 1983.
64. The Commission on Classification and Terminology of the International League Against Epilepsy. Proposal for revised clinical and electroencephalographic classification of epileptic seizures. *Epilepsia* 1981;22:489–501.
65. Treiman DM. Status epilepticus. In: Johnson RT, ed. *Current therapy in neurological disease 2*. Philadelphia: BC Decker, 1987;38–42.
66. Treiman DM, Delgado-Escueta AV. Status epilepticus. In: Thompson R, Green JR, eds. *Critical care of neurological and neurosurgical emergencies*. New York: Raven Press, 1980;53–59.
67. Treiman DM, Walton NY, Kendrick CW. A progressive sequence of electroencephalographic changes during generalized convulsive status epilepticus. *Epilepsy Res* 1990;5:49–60.
68. Treiman DM, DeGiorgio CM, Salisbury S, Wickboldt C. Subtle generalized convulsive status epilepticus. *Epilepsia* 1984;25:653.
69. Booker H, Celesia GG. Serum concentrations of diazepam in subjects with epilepsy. *Arch Neurol* 1973;29:191–194.
70. Greenblatt DJ, Divoll M. Diazepam versus lorazepam: relationship of drug distribution to duration of clinical action. In: Delgado-Escueta AV, Wasterlain CG, Treiman DM, Porter RJ, eds. *Advances in neurology, vol 34: status epilepticus mechanisms of brain damage and treatment*. New York: Raven Press, 1983;487–491.
71. Treiman DM, DeGiorgio CM, Ben-Menachem E, et al. Lorazepam vs. phenytoin in the treatment of generalized convulsive status epilepticus. Report of an ongoing study. *Neurology* 1985;35(Suppl 1):284.
72. Gunawan S, Treiman DM. Pharmacokinetics of phenytoin and its metabolite *p*-HPPH, during treatment of status epilepticus. *Neurology* 1987;37(Suppl 1):352.

73. Painter MJ. General principles of treatment: status epilepticus in neonates. In: Delgado-Escueta AV, Wasterlain CG, Treiman DM, Porter RJ, eds. *Advances in neurology, vol 34: status epilepticus: mechanisms of brain damage and treatment*. New York: Raven Press, 1983;385–393.
74. Lockman LA. Phenobarbital dosage for neonatal seizures. In: Delgado-Escueta AV, Wasterlain CG, Treiman DM, Porter RJ, eds. *Advances in neurology, vol 34: status epilepticus mechanisms of brain damage and treatment*. New York: Raven Press, 1983;505–508.
75. Walton NY, Treiman DM. Phenobarbital treatment of status epilepticus in a rodent model. *Epilepsy Res* 1989;4:216–221.
76. Lowenstein DH, Aminoff MJ, Simon RP. Barbiturate anesthesia in the treatment of status epilepticus: clinical experience with 14 patients. *Neurology* 1988;38:395–400.

Epilepsy: Current Approaches to Diagnosis and Treatment,
edited by Dennis B. Smith,
Raven Press, Ltd., New York © 1990.

9

The Role of Surgery in Therapy for Epilepsy

Allen R. Wyler

*Department of Neurosurgery, University of Tennessee at Memphis,
Memphis, Tennessee 38163;
Semmes–Murphey Clinic, Memphis, Tennessee 38103;
and EpiCare Center, Baptist Memorial Hospital,
Memphis, Tennessee 38146*

The modern era of surgery for epilepsy was introduced in the late part of the last century by a British neurosurgeon named Dr. Victor Horsely. His first reported case was operated upon in the year 1886 while he was at the National Hospital at Queen Square, London. Horsely had demonstrated that for many cases of epilepsy, a focal point could be found on the cortical surface that gave rise to the seizures, and if this focal region of brain was removed surgically the seizures would cease. Thus, the surgical therapy of epilepsy was successfully developed prior to effective anticonvulsant drug therapy. In Horsely's time, the only effective antiepileptic drug was bromide.

Horsely's observations were not fully exploited until the 1950s. At that time, Dr. Wilder Penfield began to publish his surgical results. Penfield and Jasper made a major advance in epilepsy surgery by introducing the use of electrocorticography during craniotomy. By recording directly from the surface of the patient's cortex, they were able to better localize the epileptic focus and define its margins. Thus, they were able to increase the effectiveness and utility of focal cortical excisions. Shortly thereafter, the surgery of epilepsy became an accepted alternative for selected patients who have not had their seizures controlled with medications. Unfortunately, even today, this option is not considered often enough by the physicians who treat the majority of patients with epilepsy.

There are several reasons why many patients and neurologists do not consider surgery as a therapeutic option. First, many physicians do not really know that this option is available since there are not many regional epilepsy centers where this type of specialized surgery is available. Second, the risks of surgery are often overestimated by both patient and physician. Finally, many physicians do not understand the problems faced by the patient with epilepsy, and therefore the doctors underestimate the problems that epilepsy can cause the patient who suffers from it. *The physician then may find two seizures a month quite acceptable for the patient, whereas the patient may find this degree of seizure control unacceptable.*

WHY CONSIDER SURGERY AT ALL?

There are several reasons for considering surgery when aggressive attempts to control seizures medically have failed. (a) Continued convulsive seizures have an adverse long-term effect on patients' mental capabilities. More than 100 tonic–clonic seizures per patient may be associated with a decline in I.Q. (1). (b) Active epileptic attacks will usually cause social embarrassment to the patient, which can often impair normal psychosocial development. This will have a compounding effect through young adulthood and will be reflected in the patient's long-term vocational and social outcome. (c) People with convulsive seizures have a higher incidence of sudden death in comparison to people without seizures (2). In addition, repeated seizures carry a risk of accident-related morbidity, such as broken bones, lacerations, and head injury from fall. (d) The antiepileptic medications are not without risks and side effects, especially when taken over prolonged periods of time. With successful surgery, the medications can often be reduced to monotherapy, and in some cases they can be completely eliminated.

INDICATION FOR SURGERY

The primary indication for surgery is failure to control a patient's seizures adequately with antiepileptic medication. This indication is not often debated. What is debated, however, is what defines inadequate seizure control. Unfortunately, there is no numerical threshold to define adequate and inadequate seizure control. This must be decided by considering the effect the seizures have upon the patient, his expectations, and his realistic psychosocial–vocational potentials. For example, one seizure a year could not be tolerated by a person who was making a career as an airline pilot, since that would result in the loss of his profession. On the other hand, three seizures a week might not adversely affect the psychosocial expectations of a mentally retarded and institutionalized patient. The most common mistake that most physicians make is to assume for the patient what is "acceptable control" of seizures. This is truly the patient's decision, not the physician's. In addition, the seizure's effect upon the patient's health is a consideration. For example, atonic seizures that result in abrupt falls can be much more serious in their consequences than brief absence seizures.

CRITERIA FOR CONSIDERING SURGERY

The major criterion is that the patient has undergone a reasonable trial of primary antiepileptic drugs and that they have failed to control the seizures. This criterion also assumes that the antiepileptic drugs appropriate for the patient's type of epilepsy have been tried. For example, as discussed in Chapter 5, ethosuximide, a drug used to treat true absence seizures, is not considered an appropriate drug to consider for patients with complex partial seizures and a focal electroencephalographic

(EEG) focus. Thus, for most patients who will ultimately be candidates for surgery, trials with phenytoin, carbamazepine, phenobarbital (or primidone), and valproate should have been tried. In many patients, particularly those with a well-defined EEG focus and/or anatomic lesion, "medical refractoriness" may not need to include a trial of all the major antiepileptic drugs.

Before phenytoin or carbamazepine are considered failures, they should have been administered to the point of causing toxic side effects. However, seizure control should not be obtained at the cost of chronic toxicity. In addition, it is not necessary to try secondary drugs such as diazepam in the drug trial. The length of time needed to verify the drug has had a "reasonable trial" is dependent upon the patient's seizure frequency. For example, if a patient is having four seizures a week, 2–3 weeks of treatment with phenytoin in therapeutic range may be sufficient to document success or failure. On the other hand, if the patient's seizures occur only once per month, a longer period of time is needed to make the judgment. If a seizure disorder cannot be medically controlled within 2 years of initiating aggressive medical therapy, seizure surgery should be considered seriously.

The third indication is that the patient must have a reasonable chance of benefiting from the surgery, and that the chance is better than the risks of an unacceptable surgical complication. This last criterion will largely depend on the data accumulated during the patient's work-up. For example, it would be unreasonable to consider surgery if the epileptogenic focus was located within primary speech cortex.

THE PRESURGICAL EVALUATION

The foundation of the surgical work-up is primarily dependent upon an adequate neurophysiologic evaluation. The other major components are (a) neuropsychological assessment, (b) neuroradiological investigation, and (c) a Wada test. All of these components are taken together to form a decision as to the appropriateness of elective surgery and the type of surgery best indicated. Each component will be discussed separately.

EEG Evaluation

The first stage of the work-up is an evaluation of the patient's routine electroencephalograms to correctly classify the epilepsy. If the patient has partial seizures and a non-lesion-related epilepsy, the next step is to determine where the focus resides in the brain. True primary generalized epilepsy is not well treated with any type of surgery, whereas focal or multifocal seizures can frequently be successfully treated surgically. There are two general rules concerning the selection of surgical procedures: (i) Discrete foci are best treated with focal resections; and (ii) multifocal or diffuse seizure foci may respond best to corpus callosum sectioning.

In our center we first evaluate the patient with long-term EEG/video monitoring. We do this in order to determine (a) seizure type (i.e., complex partial) and (b) location and morphology of EEG onset. We do not base surgical decisions on inter-ictal recordings.

We routinely use sphenoidal electrodes when monitoring patients with scalp elec-troencephalogram. Experience has shown that sphenoidal recordings are superior to standard scalp-only recordings for detecting discharges from mesial temporal struc-tures (3). The EEG/video monitoring should include at least two clearly recorded spontaneous seizures.

The next step in the surgical evaluation requires that the patient return for addi-tional EEG/video monitoring with intracranial electrodes. It is not within the scope of this chapter to discuss the relative merits of intracortical depth electrodes (4) or subdural strip electrodes (5,6). Both options have yielded excellent results. Spencer (7) has recently reviewed the use of depth electrodes and has emphasized that depth electrodes are needed for the more complex diagnostic cases and that their use has enabled 36% more patients to be selected for surgery by defining otherwise uniden-tifiable single epileptogenic foci. In addition, depth recordings could have pre-vented surgery for another 18% by demonstrating multifocal epilepsy, which is known to have a poor surgical prognosis. Our own experience is that scalp record-ings alone are frequently inadequate in localizing foci for surgical ablation and may result in false localization of the seizure focus. Thus, we will not consider focal resection without monitoring spontaneous typical seizures using subdural strip or depth electrodes. Since adopting this policy, our surgical success rate has improved significantly. We thus feel that the increased risk of invasive monitoring is well offset by the improved surgical outcome.

If the EEG monitoring has provided enough information to decide that surgery is an option for the patient, additional data must be obtained. A standard set of non-contrast and intravenous contrast-enhanced computed tomography (CT) scans have usually been obtained in the course of the patient's initial work-up. If several years have elapsed since the original scans, they should be repeated to ensure that the patient does not have a slow growing tumor, such as a meningioma. More recently, magnetic resonance imaging (MRI) scans have proven useful in the evaluation of surgical candidates. MRI scans are complementary to x-ray CT images because they often visualize lesions that CT will miss, such as small hamartomas (8). MRI should not completely replace CT, since the latter may demonstrate many things that MRI will miss, such as intracranial calcium associated with, for example, tuberous scle-rosis.

Neuropsychological Evaluations

It has been the practice in many epilepsy centers to use extensive neuro-psychological tests to help localize a focus. Simply stated, the rationale is that the cortical damage that caused the epileptogenic focus should also be sufficient to cause a demonstrable deficit with detailed neuropsychological testing. Thus, these test batteries can provide additional information for identifying and localizing epi-leptogenic foci. The problem is that there is no consensus as to which test batteries should be used to maximize this potential. It is clear that it is important to use a battery of tests that samples a variety of cognitive functions. For example, tests of verbal as well as visual spatial memory need to be done (9). Furthermore, the tests should have been standardized to patients with epilepsy.

Although the neuropsychological tests have been helpful, they have not been very useful in predicting the success of surgery (10).

The Intracarotid Amytal (Wada) Test

Another essential portion of the surgical evaluation is the intracarotid amytal test (11). The test is accomplished by placing a catheter into each carotid artery (from the retrograde femoral route) and injecting a bolus (approximately 100 mg) of sodium amytal, resulting in each hemisphere being "separately anesthetized." When each hemisphere is anesthetized, the patient is rapidly given a series of objects to name. Between each object the patient is also given a simple mental task (i.e., a multiplication) to serve as a distraction and then he or she is asked to recall the previously identified object. Thus, the sequence is to name an object, be distracted, and then recall the object. Because each hemisphere is tested separately, the hemisphere dominant for speech can be determined. Lateralization of memory is less predictable, but it is often used in planning surgery.

SURGICAL APPROACHES

Focal Resections

Once the cortical epileptogenic focus has been adequately localized, two surgical strategies have been used. The first approach has been termed the "tailored" resection, and the second is termed the standardized "en bloc" resection. The tailored resection was pioneered by Penfield (12). The preoperative work-up determines the location of the focus. The surgery is then usually done under local anesthesia. The cortex is explored by electrocorticography (ECoG) to determine the confines of the epileptogenic focus. If the patient is awake (under local anesthesia), the cortex is also functionally mapped using cortical stimulation. This "functional mapping" allows the surgeon to determine the location of critical neurologic function, such as the speech-related cortex. The surgeon can then "tailor" the resection to maximize removal of the epileptogenic cortex with minimal risk to obvious neurologic function. As a result, large resections can be done when needed without undue risk. In other instances, smaller resections may be mandated by the proximity of vital cortical functions or by the very focal nature of the epileptogenic "zone." This approach can maximize the chances of a good surgical result with a minimum of neurologic deficit. The problems associated with this approach are as follows: (a) The patient is awake, making the surgery difficult for most children under the age of 16 years; and (b) the time allowed for corticography and functional mapping may be limited. One solution to this problem has been developed by Goldring and Gregorie (13). Prior to ablative surgery, a craniotomy is done over the proposed resection site. A large grid of electrodes is placed over the exposed dura, and the wound is then closed. This grid can be used both for stimulation of the underlying brain and for EEG recordings. This allows the cortical region of interest to be mapped for important functions (i.e., language) and allows the regions of active spiking to be identified. After extensive study, the patient is returned to the operating room, where the cortical resection is done under general anesthesia. The obvious disadvantages to this approach are (a) the need for two separate operations and (b) the potential increased risk of infection.

When a standard "en bloc" resection is done, a craniotomy is done and a "standard" amount of cortex is removed. For example, when dealing with the temporal lobe, the resection routinely involves (a) the anterior 4.5 cm of the left (dominant) temporal lobe and (b) the anterior 5.5 cm of the right temporal lobe. This resection is done without ECoG or functional cortical mapping. The obvious advantages to this approach are as follows: (a) The surgery is done under general anesthesia; (b) the total operating time is decreased; and (c) a large block of tissue is obtained that can be studied for anatomic and neurochemical changes. The disadvantage is that without intraoperative "tailoring" of the resection site, the risk of an ensuing neurologic deficit is higher and the entire epileptogenic focus may not be removed. For example, Spencer et al. (14) found that 20% of their patients with unilateral temporal foci who were studied by depth electrodes had foci located in posterior hippocampus (i.e., caudal to the usual limits of the standard "en bloc" temporal lobectomy). Because of this, they modified their operation as follows: A standard 3.5-cm anterior lobectomy is done. Then the anterior aspect of the temporal horn is entered, and the lateral temporal cortex is elevated so that the posterior hippocampus can be removed. They feel that this provides more precise removal of the epileptogenic cortex while sparing important lateral temporal cortex. An alternative approach has been reported by Wieser and Yasargil (15). This surgical procedure has been termed the "selective amygdalohippocampectomy" because the surgeon removes the amygdala and hippocampus without removing the lateral temporal cortex. The surgery is done through a pterional approach, much the same as used by Yasargil for approaching anterior circulation aneurysms. The sylvian fissure is split, and the medial side of the temporal tip is entered. The mesial portion of the temporal lobe is then dissected in subpial fashion, removing only hippocampus and amygdala. They report excellent results in 116 patients operated upon using this technique. More impressively, they demonstrated minimal postoperative memory deficits as a result of temporal lobe surgery. In this center we have adopted this modified selective amygdalohippocampectomy for all patients with mesial temporal epileptogenic foci.

Foci occur in other lobes of the brain, but they are not as common as those in the temporal lobe. The frontal lobe is the second most common location, followed by the parietal lobe. In my own series, I have encountered only ten foci in the occipital lobe. The approach to foci outside of the temporal lobe is handled in much the same manner as described above, using a "tailored" approach.

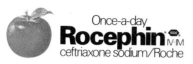

ies are combined, it will be
mporal lobectomy are sei-
esent, it is not possible to
bloc" approach is superior.
the results of resections in-
The results of surgery for
e not as good as the results
ts becoming seizure-free or
temporal epileptogenic foci

ample until recently. Meyer
ral lobe epilepsy who were
izures for an average of 7.5
e-free; 24% had occasional
eizures; and 12% were un-
and 88% benefited signifi-
nic measures for social out-
nificantly improved in most
patients whose seizures were controlled by surgery. Many epileptologists feel that
the earlier a medically refractory patient is surgically treated, the greater the improvement will be in psychosocial and vocational outcome. Thus, the trend is to
operate earlier and not to wait until adulthood (at which time the psychological
ravages of chronic epilepsy have already set in) before considering surgical intervention.

The results of any surgical series are heavily influenced by the criteria used for
selecting patients. For example, if patients are selected who have a well-defined
focus in nondominant hemisphere with no evidence of spread to the contralateral
side, who are of average intelligence, and who are between the ages of 20 and 30
years, the outcome results from surgery will be excellent. In contrast, poorer results
will be obtained from a series that includes patients with bilateral independent interictal spiking and patients with extratemporal foci.

Two points should be made. First, after a comprehensive surgical work-up, it can
usually be determined with reasonable certainty whether the patient will be likely to
have a good surgical outcome. Some patients will have a better-than-average chance
of successful surgery, whereas others will not. Second, because some patients can
be identified to be excellent candidates for surgery, they should be given this option
as soon as it is apparent that antiepileptic drugs have failed to achieve reasonable
control of their seizures.

The morbidity associated with focal excisions has been low. Ablation of the
nondominant temporal lobe can result in (a) subtle deficits in pattern recognition,
(b) subtle deficits in visual and spatial memory, and (c) some mild difficulty in
discrimination of tonal patterns. After dominant lobe resections, there may be some
mild work-finding problems. Some small field cut may result if the temporal resec-

tion is taken posterior to the tip of the ventricle. There is a small incidence of permanent hemiparesis after temporal lobectomy, but the incidence is probably less than 0.5%. The mortality rate from cortical resection is even lower. The morbidity associated with focal resections in other regions of the brain is directly related to the function subserved by cortex removed. In general, there is little morbidity with frontal resections; in fact, a patient's performance may improve some after successful removal of an active focus.

Hemispherectomy

In some patients, epileptiform activity will not be confined to one lobe or focal region but, instead, will be spread diffusely throughout an entire hemisphere. In some of these cases, a hemispherectomy may be indicated. In my own series, the most frequent indication for a hemispherectomy is medically refractory seizures that are the sequelae of infantile hemiplegia. Removal of the entire hemisphere was introduced by Krynauw in 1950 (19). However, complete hemispherectomy had as a serious complication a syndrome of superficial cerebral hemosiderosis (20) which occurred in about 25% of patients followed for 5 years. Although this complication can be treated by permanent ventriculoatrial shunt, it does increase the morbidity and mortality of the surgery. Preservation of a small portion of the hemisphere appears to prevent this complication (17). In several of my own cases of infantile hemiplegia, I have left the entire pre- and postcentral gyri.

Rasmussen (17) reported a series of patients who underwent a complete hemispherectomy: 59% of patients were seizure-free after some early attacks, 26% were markedly improved, and 15% had a less favorable result. In that series (from 1952 to 1968), two of the patients operated on early died of progressive encephalopathy. Since that complication can be minimized by leaving some cortex behind, the mortality rate of this procedure is now low.

Rasmussen (17) also reported a series of 48 patients (from 1937 to 1972) who had removal of at least three lobes of the brain. In this series of subtotal hemispherectomy, 45% were seizure-free (some after early attacks), 25% showed significant reductions in seizures, and 30% had only a "moderate or less reduction of seizure tendency." There was one postoperative death in this series. Thus, at least 70% of these patients were benefited by surgery.

Corpus Callosum Section

Van Wagenen and Herren (21) were the first to introduce the technique of corpus callosal section for treatment of epilepsy. Since then, many small surgical series have been reported in which the corpus callosum, with or without other midline tracts (such as the fornix, massa intermedia, anterior commissure, and hippocampal commissure), have been sectioned. The results in terms of morbidity and mortality have been variable (22–29). Early operations sectioned many of the midline tracts and often required more than one operation. As a result, the morbidity was high. Complications such as hydrocephalus occurred in 50% of patients. Therefore, more limited operations have recently been proposed in which only the callosum (and sometimes only the anterior two-thirds) is sectioned. Recent series with the more moderate surgical approach have demonstrated very acceptable morbidity with excellent psychosocial and cognitive function (29).

The indications for this surgery have not been clearly defined. Most published series are small and have a poorly defined group of patients. Gates et al. (26) reported a group of six epileptics with generalized discharges and falling attacks who underwent total callosal section. Although no significant change in the number of generalized discharges could be found between the pre- and postoperative electroencephalograms, there was a significant decrease in the number of falling attacks. Spencer et al. (30) have reported that they achieved "excellent" control of generalized seizures in most of 17 patients. However, in five of those patients, more intense (although not necessarily more frequent) focal seizures occurred postoperatively. This occurred primarily in patients with EEG evidence of bilateral, bifrontal, independent, and asymmetrical foci.

If one combines all reports on this procedure, the consensus is that callosal section results in a significant reduction in generalized seizures in the majority of patients. It would seem that this surgery works best for patients who suffer from atonic, tonic, clonic, or tonic–clonic seizures. In my own practice, I have retained this procedure only for patients with generalized discharges that are most prominent in the anterior scalp regions. In these patients, I have only sectioned the anterior three-quarters of the callosum. Of the patients I have operated on, only 10% are seizure-free, 80% have had a decrease in seizure severity and frequency, and 10% have not been helped by this surgery at all. However, if one considers that many of these people could not be helped at all by drugs and that their seizures carried with them a significant risk of bodily damage, these results are acceptable.

Thalamotomy

The idea that stereotactic procedures (especially thalamotomy) may help seizure disorders was put forth soon after those techniques were applied to the treatment of movement disorders. The rationale for this approach has been summarized by Ojemann and Ward (31). Although several different subcortical structures have been lesioned, there has been no consensus as to which target should be used. To date, the results have not been good enough to warrant large-scale clinical trials, and this approach is probably best kept in the experimental laboratory until more basic research is done.

SUMMARY

The previous sections have shown that there are several surgical approaches available for treating a variety of different types of partial and generalized seizure disorders. With adequate presurgical work-up, the success rate of temporal lobectomy should exceed 90%. The results of extratemporal focal resections are less favorable and are highly influenced by the presence of a focal lesion. For patients with various types of secondarily generalized epilepsies, the corpus callosum section has been refined so that it now provides modest seizure control with acceptable morbidity.

With increased use of prolonged EEG/video monitoring of patients, more precision is being obtained in localizing epileptogenic foci preoperatively. For the patients with more difficult foci to localize, the techniques of intracranial depth electrodes or of the newer, subdural "strip" electrodes are available and can provide extremely valuable data upon which rational surgical decisions can be based. The introduction of CT and MRI scanning a little over a decade ago resulted in more accurate identification of pathological structural lesions that previously would not have been diagnosed. The identification of such lesions has helped to localize many epileptogenic foci and should improve the outcome of epilepsy surgery. With increasing diagnostic accuracy for localizing and classifying epileptogenic foci, we should see an increase in postoperative success.

In addition to improved diagnostic methods, there have been many advances in surgical techniques. The increased use of the operating microscope has brought the introduction of new operative procedures such as the selective amygdalohippocampectomy, which was unknown a decade ago. The use of the microscope for routine resection of mesial temporal structures or for dividing the corpus callosum, for example, has resulted in a decrease in the morbidity associated with surgery. The use of intraoperative neuropsychological testing will allow larger resections in some dominant temporal lobes, with minimal postoperative deficits.

The mortality associated with craniotomy for epilepsy is extremely small (much less than 1%). This is due to several factors: First, the patients being operated upon are usually healthy and not suffering from an acute disease process (which is commonly the case with other neurosurgical operations). Second, the patients are usually young and do not have many secondary problems (such as hypertension and diabetes) that may predispose them to complications. Third, many of the operations are done under local anesthesia, thereby precluding a major risk factor. The mortality rate for this type of surgery is actually lower than the mortality rate for many common abdominal surgeries.

Even though the results and morbidity of surgery have been improving, there is still a reluctance by many neurologists to refer patients for surgery. The reasons are many, but most hinge around misconceptions about the risks and benefits of epilepsy surgery. Surgery is no longer a treatment option of "last resort." Good surgical candidates have a chance of an excellent result that approaches the 93% level reported by Wieser and Yasergil (15). Even for those patients in whom it is most likely that only a "palliative" resection can be done, the morbidity and mortality of modern epilepsy surgery is acceptable, and the overall results of surgery are far better than the neuropsychosocial deterioration seen with the polytherapy associated with medically intractable epilepsy.

REFERENCES

1. Dodrill CB. Correlates of generalized tonic–clonic seizures with intellectual, neuropsychological, emotional, and social function in patients with epilepsy. *Epilepsia* 1986;27:399–411.
2. Hauser WA, Annegers JF, Elveback LR. Mortality in patients with epilepsy. *Epilepsia* 1980;21:399–412.
3. Sperling MR, Mendius JR, Engle J Jr. Mesial temporal spikes: a simultaneous comparison of sphenoidal, nasopharyngeal, and ear electrodes. *Epilepsia* 1986;27:81–86.
4. Bancaud J, Talairach J, Bonis A, et al. *La stereo-electroencephalographie dans l'epilepsie*. Paris: Masson, 1965;321.
5. Wyler AR, Ojemann GA, Lettich E, Ward AA Jr. Subdural strip electrodes for localizing epileptogenic foci. *J Neurosurg* 1984;60:1195–1200.
6. Rosenbaum TJ, Laxer KD, Vessely M, Smith BW. Subdural electrodes for seizure focus localization. *Neurosurgery* 1986;19:73–81.
7. Spencer SS. Depth electroencephalography in selection of refractory epilepsy for surgery. *Ann Neurol* 1981;9:207–214.
8. Sperling MR, Wilson G, Engle J Jr, et al. Magnetic resonance imaging in intractable partial epilepsy: correlative studies. *Ann Neurol* 1986;20:57–62.
9. Ojemann GA, Dodrill CB. Verbal memory deficits after left temporal lobectomy for epilepsy: mechanism and intraoperative prediction. *J Neurosurg* 1985;62:101–107.
10. Dodrill CB, Wilkus RJ, Ojemann GA, et al. Multidisciplinary prediction of seizure relief from cortical resection surgery. *Ann Neurol* 1985;20:2–12.
11. Wada J, Rasmussen T. Intracarotid injection of sodium amytal for the lateralization of speech dominance: experimental and clinical observations. *J Neurosurg* 1952;17:266–282.
12. Penfield W, Jasper H. *Epilepsy and the functional anatomy of the human brain*. Boston: Little, Brown, 1954;748–785.
13. Goldring S, Gregorie EM. Surgical management of epilepsy using epidural electrodes to localize the seizure focus. Review of 100 cases. *J Neurosurg* 1984;60:457–466.
14. Spencer DD, Spencer SS, Mattson RH. Access to the posterior temporal lobe structures in the surgical treatment of temporal lobe epilepsy. *Neurosurgery* 1984;15:667–671.
15. Wieser HG, Yasargil G. Selective amygdalohippocampectomy as a surgical treatment of mediobasal limbic epilepsy. In: *Surgical Neurology* 1984;17:445–457.
16. Talairach J, Bancaud J, Szikla G, et al. Approache nouvelle de la neurochirurgie de l'epilepsie. Methodologie stereotaxique et resultats therapeutiques. *Neurochirurgie [Suppl]* 1974;20:1–240.
17. Rasmussen T. Surgery for epilepsy arising in regions other than the temporal and frontal lobes. In: Purpura DP, Penry JK, Walter RD, eds. *Advances in neurology*, vol 8. New York: Raven Press, 1975;207–226.
18. Meyer FB, Marsh WR, Laws ER, Sharbough FW. Temporal lobectomy in children with epilepsy. *J Neurosurg* 1986;64:371–376.
19. Krynauw RA. Infantile hemiplegia treated by removing one cerebral hemisphere. *J Neurol Neurosurg Psychiatry* 1950;13:243–267.
20. Oppenheimer DR, Griffith HB. Persistent intracranial bleeding as a complication of hemispherectomy. *J Neurol Neurosurg Psychiatry* 1966;29:229–240.
21. Van Wagenen WP, Herren RY. Surgical division of commissural pathways in the corpus callosum: relation to spread of an epileptic attack. *Arch Neurol* 1940;44:740–759.
22. Bogen JE, Vogel PJ. Cerebral commissurotomy in man. *Bull Los Angeles Neurol Soc* 1962;27:169–172.
23. Luessenhop AJ, de la Cruz TC, Fenichel GM. Surgical disconnection of the cerebral hemispheres for intractable seizures: results in infancy and childhood. *J Am Med Soc* 1970;213:1630–1636.
24. Wilson DH, Reeves AG, Gazzaniga MS. "Central" commissurotomy for intractable generalized epilepsy: series two. *Neurology* 1982;32:687–697.
25. Huck FR, Radvany J, Avila Jo Pires de Camargo CH, et al. Anterior callosotomy in epileptics with multiform seizures and bilateral synchronous spike and wave EEG pattern. *Acta Neurochir [Suppl] (Wien)* 1980;30:127–135.
26. Gates JR, Leppik IE, Yap J, Gumnit RJ. Corpus callosotomy: clinical and electroencephalographic effects. *Epilepsia* 1984;25:308–316.
27. Geoffroy GM, Lassonde F, Delise M. Cecarie corpus callosotomy for control of intractable epilepsy in children. *Neurology* 1983;33:891–897.

28. Rayport M, Ferguson SM, Corrie WS. Outcomes and indications of corpus callosum section for intractable seizure control. *Appl Neurophysiol* 1983;46:47–51.
29. Ferrell RB, Culver CM, Tucker GJ. Psychosocial and cognitive function after commissurotomy for intractable seizures. *J Neurosurg* 1983;58:374–380.
30. Spencer SS, Spencer DD, Glaser GH, Williamson PD, Mattson RH. More intense focal seizure types after callosal section: the role of inhibition. *Ann Neurol* 1984;16:686–693.
31. Ojemann GA, Ward AA Jr. Stereotactic and other procedures for epilepsy. In: Purpura DP, Penry JK, Walter RD, eds. *Advances in neurology,* vol 8. New York: Raven Press, 1975;241–265.
32. Wannamaker BB. Autonomic nervous system and epilepsy. *Epilepsia* 1985;26 (Suppl 1):S31–S39.

Epilepsy: Current Approaches to Diagnosis and Treatment,
edited by Dennis B. Smith,
Raven Press, Ltd., New York © 1990.

10

Long-Term Psychosocial Management of Epilepsy

Joseph B. Green and Rita A. Mercille

Department of Neurology, Texas Tech University Health Sciences Center,
Lubbock, Texas 79430

This chapter addresses the long-term management of patients with epilepsy whose seizures cannot be completely controlled; these are the patients who must learn to "live with epilepsy." Many suffer from complex partial seizures, whereas others have a generalized form of epilepsy often associated with myoclonic and drop attacks. Most, but not all, of this latter group are children. By definition, therefore, we are attempting to treat an incurable and chronic illness (1). The goals of treatment are to achieve (a) optimal control of seizures, (b) educational or vocational success, and (c) normal family and community relationships. Unfortunately, this is possible in a minority of those whose seizures cannot be completely controlled. There is reason to think, however, that with better long-term management, this number can be appreciably increased.

Most of the patients who require long-term management have had seizure problems since childhood. Comprehensive and vigorous treatment should be initiated early in the course of the illness. It is much more difficult to rehabilitate an immature and dependent individual who is 30 years of age than to prevent these complications from the start.

The prognosis in epilepsy is made worse by certain risk factors that increase the probability of psychiatric complications. It has been shown (2) that brain-damaged children, with or without seizures, are at a higher risk for mental disorders than children with chronic illness not involving the brain.

Although there is undoubtedly a relationship between brain lesions and emotional and psychological problems (2,3), it is inexact and limited in practical significance. There is a lack of agreement on whether there is a correlation between emotional disorders and the location of lesions, as well as between the degree of cognitive impairment and the extent of lesions (4–6). These uncertainties serve to emphasize the importance of reducing the impact of known risk factors that are susceptible to clinical management (2,7–10). For example, the use of multiple anticonvulsant drugs, especially sedatives, can be avoided. Risk factors such as mental illness of parents can be treated, and child abuse or neglect can be prevented. Seizures can be reduced in frequency and severity by effective drug therapy or timely surgery.

THE DIAGNOSTIC EVALUATION

Successful management of epilepsy depends on accurate and complete diagnosis. A complete diagnosis may require several office visits and includes (a) the classification of the seizures, (b) the etiology if known, (c) the presence of associated neurological or neuropsychological deficits, and (d) psychosocial assessment.

Practically, the potential range of a patient's problems spans many disciplines of the health and social sciences. The individual physician does not have the time or the training to address every treatment issue in depth. However, he/she should be able to identify the nature of the problem so that he/she can make an appropriate referral to other professionals and community resources. Referral to an epileptologist, psychologist, social worker, educational specialist, or vocational counselor may be necessary to acquire an adequate data base.

At the initial visit and in addition to the thorough medical and neurological work-up, the physician should perform his/her own psychosocial assessment by inquiring about the following:

school performance
employment
self-care skills
use of public transportation
social and recreational activities
family relationships

In other words, the physician needs answers to the following questions: Is a child in the age-appropriate grade, and is he/she performing at the expected level? Is an adult employed currently? What jobs has he/she held and for how long? What is the highest grade in school completed? Does the patient attend to his/her personal grooming, clothes, and meals? Does he/she use public transportation? Does the patient participate in social and recreational activities? With whom? Is a child held to the same parental expectations as his/her siblings? Is he/she disciplined in the same way? Are both parents involved in the patient's care?

THE OFFICE VISITS FOLLOWING THE INITIAL WORK-UP

At each follow-up visit, an interval history is obtained, recording the number and type of seizures as well as times of occurrence. Precipitating factors are looked for. It is helpful to get from the patient a schedule of daily activities, from the time of rising to the time of retiring. Not only may this reveal environmental triggers, but it gives information about the patient's world.

Inquiries are made about school or work, social interactions, recreation, and so on. The patient needs to know that the physician is interested in him/her as a person and that he/she is willing to listen to the report on daily activities, successes, and failures. The patient should be seen alone for part of each visit. A good time to do this is while performing the neurological examination.

It is also important to observe the patient in the presence of his/her family. Do they support his/her efforts to be an independent, competent person? Is he/she treated with respect? Does the patient behave differently and relate differently to the physician when a spouse or parent is present? Who is in control, and how are decisions made concerning medication?

The frequency and timing of patient–physician contacts should not be driven by crises. Follow-up visits should be scheduled regularly and at close enough intervals so that important treatment issues are not forgotten. Continuity of care entails follow-through and persistence in control of seizures, educational/vocational adjustment, elimination of undesirable behaviors, and so on. Although the goal is to avoid emergencies by preventive treatment at regular visits, patients do have breakthrough seizures. It is critically important for the physician to be available. Patients and families have to be educated as to what constitutes an emergency and as to what circumstances can wait for regular visits. This should be spelled out to them so that the "cry wolf" syndrome can be avoided.

TREATMENT ISSUES

In following any group of patients with epilepsy, certain psychological and emotional problems stand out. First among these is dependence, whether measured in social/psychological or economic terms (11,12). Unhealthy dependence on others, combined with lack of control over one's destiny, breeds depression and anger. Dependence can be prevented by encouraging parents and patients to take risks and to set high but realistic goals for achievement, and it can also be prevented by encouraging healthy aggression and competition.

The support of the family is often the difference between success and failure in a patient's struggle to achieve social and vocational goals (13). Risks must be taken so that a child may acquire the "normal" life experiences in order to hold his/her own with peers. The reluctance of parents and physicians to take chances may lead to undesirable prohibition of athletics, social activities, travel, and so on. An unhealthy interdependent relationship may develop; a parent may have a psychological need to keep the child dependent. Parents tend to overprotect children who are handicapped, a practice that Ounsted has called "pedophilia." One parent may exclude the other from the patient's care. Siblings may resent the special attention given to the patient.

The physician should set an example for the family. He/she should avoid condescension and should make it clear that he/she expects the patient to relate in an age-appropriate manner. Above all, he/she should treat the patient with respect and should never talk about the patient as if the patient were not in the room. The physician and the patient form an alliance. The physician is the patient's advocate with regard to family, school, and community. The patient, in turn, is willing to trust the physician and comply with his/her treatment recommendations.

The patient consents to treatment recommendations after being thoroughly informed and educated by the physician. If he/she agrees to take medication and understands the risk/benefit ratio, then he/she assumes responsibility for taking the drug. The patient must be allowed to make decisions within the limits of his/her understanding and capacity. Children, from as young as 5 years of age, should participate in the decision-making. It is expected that once a patient makes a decision about medication, he or she will begin to assume the responsibility of compliance.

Physicians may sympathize with the unpleasantness of having to take medication on a regular basis, but they must also acknowledge and reinforce that it is necessary. Patients (and families) who tend to exercise denial may "forget" to take medicine. This may happen when the painful fact of epilepsy has not been confronted early on in the illness.

The issue of compliance highlights a dilemma: How can one encourage independence and risk-taking while also stressing the importance of chronic drug-taking and regular follow-up appointments? The therapeutic alliance between patient and physician has the goal of internalizing within the patient the control of health-promoting behavior. Compliance is reinforced by physician "feedback" (directly to the patient) of regularly monitored drug levels. From the beginning, the levels are common knowledge to patient and physician so that compliance rarely becomes an issue once the therapeutic relationship is established. The physician must avoid becoming a target of the patient's angry rebellion against dependence, because the therapeutic alliance on which compliance depends will collapse. This is the rationale for empowering the patient to make the decisions about his/her treatment.

Peculiarly, persons with epilepsy and other developmental disabilities may pass through the teen-age years without overtly experiencing the turmoil of adolescence. Although normally developed physically, they show little interest in dating and have few friends of either sex. They prefer to play with younger children, and they lack intimate relationships outside the family. When they reach the third decade, they may experience a delayed and stormy adolescence, sometimes with psychotic features (14,15). These patients in their twenties resemble adolescents of 14 in their attitudes toward the opposite sex; this makes it difficult for them to attract normal persons their own age into a healthy relationship. They are needful and may be sexually exploited. They are often ignorant about sexual matters.

Persons growing up with epilepsy are often subject to social prohibitions and taboos. There may be unusual sleeping arrangements. Fear of sudden death in a seizure may lead parents to unusual degrees of observation and closeness which inhibit normal psychosexual development. They may sleep with a child. Parents may be afraid to leave a child for fear that he/she may be abused while having a seizure. The physician must be sensitive to these fears and allow them to surface in conversation when presented during an appropriate moment. Parents and patients may have inaccurate information about the genetics of epilepsy, and they may utilize denial or repression of sexual needs rather than discuss contraceptive methods with the physician. The physician should ascertain whether the patient has age-appropriate social and sexual relationships.

Although too much stress cannot be put on the syndrome of dependence, depression, and anger, patients with epilepsy do develop other psychiatric complications. Disabling anxiety may be couched in terms of fear of having a seizure. Panic reactions may coexist with an epileptic disorder. The use of antidepressant or anxiolytic drugs may be unavoidable (16).

Patients with epilepsy may become psychotic, usually in young adulthood, after many years of incompletely controlled seizures and chronic invalidism (14,15,17). Although this may be explained by a limbic kindling of abnormal behavior and affect, it seems as likely that psychosis may result from (a) a stunting of human development, (b) depression, and (c) chronic drug toxicity.

The physician can often obtain helpful clues to psychosocial problems by observing the interaction of patients and families with each other and with himself. Some examples may be cited:

The patient is asked how many seizures he/she has had and the parent answers, before the patient can speak, "We have had five seizures, Doctor." The "we" is a significant part of the response and indicates a problem of separation and overdependence. "Our seizures are better" or "We are feeling better" are not appropriate responses for a parent, and they are particularly bizarre when the child is an adolescent or an adult.

One must also be wary of the condescending or patronizing parent. While the physician engages the patient in serious conversation about his/her goals and ambitions, this parent can be seen smirking in the background, making various gestures, shaking his/her head, and so on. Chances are that the patient is having his/her plans undermined.

Then there is the elderly and burdened parent who has been through it all and is long-suffering—perhaps with a 40-year-old "child" who has never been employed and who has never had the seizures completely controlled. The "child" is completely dependent on the parent and has outbursts of rage, which the elderly parent cannot handle. This tragic situation could have been avoided by earlier placement of the patient in independent or semidependent living arrangements and socialization with peers and adults outside of family.

There is the spouse-parent, that is, the spouse of the patient with epilepsy who is often revealed by the patient's reply, "Gosh, I don't know what I do during a seizure. I really don't know anything about it, and I don't know about my medications—she takes care of all of that," pointing to his wife. It is not unusual for a spouse to take responsibility for his or her partner with regard to medications, reporting of seizures, and so on. In these cases, almost always the spouse is merely continuing the role of the patient's parents. The physician should insist that the patient take responsibility for him/herself and that the patient, not the spouse, telephone in the event of problems.

Some patients who are parents involve their children in their epilepsy in a reversal of roles. The children run to them when they have seizures, call the physician, and so on, even though the children may be as young as 8 or 9 years old. The patient tells you how concerned he/she is about the children's future and how this might affect them. At the same time, the parent continues to foist this dependence upon them.

There is the "seductive" patient who attempts to play out fantasies with the physician. In these cases, the physician should insist that the spouse or family come with him/her for the visits. In this way the patient is forced into the mature role and behavior expected in the real world.

There is the "retired" patient who has been through all the possible referrals to community and state agencies and has seen many physicians and has been on every medication. He/she is content sitting at home watching television. He/she continues to have occasional seizures, but he/she is passive enough to agree to still another attempt at rehabilitation.

There is the "professional" epileptic—a patient who attributes every problem he/she has to his/her epilepsy. Some of these patients have pseudoseizures (6,18).

Finally, there is the "survivor." This is the patient who has occasional seizures but has learned to work the system. He/she has secured disability income, has gotten all the possible benefits from voluntary agencies, and has managed also to obtain free medical care and subsidized medication.

Beware of the "pharmacologist" patient or parent who wants to know all the possible side effects of medication. He/she will get them with any medication prescribed. When the patient (or parent) does not accept the diagnosis of epilepsy, there is no safe or satisfactory antiepileptic medication. Then there is the patient who asks if his/her medication can be decreased or discontinued. Always do a drug level on this patient since he/she has probably already done what he/she is asking the physician to do. And finally with this patient, confront the issue squarely— maybe the medication is not helping, maybe the patient is right, and maybe it would be better if the patient were not taking the drug. Some patients are better off on no medication at all.

The physician should advocate for his/her patient in school and work settings. His/her patient is not an "epileptic" but is, instead, a citizen who is entitled to educational and employment opportunities and who has the misfortune of having epilepsy. Teachers and school nurses are an important source of useful clinical information. Occasionally, teachers are the first to suspect a seizure problem. They can help determine the frequency and severity of seizures. Teachers are key persons in obtaining remedial help for learning disabilities, common in patients with epilepsy (14,19). Observations by teachers may corroborate or contradict information obtained from parents. Teachers and school nurses may help with problems in compliance. The physician, in turn, may help the teacher by advising on proper emergency care of seizures, seizure types, and symptoms of drug toxicity.

Helpful discussions can be held on (a) how to deal with the reactions of the other children to the patient's seizures and (b) how best to facilitate return to the status quo and classroom routine.

Preparation for employment begins with early setting of realistic educational and vocational goals. This requires thorough evaluation of cognitive and adaptive abilities. Neuropsychological testing and vocational counseling are highly desirable and may be arranged through the school, the vocational rehabilitation agency, or a specialized clinic. Preparation for employment includes the establishment of good work habits in childhood. Parents must insist that the child measure up with regard to standards set for siblings in attending to his/her personal grooming, clothes, and room and in doing his/her share of the household chores. School assignments must be done punctually and completely. The child should learn to accept criticism and to follow directions. In a survey of rehabilitation failures, inability to accept and use supervision was a much more important obstacle to success than were seizures (L. C. Hartlage and J. B. Green, *unpublished data*).

SUMMARY

Long-term management of epilepsy is founded on a therapeutic alliance between physician and patient. The physician supports the patient's drive for self-realization and independence, and the patient trusts the physician by complying with his/her recommendations.

REFERENCES

1. Rodin EA. *The prognosis of patients with epilepsy*. Springfield, Ill: Charles C Thomas, 1968.
2. Graham P, Rutter M. Organic brain dysfunction and child psychiatric disorder. *Br Med J* 1968;3:695.
3. Gudmundsson G. Epilepsy in Iceland. *Acta Neurol Scand [Suppl]* 1966;25:43.
4. Herman BP, Dikmen S, Wilensky AJ. Increased psychopathology associated with multiple seizure types: fact or artifact? *Epilepsia* 1982;23:587.
5. Waxman SG, Geschwind N. The interictal behavior syndrome of temporal lobe epilepsy. *Arch Gen Psychiatry* 1975;32:1580.
6. Whitman S, Hermann B, Gordon AC, Berg BJ. Do people with epilepsy have more psychological problems? *National Spokesman* 1982; Jan/Feb:1–10.
7. Dikmen S, Matthews CG. Effects of major motor seizure frequency upon cognitive–intellectual functions in adults. *Epilepsia* 1977;18:21.
8. Reynolds EH, Shorvon SD. Monotherapy or polytherapy for epilepsy? *Epilepsia* 1981;22:1.
9. Shorvon SD, Reynolds EH. Reduction of polypharmacy for epilepsy. *Br Med J* 1979;2:1023.
10. Theodore WH, Porter RJ. Removal of sedative–hypnotic antiepileptic drugs from the regimens of patients with intractable epilepsy. *Ann Neurol* 1983;13:320.
11. Hartlage LC, Green JB. The relation of parental attitudes to academic and social achievement in epileptic children. *Epilepsia* 1972;13:21.
12. Hartlage LC, Green JB. Dependency in epileptic children. *Epilepsia* 1972;13:27.
13. Ziegler RG. Impairments of control and competence in epileptic children and their families. *Epilepsia* 1981;22:339.
14. Pritchard PB, Lombroso CT, McIntyre M. Psychological complications of temporal lobe epilepsy. *Neurology* 1980;30:227.
15. Slater E, Beard AW, Glithero E. The schizophrenia-like psychoses of epilepsy. *Br J Psychiatry* 1963;109:96.
16. Ramani V, Gumnit RJ. Intensive monitoring of interictal psychosis in epilepsy. *Ann Neurol* 1982;11:613.

17. Glaser GH. The problem of psychosis in psychomotor temporal lobe epileptics. *Epilepsia* 1964;5:271.
18. Ramani V, Gumnit RJ. Management of hysterical seizures in epileptic patients. *Arch Neurol* 1982;39:78.
19. Stores G, Hart J, Piron N. Inattentiveness in school children with epilepsy. *Epilepsia* 1978;19:169.

Epilepsy: Current Approaches to Diagnosis and Treatment,
edited by Dennis B. Smith,
Raven Press, Ltd., New York © 1990.

11

Diagnosis and Treatment of Psychiatric Problems Associated with Epilepsy

Dietrich Blumer

Department of Psychiatry, University of Tennessee at Memphis, Memphis, Tennessee 38146

Our understanding of the neurologic aspects of seizure disorders has greatly increased over the last four decades. The notion of epilepsy as a psychiatric disorder has long faded, and epilepsy is recognized as a major neurologic disorder. Concomitantly, psychiatrists have shown limited interest in epilepsy. The understanding of the psychiatric complications that may be associated with seizure disorders has suffered, and guidelines for their treatment—beyond common-sense psychosocial considerations—have been notably absent.

Since epilepsy often involves the neural substrate of cognitive, emotional, and behavioral functions, it is evident that neuropsychiatric considerations may be of major importance in the treatment of some forms of epilepsy. The recognition of complex yet characteristic psychiatric syndromes associated with epilepsy indeed has led to the recent development of an effective pharmacologic intervention for these disorders (1–3).

NATURE OF THE PSYCHOPATHOLOGY ASSOCIATED WITH EPILEPSY

A set of frequently debated personality and behavior changes has been ascribed to the interictal phase of temporal lobe epilepsy. It consists, in essence, of a deepened and labile emotionality, with irritability and hyperethical trends, slowness–viscosity, and a global hyposexuality (4–8). These traits tend to be subtle, are not consistently present, and, with the exception of episodes of excessive anger, rarely prompt psychiatric intervention. It has become recognized that depressive episodes are the predominant disorder requiring psychiatric treatment among patients with epilepsy (3,9–11). The suicide rate among patients with epilepsy tends to be five times higher than in the general population (12,13). Furthermore, anxiety has been cited as a problem perhaps as frequent as depression among patients with epilepsy (14–16). Surveys have indicated that about 7% of patients with epilepsy may suffer at one time or another from a psychosis (17). Psychoses with paranoid, delusional, and/or hallucinatory symptoms have been described as the schizophrenia-like episodes of epilepsy (18). In 1978, the Commission for the Control of Epilepsy and Its Consequences noted that 12% of institutionalized mental patients had epilepsy (19).

The confusing wealth of psychopathology reported in association with epilepsy has led many observers to doubt the existence of mental changes that could be specifically related to seizure disorders. Furthermore, it appeared impossible to sort out the respective roles of psychosocial factors, brain damage, medication, and the seizure condition per se. The role of these factors will be discussed before we define the psychiatric syndromes that tend to be associated with certain forms of epilepsy.

Role of Psychosocial Factors

Since ancient times, it has been appreciated that the recurrent sudden loss of control with display of peculiar behavior experienced by patients with epilepsy tends to result in embarrassment and shame for these patients. Patients with epilepsy were often shunned, although they may also have inspired awe, as the old term "sacred disease" suggests (20). Our more enlightened era has brought a better understanding of the illness and has also brought hope for control of the attacks in the great majority of patients. Support groups are available through many chapters of the Epilepsy Foundation of America, and the prejudices of employers, schools, and the general public are receding. A seizure disorder, nevertheless, still may represent a major handicap.

Modern psychiatric thinking assumes that stress, while obviously of importance, is a mere precipitating factor and does not explain the nature of the psychiatric disorder that occurs. The latter is determined by the individual biologic factors, such as the genetic vulnerability and the state of the central nervous system (CNS). The particular vulnerability of patients with epilepsy toward depression is highlighted by a recent study which showed that patients with epilepsy were depressed twice as often and had a fourfold increase of suicide attempts, when compared with a matched group of individuals with other handicaps (9).

Role of Brain Damage

Modern neuroradiologic procedures can detect brain lesions in only a minority of patients with epilepsy. Once detected, neuropsychologic measures and the psychiatric evaluation can provide a fair assessment of the impact of a cerebral lesion on mental functions. The experience with the subtle lesions of the limbic–temporal zones suggests that it is not the lesion per se but, instead, the secondary discharging focus that may be associated with reversible emotional changes (3). Thus, the role of static cerebral lesions in the highly variable psychiatric disorders associated with epilepsy probably does not represent a significant confusing factor for our understanding of the psychiatric complications of epilepsy.

Role of Medication

Like that of brain damage, the role of the antiepileptic drugs on the mental functions of the patient is presently rather well understood and is of broad significance (3,21). Antiepileptic polypharmacy and the use of sedative antiepileptic drugs (phenobarbital and primidone) tend to exert a damaging effect on cognitive and emotional functions. Conversely, carbamazepine and valproate have psychotropic properties and are the antiepileptic drugs of choice for patients with both epilepsy and emotional disorders. The important issue of the proper use of antiepileptic drugs will be further discussed in the section on treatment.

Role of the Seizure Disorder

Patients with idiopathic, nonlocalization-related epilepsy tend to have a favorable outcome. No significant psychiatric complications have been linked to this group of epilepsies. In contrast, symptomatic generalized epilepsies such as infantile spasms and the Lennox–Gastaut syndrome still carry a bleak prognosis, since their multiple seizure types tend to be uncontrollable and because intellectual deterioration is associated in the majority of cases.

Patients with seizures of temporal lobe origin represent the majority of adult patients with epilepsy. Their seizures are often difficult to control, and the course of the illness tends to be chronic. Psychiatric complications have been specifically ascribed to temporal lobe epilepsy. However, it has been shown that some patients diagnosed as suffering from apparently generalized seizures may show similar psychiatric changes, presumably from secondary involvement of the temporal–limbic zones (3).

Gastaut has pointed out that the traits characteristic for temporal lobe epilepsy—heightened emotionality, slowness–viscosity, and global hyposexuality—represent the very opposites of the placidity, fleeting attention, and hypersexuality observed after bilateral temporal ablation (Klüver–Bucy syndrome) and may be considered the effect of a discharging lesion in the temporal–limbic system (6,22). It is evident that the heightened emotionality not only includes an exceptional ethical–religious fervor and a trend to react at times with explosive anger but also includes intensified and labile moods with prominent depression, anxiety, and paranoid, delusional, and hallucinatory experiences. Indeed, the full range of psychiatric symptoms may be present in a highly episodic, atypical, and often polysymptomatic (pleomorphic) pattern. These emotional disorders are neuropsychiatric in nature and, like the seizures themselves, tend to be responsive to proper pharmacologic treatment (3). We have termed this complex psychiatric disorder related to epilepsy the "paroxysmal neurobehavioral disorder" or "temporal lobe syndrome."

The peri-ictal (preictal, ictal, and postictal) mental changes are directly related to clinical seizures and clearly demonstrate the effects of epileptic disorders on emotionality and cognition. They are reviewed before discussing the important psychiatric changes that may occur during the interictal phase of epilepsy.

Ictal Mental Changes

While everybody will recognize a generalized convulsion, partial seizures ("auras") will often escape medical attention, since they are not followed by a more ostensible event with loss of consciousness. On rare occasions there may be a "continuous aura" or partial seizure status, but typically the aura is sudden and brief (measured in seconds). On careful exploration, the aura frequently consists of a complex experience with various sensory, affective, cognitive, autonomic, and somatic elements, and it is characteristically reported as a unique yet indescribable experience. The observable events that may follow the subjective aura are similarly complex, are usually not recalled by the patient, and have to be reported by an observer. While the seizure events tend to be highly individual, they typically reoccur in a stereotyped manner in a given patient. Proper inquiry is required, since temporal lobe seizures often remain undiagnosed.

Epidemiologic studies have shown that as many as 25% of individuals with epilepsy remained undiagnosed; most of these patients had simple partial seizures (23,24). A recurrent peculiar feeling in the stomach which may rise upward and lead to the experience of a near-faint may be rationalized by the patient ("everybody has such experiences"). If the experience is bizarre (e.g., consists of a peculiar hallucination), the event is so embarrassing that it may remain concealed. Simple and complex partial seizures of temporal lobe origin indeed present with a wide range of "psychopathology" (altered mood, fear, sexual arousal, paranoid ideation, compulsive thought disorder, illusion or hallucination, depersonalization, or peculiar somatic experiences) and tend to be followed by a confusional–amnestic state. It should be no great surprise that any such mental changes can occur, in a less stereotyped and more protracted form, as a result of interictal or subictal discharges in the temporal–limbic zones, resulting in the characteristic atypical, episodic, and pleomorphic psychopathology.

Preictal and Postictal Psychiatric Complications

A minority of patients experience a prodrome that is fairly consistent for a given patient. Increased moodiness, irritability, and headaches tend to be particularly common. The prodrome lasts from hours to days, and the seizure may bring welcome relief. The characteristic confusional–amnestic postictal state of the complex partial seizure, though sometimes imperceptible, lasts for minutes, or it may be prolonged for as long as an hour after marked bitemporal discharges. The confusion may clear while the amnesia still persists, and the patient may carry out routine coherent acts for which he/she will have no recollection.

A particular entity is the postictal psychosis, which follows upon a flurry of major or minor seizures. This is an acute confusional state that may last for days to as long as 2 weeks. Its relationship to a preceding flurry of seizures may be overlooked if the seizures were minor or not observed or if there was an interval of relative lucidity of 12–24 hours between the last seizure and the onset of the psychotic state.

A prolonged postictal psychosis may require intervention with tranquilizing medication. In some patients, a significant depressive state occurs following a seizure, lasting hours or days. For both the postictal psychosis and the postictal depressive episodes, control of the seizures is of obvious importance.

Differential Diagnoses of the Interictal Psychiatric Syndromes

The biologically based psychiatric complications of epilepsy, referred to as "paroxysmal neurobehavioral disorder," consist of highly episodic, atypical, and pleomorphic syndromes. This fluctuating and often complex psychopathology cannot be placed properly in any of the traditional psychiatric categories. A marked lability of moods, changing within hours, days, or weeks, is the most prominent characteristic of this disorder. The depressive trend is predominant, though a number of patients will also experience brief periods of elation. The depressive mood is often associated with an angry or even explosive mood—a state of mind that has been termed "dysphoric mood." The intensity of the depressive mood may carry a suicidal risk. The rapidity of the mood shifts and the admixture of an intense angry affect (and of other mental changes) clearly distinguish these psychiatric complications from manic–depressive disorders.

Schizophrenia-like traits are frequently admixed to the mood changes. Paranoid, hallucinatory, or delusional symptoms may be the predominant mental changes. Their usually more fleeting nature and the intactness of affect, rapport, and judgment are characteristic and distinguish these traits from those observed in schizophrenic disorders.

Anxiety may be frequently present as well, rarely as a chronic state but rather in acute episodes that may need to be differentiated from panic attacks. Any of the well-known psychiatric symptoms—from abuse of alcohol and drugs to obsessive–compulsive traits—may appear, out of their customary context, as part and parcel of a psychiatric syndrome associated with epilepsy. This atypical and pleomorphic psychopathology is highly episodic; only rarely a trait may be chronically present. However, a depressive baseline is often present.

Highly conscientious, spiritually oriented, and at times hyperreligious personality trends tend to be present and represent a very positive aspect in many individuals, contrasting sharply with the angry–dysphoric episodes that may occur in the same individuals. The detail-bound, circumstantial, slow and persevering trends, once considered a mainstay of the old "epileptic personality," may be present in various degrees. Patients tend to be very cooperative and loyal as long as they feel that they are being treated fairly.

The listed psychiatric complications of epilepsy are problems of the interictal phase. Though they are complex in nature, their pharmacologic treatment is relatively simple and, in our experience, has been generally effective. *It is of primary importance to recogize the emotional disorders as related to epilepsy; treating the patient as if he/she suffered from an independent psychiatric disorder results in ineffective treatment.*

THE RECOGNITION OF EPILEPSY

The large number of patients with epilepsy who have remained undiagnosed tend to suffer from simple and/or complex partial seizures of temporal lobe origin (23,24). Some of these patients may present to the physician with vague physical complaints (such as aches and pains) or with various complaints of nervousness (such as labile moods, irritability, anxiety, or forgetfulness). A careful exploration is required in order to detect the presence of subtle seizure events. The patient must be asked about sudden stereotyped peculiar and often complex experiences of brief duration, ranging from a funny feeling in the stomach or the head to scary hallucinatory experiences. Such events may have been brushed off by the patient as insignificant or may have been anxiously concealed for years as the stigma of an unsound mind. Many patients do not experience an aura, and it is important to inquire about lapses of awareness, episodes of failing concentration, and forgetfulness. For a complete inquiry, a next of kin must be questioned about the observation of sudden lapses of attention with or without peculiar behavior, followed by a brief period of confusion and amnesia. Since the patient can only report the aura of his seizure and some of its aftermath, the observation by others of sudden, brief, and stereotyped changes of appearance and behavior should always be ascertained. Such observations range from sudden arrest of ongoing activity, a vacant stare, changes of facial complexion, grimacing, other muscular spasms, and respiratory changes to the highly pathognomonic oral automatisms of lip smacking, chewing, swallowing, or salivating.

An electroencephalogram (EEG) after 24 hours of sleep deprivation is indicated for every patient with suspected epilepsy (see Chapters 2, 3). The sleep deprivation serves as provocative stress and secures the recording of a period of drowsiness and sleep. Sphenoidal or nasopharyngeal leads may occasionally contribute positive electroencephalographic findings. It may be indicated to record an EEG under the condition of any stress that reportedly provokes an attack. Even perfectly executed repeat EEGs, however, may be silent. This fact, often ignored, emphasizes the significance of the clinical events that tend to be pathognomonic in many cases.

An inquiry has to be carried out for preceding cerebral impairments, including perinatal insults, protracted febrile convulsions, head injuries, and meningoencephalitis. The family history may be positive for seizure disorders or migraine. A neurological evaluation with computed tomography (CT) scan and magnetic resonance imaging (MRI) scan is mandatory in suspected cases.

TREATMENT

Use of Antiepileptic Drugs

The sedative antiepileptic drugs (barbiturates and, to a lesser extent, primidone) tend to be psychotoxic even at a "therapeutic" range, resulting in excessive sedation, in dependence, and in negative emotional effects: (a) hyperactivity and temper outbursts in children and (b) depression and emotional lability in adults. Sedative antiepileptic drugs should only be prescribed as a last resort. If a patient treated with phenytoin has emotional difficulties, the drug should be replaced by carbamazepine, or by valproate if primary generalized seizures are present.

Psychotropic effects have been ascribed to carbamazepine since its earliest use more than 25 years ago (25). It appeared to be beneficial for the following symptoms exhibited by many patients with epilepsy: slowness and viscosity; emotional intensity and lability; apathy; depressed mood; and anxiety (26). The emotional improvement, however, was ascribed (by some) to better seizure control or to the relief from toxic effects of the traditional anticonvulsants, and the issue remained controversial. The increasingly wide use of carbamazepine over the past 10 years for patients with a wide variety of psychiatric disorders in the absence of any seizures has established the psychotropic effects of carbamazepine beyond any doubt (27). There is good evidence that excellent responders to carbamazepine among psychiatric patients may suffer from atypical, highly episodic, pleomorphic syndromes of organic origin, which may be considered formes frustes of epilepsy (2).

More recently, there has been similar evidence that valproate can be effective for many psychiatric patients (28). The majority of the psychiatric patients responding to carbamazepine and valproate are diagnosed as "affective disorders" and are simultaneously treated with an antidepressant or with lithium.

Adjunct Use of Antidepressants or Lithium

Once it was evident that many psychiatric patients with atypical disorders showed syndromes that were characteristic for certain patients with epilepsy, and indeed at times had subtle seizures themselves (1,2), it was logical to treat patients presenting with epilepsy and psychiatric complications by an identical pharmacologic method. Carbamazepine or valproate, enhanced if necessary with a modest amount of an antidepressant drug or with lithium, proved to be effective for the full range of psychiatric disorders associated with epilepsy—not only for depressive and labile moods but also for anxiety, irritability, and even for the schizophrenia-like syndromes presenting with paranoid, delusional, and/or hallucinatory symptoms (2,3).

As co-medication to the anticonvulsant, most tricyclic antidepressants are prescribed at a dose of 75–125 mg at bedtime. We prefer to start with imipramine, but it may be best to first prescribe desipramine if a patient lacks energy and has no problem with insomnia. Desipramine has the least anticholinergic side effects among the tricyclic antidepressants and tends to be activating, but it may sometimes interfere with the sleep and should therefore be best prescribed at 25 mg three times daily, with increases added to the early doses. A marked insomnia may require the prescription of a sedative drug (75–125 mg of either amitriptyline or doxepine) at bedtime. Trazodone tends to be less effective, but monoamine oxidase (MAO) inhibitors (phenelzine or tranylcypromine) may be alternative adjuncts to the anticonvulsant drugs in some cases. Lithium is an alternative adjunct when the antidepressants have not been effective. Again, a low therapeutic blood level is required in combination with the anticonvulsant drug.

A lowering of the seizure threshold with the prescription of modest doses of a tricyclic antidepressant is very rarely of clinical significance. The seizure threshold appears to be merely affected upon rapid introduction of the drug and by doses of over 200 mg daily (29).

Illustrative Cases

Case 1

This 29-year-old housewife had been somewhat anxious and easily depressed from an early age on. In her teens she had suffered from headaches and intermittent left shoulder pain, and she also experienced episodes of feeling hot, nauseated, and faint, accompanied by perspiring and getting flushed in the face. At age 20 she experienced the first of three generalized tonic–clonic seizures, which were always preceded by a strange thought in her head. The diagnosis of epilepsy was now made in spite of negative EEGs. Following the birth of her first child, she was very depressed; 3 years later, at age 25, following the birth of her second child, she had to be hospitalized for a severe depression. She remained on an antidepressant (trazodone) and on anticonvulsant polytherapy.

When seen, she was anxious and mildly depressed. She experienced an average of three complex partial seizures per week, consisting of a fear, a funny feeling in the stomach, and tingling all over her body; her husband observed her staring and smacking her lips. She was taking phenytoin, carbamazepine, valproate, and trazodone. Phenytoin was the only anticonvulsant in therapeutic range. During brief hospitalization, an EEG after 24 hours of sleep deprivation showed a right temporal paroxysmal focus; monotherapy with carbamazepine was established and the antidepressant was discontinued. With carbamazepine at therapeutic range, she has remained emotionally stable, has not required an antidepressant drug, and has only occasional auras without any loss of consciousness.

Comment. After belated diagnosis of epilepsy, this patient was treated with inappropriate anticonvulsant polypharmacy. Her anxiety and occasional severe depression may have been controlled from early on if she had been treated with carbamazepine at the time of onset of her simple partial seizures of temporal lobe origin. She may need the addition of an antidepressant at a later time, but she is presently doing well on carbamazepine monotherapy.

Case 2

This 26-year-old single female, a clerk in a drugstore, had suffered a linear skull fracture with a period of unconsciousness at the age of 18 months. At age 13 she began to have absences, with gradually increasing frequency. An EEG at age 13 showed left anterior temporal sharp waves and generalized bursts of 5-per-second spike-and-waves on hyperventilation. She was treated with a variety of anticonvulsants, without achieving seizure control. Phenytoin had been prescribed fairly persistently over the years, and recently valproate had been added. She still had nocturnal seizures.

She had a problem with her temper since the age of 2 or 3 years, and over the last few years her mother had become afraid of her because of her rages. She attended church regularly and read the Bible daily, yet she was prone to explode in a rage over minor matters at home, did not help around the house, and was in jeopardy of losing her job because she was sometimes very brusque with customers. She experienced rapid mood shifts and was often listless and depressed.

A repeat EEG revealed generalized spike-and-wave and polyspike bursts. The phenytoin was discontinued, and monotherapy with valproate was established. She made a complete turnaround: Her seizures, her temper, and moodiness ceased and she became congenial at home and at work. A small amount of norpramine had been initially prescribed with the valproate, because of the severity of her behavior problem, but had to be discontinued after a couple of days because of a skin rash; the norpramine was obviously not needed.

Comment. Correct diagnosis of the primary generalized seizure disorder led to the choice of valproate. This case again demonstrates the effectiveness of monotherapy with a psychotropic anticonvulsant for a marked emotional disorder.

Case 3

A 35-year-old housewife and writer had experienced a few seizures between the ages of 1 and 4. During a certain week in her seventh grade of schooling she became unable to concentrate steadily. She began to experience, for brief moments, a recurrent cosmic–spiritual sensation that exerted a magnetic fascination. She learned only later that she was nicknamed "Spacey" by her schoolmates because she would often not respond when spoken to. By the tenth grade, bad days began to alternate with good days. Despite her intelligence, she began to fail in school. When sent to a boarding school, she became increasingly depressed and made a suicide attempt. She attempted college but soon dropped out, and then she entered a psychiatric hospital for a prolonged stay and was in psychotherapy over a few years. She began to work; then, aided by an antidepressant drug (imipramine), she was able to resume college with success. She married and had two children. Prior to her first pregnancy she stopped the antidepressant.

After her first pregnancy, at age 24, she suffered the first of a few generalized seizures, preceded by a smell and a sense of déjà vu, and epilepsy was diagnosed. She didn't like to take anticonvulsants, since phenytoin made her depressed and carbamazepine didn't control her attacks. An understanding husband, her strong spiritual orientation, and an angry defiance against being judged insane pulled her through her persistent emotional difficulties—episodic depressions, anxiety attacks, and a marked postmenstrual irritability.

One year before she was first seen she had been advised to resume carbamazepine, and at therapeutic levels her seizures were controlled. However, she had become recently so depressed that she was unable to work. Her emotions were very intense and labile; she was often very angry and explosive, or fearful to the point of paranoid sensitivity. Though highly intelligent, she tended to get bogged down with little details. Upon the addition of 100 and then 150 mg of imipramine daily to the carbamazepine, she made an excellent recovery. With the exception of some feelings of depression for a couple of days subsequent to her menses, she has remained emotionally stable and successful in her career. She feels "liberated."

Comment. This young woman's epilepsy was diagnosed after a delay of 10 years once she suffered a major seizure. She presented with a labile depression and a characteristic admixture of various emotional changes—anxiety, anger, paranoid sensitivity—and responded when an antidepressant was added to the carbamazepine. An early diagnosis and proper treatment of the epilepsy could have made a marked difference in the life of this woman over the preceding 20 years.

Case 4

A 37-year-old housewife had experienced a total of five generalized tonic–clonic seizures over the past 4 years. She also experienced, a few times each month, peculiar episodes of feeling dizzy, like floating, with everything around her getting bigger, and she would get weird jerks from her feet and goose flesh. Thereafter she would feel cloudy and weak for a moment and would sleep for 2 hours. At times she would briefly get a cloudy sensation and would feel like she was leaving her body.

Emotional problems had become increasingly prominent over the past 2 years: She was persistently depressed, with a marked depression lasting for days until it would lift for a couple of days; furthermore, she suffered from episodes of feeling mean and angry, had lost her sexual desire, had frequent headaches and insomnia, and was forgetful. Her active and outgoing lifestyle had become one of isolation, and she was fearful of leaving the house; moreover, after having been very neat her entire life, she had become somewhat sloppy. Phenytoin, prescribed at high doses over the past couple of years together with diazepam, had merely resulted in excessive sleepiness. After her medications were replaced by carbamazepine with the addition of imipramine (75 mg) at bedtime, she felt bright, less depressed, and calmer. She continued to have frequent simple partial seizures and myoclonic jerks during her sleep, and she required higher doses of carbamazepine and finally the addition of 1 mg of clonazepam at bedtime. After 11 months of treatment, the following changes were reported: She was greatly improved, with depressive moods reduced to few hours at a time; her irritability had ceased and she again felt affectionate toward her husband; she had become active and outgoing again; her headaches and insomnia were gone.

Comment. This patient improved initially upon treatment with carbamazepine and an antidepressant, but she only made a substantial recovery once the anticonvulsant medication was sufficiently raised. She had been constantly encouraged to overcome her phobic state, and this support may well have facilitated the recovery.

Case 5

Ten years ago, this 64-year-old business executive began to suffer from occasional vague complaints consisting of sudden dizziness, headaches, and numbness. Neurologic findings were absent, but an abnormal EEG with left temporal sharp activity was discovered, and he was treated with various anticonvulsants. Four years ago he began to suffer from increasing forgetfulness. His memory impairment increased, and he would repeat himself at work. A diagnosis of dementia was made, and he had to give up his business. Upon careful review of his condition, it was evident that he suffered from frequent flurries of complex partial seizures with staring, lip smacking, and swallowing as often as six times daily. Repeat seizures were followed by marked confusion and amnesia, and improvement of his organic mental impairment would follow, until the next series of seizures. He was, in fact, unable to take care of more than routine matters, and his family suffered the agony of awaiting gradual further deterioration.

Once the relationship of his frequent complex partial seizures with the memory impairment was recognized, a course of treatment with carbamazepine was begun. He tolerated only a small amount of carbamazepine because of dry mouth and urinary hesitation. At 50 mg of carbamazepine three times daily, a blood level of 4.2 was measured. However, his recovery was prompt and complete. He was seizure-free, reported an excellent memory, felt "reborn," and resumed an active lifestyle.

Comment. In this patient the presence of seizures was suspected, but their impact was not appreciated. A severe memory impairment is more likely to be associated with temporal lobe seizures in the elderly.

Case 6

A 12-year-old girl had experienced febrile convulsions at 17 months of age, followed by isolated generalized tonic–clonic seizures at ages 6, 7, and 9, for which she was treated with phenytoin.

Six months prior to our evaluation she developed (a) unexplained episodes of marked fear, (b) increasing irritability, and (c) a severe lability of moods. When hallucinations occurred, she was hospitalized and treated unsuccessfully with antipsychotic drugs. Her condition fluctuated markedly but did not remit. The diagnoses of schizoaffective disorder or borderline personality were entertained during 3 months of psychiatric hospitalization, and the parents were given a bleak prognosis for the girl's future. When the mother observed recurrent episodes of chewing motions during a confusional state lasting for 2½ days, she insisted on a transfer to an epilepsy center.

Prolonged electroencephalographic monitoring was negative; however, in view of the characteristic history, the diagnosis of temporal lobe syndrome was made and she was promptly treated with carbamazepine. Upon the addition of 50 mg of imipramine, her emotional disorder remitted completely and she was able to return to school after 2 weeks of evaluation and treatment. Her disposition has become gentle and even-tempered; in fact, it is now better than it had been for years preceding the acute emotional illness.

Comment. Patients with psychiatric disorders of psychotic proportions may require inpatient treatment in a specialized center. In this case, the presence of a seizure disorder was known, but its role in producing a characteristic and severe atypical, variable, and pleomorphic psychiatric disorder was first only suspected by the mother.

PSEUDOSEIZURES

Two monographs provide valuable information on the topic of pseudoseizures (30,31). We summarize here the more recent findings and relate our own experience with this difficult topic.

Definition

The term "pseudoseizures" refers to paroxysmal episodes for which an epileptic origin was suggested but can be ruled out. The terms "hysterical seizures" or "psychogenic seizures" are often used as synonyms for "pseudoseizures" but suggest an origin of the attacks which is too narrow or too vague, respectively. We prefer the term "pseudoseizures," since we do not clearly understand the more precise nature of the events. Certain cardiovascular episodes, as well as transient cerebral ischemia, inner ear disturbances, and hypoglycemic episodes, though sometimes classified as "seizures" in a broad use of the term, have an identifiable somatic origin other than epilepsy and are usually not referred to as "pseudoseizures." Similarly, panic attacks represent a well-defined psychiatric disorder with prolonged duration and maintained consciousness, and they are not termed "pseudoseizures." Seizures that are consciously faked for a specific purpose appear to be rare nowadays; the seizure skillfully executed by Thomas Mann's Felix Krull, before the draft board of the Imperial German Army, is an illustrious example of a factitious seizure.

Prevalence

Pseudoseizures are frequently encountered and occur more often among females. One study has shown that 22% of patients treated for epilepsy actually had nonepileptic seizures (32). It has been suggested that 5–36% of patients with pseudoseizures also have true epileptic attacks (33). *For proper diagnosis, patients with possible pseudoseizures may have to be referred to a center where intensive simultaneous monitoring with closed-circuit television and electroencephalography can be carried out* (see also Chapter 3).

The study of patients after implantation of subdural strip electrodes revealed that a majority of the same patients in whom previously partial seizures without changes on scalp EEG had been recorded showed now restricted discharges from within basal limbic structures associated with similar episodes (34). This finding casts doubt on the prevalence figures for pseudoseizures and for the combined diagnosis of epileptic and pseudoepileptic seizures, as far as complex partial seizures are concerned.

The diagnosis of generalized tonic–clonic seizures versus pseudoseizures can be usually clarified, because both the clinical presentation and the ictal EEG are usually revealing. The recognition of true complex partial seizures, on the other hand, tends to be more difficult. The two diagnostic problems are therefore discussed separately.

Diagnosis of Generalized Tonic–Clonic Seizures

Recognition of the nature of a generalized tonic–clonic attack is of particular importance if a patient seems to present with threatening status. With increased antiepileptic medication, pseudoseizures may become more frequent and may subside with detoxification from the drugs (35).

The stereotyped nature of the generalized epileptic tonic–clonic seizure and the uncoordinated motor activity of pseudoseizures permit a differential diagnosis in a majority of the cases. Incontinence or self-injury are often absent in genuine seizures and may occasionally occur in pseudoseizures. The following observations have been listed as characteristic for pseudoseizures (36): out-of-phase upper-extremity movements and out-of-phase lower-extremity movements; no vocalization or vocalization at the start of the event (in genuine generalized seizures the vocalization tends to occur in the middle of the seizure); pelvic forward thrusting; lack of total body rigidity; turning of the head from side to side (in genuine seizures the head is likely to turn to one side); absence of staring; duration of the seizure beyond 2 minutes (genuine generalized tonic–clonic seizures show a tight distribution of duration, ranging from 50 to 90 seconds).

Intensive video/EEG monitoring for recording of an attack may be necessary. The ictal and postictal EEG will show (a) significant changes with generalized tonic–clonic seizures of epileptic nature and (b) absence of any significant changes with pseudoseizures.

Diagnosis of Complex Partial Seizures

Complex partial seizures are peculiar and highly individual events. They may present with a wide variety of subjective events (aura) and subsequent observable events for which the patient has no memory. In a given patient, the events tend to reoccur in a stereotyped fashion with each seizure, lasting for less than 90 seconds, and are usually followed by a more prolonged and less stereotyped period of confusion, during which there may be increasing interaction with the environment; amnesia may extend beyond the confusional state. Although a characteristic complex partial seizure can be well recognized, this type of seizure tends to lead to misdiagnosis. Pseudoseizures may also present in a rather stereotyped pattern. Desai et al. (37) determined the diagnosis of pseudoseizures by the assessment of four criteria: (i) deviation of seizures from characteristics of known seizure types; (ii) absence of epileptiform activity in the ictal EEG; (iii) absence of slowing in the postictal EEG; and (iv) relation of seizure frequency to decreasing plasma concentrations of antiepileptic drugs. They concluded that no single criterion was sufficient for an unequivocal diagnosis.

Wyler et al. (34) have documented the presence of true complex partial seizures in nine of 15 patients who had carried the diagnosis of pseudoseizures and underwent long-term video/EEG monitoring after implantation of subdural electrodes. All patients previously had normal scalp EEGs recorded during their attacks. It is generally agreed, though not widely known, that the ictal activity of a complex partial seizure can escape detection when monitored with sophisticated procedures such as prolonged video/EEG monitoring with scalp electrodes or the less reliable procedure of 24-hr ambulatory cassette recording. The difficulty of documenting frontal lobe seizures by scalp EEG monitoring has been emphasized by Williamson et al. (38).

Of diagnostic value is a comparison between (a) the serum prolactin level obtained within 20 minutes after a generalized tonic–clonic or complex partial seizure and (b) the patient's baseline level (39). Significant increases are indicative of a genuine seizure. The provocation of a seizure (and its termination) by injection of saline with appropriate suggestions will only be successful with a pseudoseizure.

Psychological Aspects

The psychiatric status of patients with pseudoseizures is not clarified by the existing literature. Gumnit and Gates (40) divided 65 patients discharged with a diagnosis of psychogenic seizures into five subgroups: (i) psychological distress; (ii) inappropriate coping mechanisms; (iii) misinterpretation of normal physiological stimuli; (iv) psychotic behavior; and (v) a true aura or seizure followed by a psychogenic seizure. Wilkus et al. (41) compared 25 patients with pseudoseizures to 25 patients with epilepsy and reported an MMPI pattern like that frequently seen in conversion hysteria (Hs and Hy elevated and higher than D) for the pseudoseizure group and exactly the reverse for the epilepsy group, allowing a correct classification of 80–90% of the cases by MMPI rules alone. Both groups exhibited evidence for brain damage or impairment of brain functions by neurologic history; on neuropsychologic testing, this evidence was exhibited at an equally high frequency. This finding confirmed earlier reports of the presence of organicity in patients with pseudoseizures, and it pointed at a handicap for their adaptive abilities.

Our own experience supports the finding that a mild degree of organicity may be often present in patients with pseudoseizures (34). We have been further impressed by the similarity of many patients with pseudoseizures to patients who are prone to somatize. They may present with chronic pain in addition to the pseudoseizures, and, like chronic-pain patients, they may present a stoic facade and show little ability to verbalize emotional conflicts, which are denied and somatized. Other patients may be highly emotional, with labile moods and irritability, and may indeed present the traits of the temporal lobe syndrome in the absence of any genuine seizures.

The frequent finding of early sexual abuse among patients with pseudoseizures is undoubtedly of significance, and it needs to be addressed in the treatment (42).

Treatment

The results of treatment of patients with pseudoseizures are not well known. Ramani et al. (43) reported on the treatment efforts in nine patients with epilepsy and pseudoseizures; the results were satisfactory for most of the patients at a 4-year follow-up. Gumnit and Gates (40) reported on the 2-year follow-up of an initial group of 32 of their 65 patients with psychogenic seizures: 63% became seizure-free, and an additional 18% were greatly improved. They noted that brief treatment was often very effective in patients who simply had a misinterpretation problem or an inappropriate coping mechanism, whereas treatment of patients with deep-seated emotional conflicts tended to be time-consuming and frustrating.

If a patient is found to have pseudoseizures, it needs to be explained that he/she does not have epilepsy but that, nevertheless, there is a reason for the spells, that stress appears to play a significant role, and that proper treatment is available. Ideally, the treatment should be carried out by the evaluating psychiatrist who will have some experience with this often difficult group of patients.

Pseudoseizures may be symptoms of a depressive somatization disorder, and the patient may show signs of masked depression—a stoic comportment with lack of energy, insomnia, inability to enjoy life, aches, and pains. For such a patient the use of antidepressants with psychotherapy is indicated. For the contrasting group of patients with pseudoseizures who tend to be highly emotional and present with traits of a temporal lobe syndrome, we may continue the prescription of an anticonvulsant with psychotropic properties (carbamazepine or valproate), with the clear specification that the drug is not employed for epileptic seizures. As with any patient with a temporal lobe syndrome, the antiepileptic drug may have to be combined with an antidepressant drug (or with lithium), at a modest dose.

CONCLUSION

For many practicing physicians, there appears to be a remarkable difficulty in recognizing epilepsy. Perhaps one-fifth of the patients diagnosed as being epileptic may not have a true seizure disorder, and as many as one-fourth of all individuals with epilepsy remain undiagnosed because of the subtle and subjective nature of their seizures. The problem appears to be compounded by a failure to refer patients with pseudoseizures or difficult diagnostic problems to an epilepsy center. Many physicians evidently are not aware of the resources available to them for the clinical assessment of seizure disorders.

The psychiatric aspects of epilepsy are still widely ignored. Recognition of the characteristic atypical, variable, and pleomorphic psychopathology that may be associated with certain forms of epilepsy (temporal lobe epilepsy in particular) is essential because this paroxysmal neurobehavioral syndrome ("temporal lobe syndrome") requires specific treatment. The treatment consists, whenever possible, of antiepileptic drug monotherapy with a psychotropic agent (carbamazepine or valproate), aided if necessary by the addition of a modest amount of antidepressant drug or of lithium.

The pharmacologic treatment is identical for the various manifestations of the paroxysmal neurobehavioral syndrome—mood changes, excessive temper, anxiety, suicidal impulses, and psychotic manifestations. Psychiatric treatment of the patients as if they had a mental disorder independent of epilepsy results in ineffective treatment.

REFERENCES

1. Himmelhoch JM. Major mood disorders related to epileptic changes. In: Blumer D, ed. *Psychiatric aspects of epilepsy*. Washington, DC: APA Press, 1984;271–294.
2. Blumer D, Heilbronn M, Himmelhoch J. Indications for carbamazepine in mental illness: atypical psychiatric disorder or temporal lobe syndrome? *Compr Psychiatry* 1988;29:108–122.
3. Blumer D, Zielinski JJ. Pharmacologic treatment of psychiatric disorders associated with epilepsy. *J Epilepsy* 1988;1:135–150.
4. Bear DM, Fedio P. Quantitative analysis of interictal behavior in temporal lobe epilepsy. *Arch Neurol* 1977;43:454–467.
5. Blumer D, Benson DF. Psychiatric manifestations of epilepsy. In: Benson DF, Blumer D, eds. *Psychiatric aspects of neurologic disease*, vol 2. New York: Grune & Stratton, 1982;25–48.
6. Gastaut H. Interpretation of the symptoms of psychomotor epilepsy in relation to physiological data on rhinencephalic function. *Epilepsia* 1954;3:84–88.
7. Waxman SA, Geschwind N. The interictal behavior syndrome of temporal lobe epilepsy. *Arch Gen Psychiatry* 1975;32:1580–1586.
8. Bear DM, Freeman R, Greenberg M. Behavioral alterations in patients with temporal lobe epilepsy. In: Blumer D, ed. *Psychiatric aspects of epilepsy*. Washington, DC: APA Press, 1984;197–228.
9. Mendez MF, Cummings JL, Benson DF. Depression in epilepsy. *Arch Neurol* 1986;43:766–770.
10. Betts TA. A follow-up study of a cohort of patients with epilepsy admitted to psychiatric care in an English city. In: Harris P, Maudsley C, eds. *Epilepsy: proceedings of Hans Berger centenary symposium*. Edinburgh: Churchill Livingstone, 1974:326–338.
11. Robertson MM, Trimble MR. Depressive illness in patients with epilepsy: a review. *Epilepsia* 1983;22:515–524.
12. Zielinski JJ. Epilepsy and mortality rates and causes of death. *Epilepsia* 1974;15:191–201.
13. Matthew WS, Barabas G. Suicide and epilepsy: a review of literature. *Psychosomatics* 1981;22:515–524.
14. Currie S, Heathfield KWG, Henson RA, Scott DF. Clinical course and prognosis of temporal lobe epilepsy: a survey of 666 cases. *Brain* 1971;94:173–190.
15. Betts TA. Depression, anxiety and epilepsy. In: Reynolds EH, Trimble MM, eds. *Epilepsy and psychiatry*. Edinburgh: Churchill Livingstone, 1981;60–71.

16. Trimble MR, Perez MM. Quantification of psychopathology in adult patients with epilepsy. In: Kulig BM, Meinardi H, Stores G, eds. *Epilepsy and behavior '79*. Lisse: Swets and Zeitlinger, 1980;118–126.
17. Gudmundsson G. Epilepsy in Iceland: a clinical and epidemiological investigation. *Acta Neurol Scand* 1966;25(Suppl 43):1–124.
18. Slater E, Beard AW. The schizophrenia-like psychoses of epilepsy. *Br J Psychiatry* 1963;109:95–150.
19. Masland RL. Commission for the control of epilepsy. *Neurology* 1978;28:861–862.
20. Temkin O. *The falling sickness*. Baltimore: The Johns Hopkins Press, 1971.
21. Trimble MR. Anticonvulsant drugs: mood and cognitive function. In: Trimble MR, Reynolds EH, eds. *Epilepsy, behavior and cognitive function*. New York: John Wiley & Sons, 1987;135–143.
22. Blumer D. The psychiatric dimension of epilepsy: historical perspective and current significance. In: Blumer D, ed. *Psychiatric aspects of epilepsy*. Washington, DC: APA Press, 1984;1–65.
23. Zielinski JJ. People with epilepsy who do not attend doctors. In: Janz D, ed. *Epileptology, Proceedings of the seventh international symposium on epilepsy*. Stuttgart: Georg Thieme, 1976;18–23.
24. Zielinski JJ. Epileptics not in treatment. *Epilepsia* 1974;15:203–210.
25. Lorgé VM. Klinische Erfahrungen mit einem neuen Antiepilepticum Tegretol (G 32 883), mit besonderer Wirkung auf die epileptische Wesensveränderung. *Schweiz Med Wochenschr* 1963; 93:1–16.
26. Dalby MA. Antiepileptic and psychotropic effect of carbamazepine (Tegretol) in the treatment of psychomotor epilepsy. *Epilepsia* 1971;12:325–334.
27. Post RM, Uhde TW. Carbamazepine in psychiatric disorders. *Psychopharmacol Bull* 1985;21:10–17.
28. McElroy SL, Pope HG Jr. *Use of anticonvulsants in psychiatry: recent advances*. Clifton, NJ: Oxford Health Care, Inc., 1988.
29. Dessain EC, Schatzberg AF, Woods BT, Cole JO. Maprotiline treatment in depression: a perspective on seizures. *Arch Gen Psychiatry* 1986;43:86–90.
30. Riley TL, Roy A, eds. *Pseudoseizures*. Baltimore: Williams & Wilkins, 1982.
31. Gross M, ed. *Pseudoepilepsy*. Lexington, MA: Lexington Books, 1983.
32. Mattson RH. Value of intensive monitoring. In: Wada JA, Penry JK, eds. *Advances in epileptology: the Xth Epilepsy International Symposium*. New York: Raven Press, 1980;43–51.
33. Ramani V. Intensive monitoring of psychogenic seizures, aggression, and dyscontrol syndromes. In: Gumnit RJ, ed. *Advances in neurology*, vol 46: *intensive neurodiagnostic monitoring*. New York: Raven Press, 1986;203–217.
34. Wyler AR, Hermann BP, Blumer D, Richey ET. Pseudoseizures. Submitted for publication, 1989.
35. Niedermeyer E, Blumer D, Holscher E, Walker BA. Classical hysterical seizures facilitated by anticonvulsant toxicity. *Psychiatr Clin* 1970;3:71–84.
36. Gates JR, Ramani V, Whalen S, Loewenson R. Ictal characteristics of pseudoseizures. *Arch Neurol* 1985;42:1183–1187.
37. Desai B, Porter RJ, Penry JK. Psychogenic seizures: a study of 42 attacks in six patients, with intensive monitoring. *Arch Neurol* 1982;39:202–209.
38. Williamson PD, Spencer DD, Spencer SS, Novelly RA, Mattson RH. Complex partial seizures of frontal lobe origin. *Ann Neurol* 1985;18:497–504.
39. Dana-Haeri J, Trimble MR, Oxley J. Prolactin and gonadotrophin changes following generalized and partial seizures. *J Neurol Neurosurg Psychiatry* 1983;46:331–335.
40. Gumnit RJ, Gates JR. Psychogenic seizures. *Epilepsia* 1986;27(Suppl 2):S124–S129.
41. Wilkus RJ, Dodrill CB, Thompson PM. Intensive EEG monitoring and psychological studies in patients with pseudoseizures. *Epilepsia* 1984;25:100–107.
42. Gross M. Hysterical seizures: a sequel of incest. In: Gross M, ed. *Pseudoepilepsy*. Lexington, MA: Lexington Books, 1983;119–128.
43. Ramani SV, Quesney LF, Olson D, Gumnit RJ. Diagnosis of hysterical seizures in epileptic patients. *Am J Psychiatry* 1980;137:705–709.

Epilepsy: Current Approaches to Diagnosis and Treatment,
edited by Dennis B. Smith,
Raven Press, Ltd., New York © 1990.

12

Epilepsy and Aggression

David M. Treiman

Neurology and Research Services,
West Los Angeles VA Medical Center, and
Department of Neurology, UCLA School of Medicine,
Los Angeles, California 90073

> Whenever a murder has been committed suddenly, without premeditation, without malice, without motive, openly and in a way quite different from the way in which murders are commonly done, we ought to look carefully for evidence of previous epilepsy. . . .
>
> Maudsley, 1873 (1)

As the quotation above indicates, there has been a long-standing assumption of a relationship between epilepsy and violent and aggressive acts, particularly in the psychiatric literature. This attitude has persisted so that even modern psychiatric texts make statements with regard to complex partial epilepsy such as ". . . clinically the clouded state suggests a delirium with liberation of aggressive and occasionally self-destructive impulses. Acts of violence may be committed in the automatisms and may be of a strikingly brutal nature, the patient pursuing his crime to a most revolting extreme" (2). Such attitudes are sufficiently pervasive in the psychiatric and general medical community that a common reaction of most non-neurological physicians is to refer any patient who exhibits episodic violent behavior for a neurological consultation and for an evaluation for possible complex partial epilepsy.

These attitudes are held widely by members of the lay population as well and have led to the frequent use of the "epilepsy defense" by attorneys defending individuals accused of violent and aggressive crimes. The resultant publicity associated with the use of such a defense has had the unfortunate result of reinforcing the negative stereotype and social stigmata suffered by people who have epilepsy. This, in turn, has led to an effort by the Epilepsy Foundation of America and others involved in the care and treatment of patients with epilepsy to resist consideration of the possibility of a relationship between violence and epilepsy. Although a number of the studies that suggest the presence of interictal behavioral disturbances in patients with epilepsy have been seriously flawed, and thus have been strongly criticized because of their potential to exacerbate the social stigmata of having epilepsy, Engel et al. (3) have suggested that to deny that such a relationship might exist may result in failure to search for a preventable or treatable cause of considerable disability among patients with epilepsy. Engel et al. have thus suggested careful and cautious study of the neurobiology of possible interictal behavioral disorders in patients with epilepsy. Such an approach can be focused on the specific question of whether or not there is a relationship between epilepsy and violence or aggressive behavior.

The remainder of this chapter will be devoted to a consideration of a relationship between epilepsy and aggression in four areas: (i) What is the neurobiology of aggression, particularly as ascertained from animal studies? (ii) Is there any evidence of a relationship between epilepsy and violence from clinical studies? Specifically, is epilepsy more common in violent and aggressive individuals, and is violence or aggressive behavior more common in epileptics? (iii) What is the differential diagnosis of episodic violence? (iv) How should individuals who have episodes of violent behavior be evaluated?

NEUROBIOLOGY OF VIOLENCE

The neurobiology of violence and aggression has been extensively studied in both experimental animals and in humans. In 1973 a workshop was held at the National Institute of Neurological Diseases and Stroke on the biomedical research aspects of brain and aggressive violent behavior. That conference was divided into four workshops: (i) neuroanatomical and neurophysiological studies, (ii) neurochemical and pharmacological and genetics studies, (iii) behavioral studies, and (iv) clinical studies. A detailed report of the results of the conference was published by Goldstein in 1974 (4) and is summarized below.

The consensus of the conference was that derangements of behavior predominately involve brain structures rostral to the rhombencephalon, particularly the limbic lobe and limbic system including the hypothalamus. The reticular and raphe systems as well as nigrostriatal systems may also be physiologic substrates for aggressive behavior.

Two general types of aggressive behavior have been investigated in animal models utilizing a variety of neurochemical and pharmacological studies: affective aggression and predatory aggression. "Affective aggression" refers to the aggressive behavior seen in several animal models in which a change in the apparent affect of the experimental animal is also seen associated with the aggressive behavior. Affective aggression includes sham rage behavior in cats, aggression induced by foot shock in rats, isolation-induced aggression in mice, and the spontaneous aggression seen in a number of experimental animals following the administration of drugs or the placement of cerebral lesions. The term "predatory aggression" is applied to behavioral models such as the mouse-, frog-, or turtle-killing behavior of rats and the quiet biting attack of cats. Such behaviors tend to be highly stereotyped and are not associated with increased irritability or other behavioral changes in the animals at the time of the attacks or shortly before.

Norepinephrine appears to facilitate the expression of affective aggression and sometimes may trigger it, whereas the same transmitter appears to inhibit predatory aggression. On the other hand, cholinergic mechanisms appear to be primarily involved in facilitating or triggering predatory aggression. Acetylcholine may also facilitate affective aggression. Dopamine appears to act like norepinephrine in that it facilitates affective aggression and inhibits predatory aggression, whereas serotonin is probably inhibitory for both classes of aggression.

Although it has been possible to elicit several different kinds of stereotypic aggressive behavior in the animal models described above, utilizing a variety of different ablation, stimulation, and pharmacological procedures, *none of these models exhibit behavior that approximates the behavior of animals or humans undergoing an epileptic seizure.* A common feature of most types of epileptic seizures (with the exception of a brief absence seizure seen in petit mal epilepsy) is a progression through a predictable and stereotyped sequence of behavioral events. In addition, most models of aggressive behavior require some kind of exogenous stimulus to elicit a rage reaction. Thus in general it can be said that at present there is no evidence from animal models that directed aggression may occur as an initial behavioral manifestation of an epileptic seizure. Postictal aggression has been observed in some animal models of epileptic seizures, just as "resistive" violence is sometimes seen in humans during the period of reactive automatisms or of postictal confusion following a complex partial or generalized tonic–clonic seizure. Such postictal behavioral disturbances, when they are violent, consist of nondirected violence and are probably best explained, as least in humans, as a Todd's phenomenon in which there is a transient postictal paralysis of frontal lobe function. Engel et al. (3) have suggested that such postictal automatisms most likely reflect behaviors released from higher cortical control. Pinel et al. (5) have reported nondirected reactive biting following amygdaloid kindling in rats. Such reactive biting rarely occurs spontaneously, but it is easily provoked during the postictal phase by touching or rough handling (6).

Griffith et al. (3) have recently described an experimental model for limbic-epilepsy-induced disturbances in interictal defensive reactivity. In this model, epileptic seizures are produced in cats by microinjection of kainic acid into the dorsal hippocampus. This induces an acute phase lasting 2–3 days characterized by recurrent partial onset seizures, some of which secondarily generalize. Between seizures, during this acute phase, the cats demonstrate an exaggerated defensive rage response to mild threat or handling. Spontaneous seizures cease after 2–3 days and are followed by a latent period of several weeks during which time the cats exhibit normal behavior. After several weeks, spontaneous seizures reoccur at irregular and widespread intervals; once they return, however, the cats again become difficult to handle and display exaggerated defensive responses to mild threat. No epileptiform electroencephalographic (EEG) changes are observed in the amygdala or middle to lower hippocampus associated with the exaggerated defensive responses. Thus Engel et al. (3) have suggested that such behavior is interictal and that this enhanced defensive rage in cats should be viewed as epilepsy-induced alteration in affective display rather than as an ictal phenomenon. Although a number of animal models should prove useful in studying the neurobiology of violence and aggression, thus far none have exhibited aggressive behavior associated with a definitely ictal epileptiform event. Clearly, more research is needed regarding the neurobiology of violence and aggression and of the relationship, if any, to epilepsy.

EPILEPSY AND VIOLENCE: IS THERE A RELATIONSHIP?

We need now to consider the question of whether there is a relationship between epilepsy and violence and aggressive behavior. This question can be addressed in three ways: (i) Is epilepsy more common among violent and aggressive people? (ii) Are violence and aggression more common among people with epilepsy? If so, are these behaviors ictal or interictal? (iii) Does ictal violence occur? Can epileptic automatisms be organized such that they result in acts of directed aggression? If so, can such acts be precipitated by external stimuli?

There are two ways to address the question of whether epilepsy occurs more frequently in criminals and violent people. The first is to look for evidence of epilepsy in EEG studies of such persons. The second and more direct way is to look at the incidence of epilepsy among prisoners, specifically those identified as perpetrators of violent crimes.

EEG Studies

Between 1949 and 1969, four EEG studies of murderers or other criminally aggressive individuals were published in Great Britain (7–10). All of these studies were marred by the inclusion of benign variants such as 14- and 6-per-second positive spike bursts, small sharp spikes, and rhythmic midtemporal bursts of drowsiness ("psychomotor variant") as abnormal patterns. Although such patterns have been considered abnormal in the past and have been reported more frequently in children with behavioral problems than in normal controls, most electroencephalographers now view them as variant patterns that have no specific diagnostic implications (11) (see also Chapter 2).

The best EEG study of violent individuals is that of Riley and Niedermeyer (12). These investigators studied 229 electroencephalograms in 212 patients who had been referred specifically because of episodes of violence, recurrent aggressive behavior, destructive behavior, or outbursts of anger without provocation. Fourteen of the 212 (6.6%) patients had minimally or slightly abnormal electroencephalograms. None of the abnormalities were epileptiform, and the percentage of patients with abnormalities and the type of abnormalities seen were similar to those observed in samples of the normal population. These authors concluded that there was no EEG evidence for an increased incidence of epilepsy in nonincarcerated patients who had been referred specifically because of episodic violent behavior.

Prevalence of Epilepsy in Prisoners

For the last 20 years, Gunn (13) has carried out a series of studies of epilepsy in the British prison system which have been detailed in a monograph. Gunn summarized the results of a number of previous studies that demonstrated a two- to fourfold increase in prevalence of epilepsy in prisoners compared with the normal population of Great Britain. Many of these studies had suggested a higher prevalence of epilepsy in young offenders, especially violent offenders. To verify these observations, Gunn and Bonn (14) carried out two census surveys. The first examined receptions to all prisons and borstals in England and Wales during the month of November 1966. The second was a review of all epileptic residents at the same institutions on the night of December 13, 1966. During the 1-month survey of admissions, a total of 5096 men were incarcerated; 46 of these prisoners were epileptic, a prevalence rate of 9/1000. Of the 46, eight (17%) were committed for acts of violence, compared with 11% of the nonepileptics sentenced. This difference was not statistically significant. Furthermore, there were no differences between the epileptic and non-epileptic populations in any of the categories of offenses for which the men were convicted. The prevalence rate for epilepsy in the prison population was twice the 4.5/1000 figure reported for Great Britain in a survey of the College of General Practitioners (15).

A number of American studies have investigated the prevalence of epilepsy in various prison populations. Prisoners in New York City (16), in North Carolina (17), and in Illinois (18) all have been found to have a prevalence of epilepsy of 1.8–1.9%. This rate is more than three times the prevalence of 0.59% found by Hauser and Kurland (19) in their comprehensive survey of the Rochester, Minnesota, population.

One of the problems in prevalence studies of seizure disorders is defining what constitutes epilepsy. Differences in the criteria used for diagnosis and the method of data collection can result in both under- and overestimates of prevalence. King and Young (18), in their study of epilepsy in Illinois prisoners, used prescription rates for antiepileptic medication as the basis for the diagnosis of epilepsy in their review of 12,030 prisoners. In order to ascertain the validity of this estimate of prevalence rates, members of the same research group, in a follow-up study, investigated the prevalence of epilepsy in the Illinois prison system by carrying out a detailed medical examination of all of the men alleged to have epilepsy of the 3652 men who entered the system from September 1980 through February 1981 (20). Each suspected case was evaluated by both an internist and a neurologist. Based on their detailed examinations, these investigators reported a 2.4% prevalence of epilepsy in the Illinois prison system. In this population there was no greater prevalence of epilepsy among those convicted of serious crimes, and there was no greater prevalence of serious crimes among the epileptic prisoners when compared to age- and race-matched control prisoners or crimes. Rather, the two- to fourfold increase in prevalence of epilepsy among incarcerated individuals most likely reflects a prevalence of epilepsy among economically deprived urban populations rather than an increased frequency of criminal activity among epileptics. A higher incidence of head trauma may also account for the greater prevalence of epilepsy in the prison population.

VIOLENCE IN PEOPLE WITH EPILEPSY

Interictal Violence

A number of studies have reported an increased prevalence of violent and aggressive behavior in patients with epilepsy. Most of these studies have concentrated on selected small populations of patients with severe intractable seizure disorders and thus do not reflect the prevalence of violence in the general epilepsy population. Ounsted (21), working at Park Hospital for Children in Oxford, evaluated 100 children with temporal lobe epilepsy. Thirty-six had outbursts of "catastrophic rage." Most of the children with rage outbursts suffered their first seizures early in life, had low intelligence, and exhibited hyperkinetic behavior. Children who had no evidence of neurological dysfunction other than temporal lobe epilepsy did not exhibit violent behavior or catastrophic rage.

Similar results have been published in three separate reports of adults with intractable temporal lobe epilepsy who underwent temporal lobectomies at the Maudsley Hospital in London. James (22) reviewed 72 patients and found 20 of them to have shown aggression. Serafetinides (23), who studied the first 100 patients in that series and thus overlapped James' review, found 36 patients with aggressive behavior. Most of the aggressive patients were men who had onset of seizures before the age of 10. Taylor (24) studied another 100 patients who partially overlapped with the series reported by Serafetinides. He considered 27 of them to be aggressive. Although James, Serafetinides, and Taylor used different operational definitions of aggression, they each concluded that roughly one-third of the patients exhibited aggressive behavior. In this highly selected sample of intractable temporal lobe epileptics with severe psychiatric symptoms, the patients who were considered violent or aggressive shared common characteristics with the violent children at Park Hospital. Aggression tended to occur with epilepsy that had its origin in childhood or adolescence; it also tended to occur more frequently in men as well as in patients of low intelligence who required institutionalization.

Rodin (25) conducted a similar survey of 700 patients with epilepsy from the Lafayette Clinic and Epilepsy Center in Michigan. In this group of unselected, noninstitutionalized epileptics, 34 patients (4.9%) were coded as "destructive–assaultive" during their initial evaluation. Young men with below-average intelligence had more behavioral and psychiatric problems, poorer employment records, and more evidence of organic brain disease on neurological examination than did a control group matched for age, sex, and intelligence.

Rodin (25) found no relationship between seizure type and violence, and he specifically found no increase in the prevalence of violence or aggression in patients with temporal lobe epilepsy. Currie et al. (26) studied 666 patients who had temporal lobe epilepsy seen at the London hospital between 1949 and 1967 and found 7% to have exhibited an aggressive effect on mental status examination. However, there was no documentation of aggressive behavior on the part of these patients. When patients with neurological deficits (27,28) or with I.Q.s below 70 (29,30) have been excluded, no relationship between temporal lobe epilepsy and aggressive acts has been found. Juul-Jensen (31) found no greater predilection for violent behavior in patients with temporal lobe epilepsy than in patients with other types of epilepsy in a survey of 1020 unselected adult patients followed in an outpatient clinic.

Several studies of aggressive personality traits have been carried out in epileptics using a variety of psychological tests. Hermann et al. (32) compared 153 patients with temporal lobe epilepsy and 79 with generalized epilepsy on measures of aggression from the Minnesota Multiphasic Personality Inventory. Analysis of covariance indicated that seizure type was not related to aggression. The same population was studied by Hermann and Riel (33) using the "TLE personality scales" developed by Bear and Fedio (34). Neither anger nor aggression differed as a function of seizure type. Whitman et al. (35) found no difference between 35 children with temporal lobe epilepsy and 48 children with primary generalized epilepsy in terms of standardized measures of social competence, aggression, and overall behavior disorder. On the basis of standardized neuropsychological tests, Hermann (36) classified 50 children with epilepsy into two groups: good neurological functioning and poor neurological functioning. He found significantly more aggression, overall psychopathology, and less overall social competence in the poorly functioning group. He concluded that aggressive behavioral traits were related to other neuropsychological deficits and not to seizure type.

The aforementioned studies have dealt with the occurrence of interictal violent behavior or aggressive personality traits in epileptics. Many of the studies have been biased toward severe intractable forms of epilepsy and have been carried out in groups of patients with a high incidence of concomitant psychiatric symptoms and neurological deficits. A common finding is that interictal violence tends to occur in young men with low I.Q.s and with a history of early and severe epilepsy who also have associated neurological deficits. When unselected populations of patients with epilepsy are studied, there is no increased prevalence of violent behavior. When patients with severe psychiatric disorders, low I.Q., or other neurological deficits have been removed from series of patients with temporal lobe epilepsy, there is no increased prevalence of violence. Thus, the evidence to date does not point to an increased prevalence of violent behavior in patients with epilepsy in general and temporal lobe epilepsy in particular. All the violent and aggressive personality traits that occur in such groups can be accounted for by other neurological and psychiatric deficits.

Ictal Violence

The question of whether or not violence can occur as an ictal manifestation is of particular importance because of the increased frequency with which epilepsy has been used as part of the "diminished legal responsibility" and "insanity" defenses for crimes of violence, particularly in the United States. Because of this approach to legal defense, it is essential to try to establish, on the basis of objective data, whether violence or aggression can occur as a part of an epileptic seizure and to determine appropriate criteria for the use of the epilepsy defense if violence or aggression does occur under such circumstances.

Two lines of inquiry may help address the question of ictal violence. The first is to consider each individual case thus far reported in which an act of violence is alleged to have been due to an epileptic seizure. The second is to review the behavioral characteristics associated with complex partial seizures and to analyze the nature of violence or aggression that might possibly occur during an epileptic attack.

HISTORICAL ACCOUNTS OF VIOLENCE ALLEGEDLY DUE TO A SEIZURE

Review of the Medical Literature

Treiman and Delgado-Escueta (37) published a detailed review of 29 cases reported in the medical literature from 1872 to 1981 in which violent events were reported to be due to a seizure. Table 1 summarizes a number of features of these cases. In only three of these cases was the evidence strongly suggestive of a relationship between ictal epileptic attacks and violent automatisms. East, in a 1927 textbook of forensic psychiatry (38), described two cases of violent behavior which might have been associated with a seizure. In the first case, a 20-year-old man strangled his pregnant wife while in bed with her. He attempted suicide afterwards and had no memory of the event. In the other case, two policemen and an ambulance attendant were involved in a struggle with a patient who was seen to have had a seizure shortly beforehand but who continued to be antagonistic on examination, long after the seizure. Gunn and Fenton (39) collected 17 cases of epileptic prisoners who experienced a seizure within 12 hours of their crime. In only one of these was the violence clearly related to a seizure. The patient was a 32-year-old man who developed generalized tonic–clonic seizures at the age of 18. At age 20 he had a generalized tonic–clonic seizure early in the morning while staying at his girlfriend's house. While still in a postictal and confused state, he violently attacked a man who lived in the house, and then he subsequently attacked his girlfriend and the man's wife. On admission to the hospital shortly thereafter, he was mentally confused and amnesic for all events. He was sent to Broadmoor Hospital for the Criminally Insane. Thereafter, he had a generalized tonic–clonic seizure every 1–2 years during which he would become perplexed, frightened, and, if restrained in any way, dangerously aggressive.

The last two cases are both examples of "resistive violence" in which attempts to restrain patients still in a postictal confusional state produced violent reactive automatisms and amnesia. Knox (40) reviewed 43 cases of patients who had episodes of automatic behavior during their seizures. Six exhibited resistive automatisms. However, none showed directed violence or aggression toward other objects or individuals unless they were restrained at the end of the seizure. One patient, a 50-year-old man with a well-documented 5-year history of complex partial epilepsy, had several episodes of resistive automatisms while under observation. During these episodes

TABLE 1. *Summary of 29 reported cases of violence allegedly due to a seizure: medical literature*

20 of 29:	Diagnosis of epilepsy before event
3 of 21:	Premeditated
9 of 15:	Provoked
3 of 25:	Associated with alcohol
13 of 17:	Amnesia for event
7 of 13:	Definite epileptiform EEG abnormality
8 of 21:	Convicted
11 of 21:	Committed
2 of 21:	Acquitted

he would stagger about, but if anyone attempted to assist him he would shout "leave me alone!" On one occasion he caught an orderly by the throat, held him for several minutes, and yelled "I'll kill you." He kicked the doctor on another occasion. He frequently exhibited primitive postictal aggressive behavior when restrained or assisted at the end of an epileptic attack. If he had an attack at work, his colleagues knew not to approach him: "It seems I don't attack them if I am not touched."

In each of these cases, nondirected aggressive or violent behavior has occurred in response to restraint at the end of an unequivocal generalized tonic–clonic seizure at a time when the patient was still confused. It would appear that most, if not all, ictal violence that has been observed in patients or legal defendants is "resistive violence" that occurs at the end of an unequivocal stereotypical seizure. The phenomenon of "resistive violence" had been observed in experimental animal seizure models. It is probable that such resistive violence occurs as a result of differential recovery of functional areas of the brain such that there is a relative delay in the recovery of frontal lobe function compared with the recovery of pure motor functions. Thus a patient may act with a primitive lack of restraint or disinhibition similar to that of an individual whose social restraint is compromised by alcohol or other centrally active drugs.

Review of the Legal Literature

Treiman (41) has recently provided details of the 75 crimes of violence where epilepsy has been used as a defense that have been reviewed in the appellate literature from federal and state courts in the United States.

In 56 of 72 cases the diagnosis of epilepsy had been made before the crime, although in most cases not by an epileptologist or even a neurologist. EEG data were rarely provided. Nine cases occurred before the availability of the clinical electroencephalogram. Of the remaining 66 cases, EEG data were cited in 23 reports. Only eight of these 23, however, demonstrated a definite epileptiform EEG abnormality. In six other cases, the electroencephalogram was said to be abnormal, but the nature of the abnormality was not specified. In only 12 of 50 cases was there any evidence for amnesia for the criminal event, and in many of these cases there had also been heavy consumption of alcohol around the time of the crime. In some of the cases the only evidence for amnesia was the defendant's subjective claim that he could not remember the events in question. In 27 of 57 cases where this information was available, the defendant has been drinking heavily when the crime was committed. In 26 of 60 cases the crime was premeditated and planned beforehand. In 36 of 57 cases the violent episode was provoked by anger. Forty-five of the cases involved first- or second-degree murder. In 11 cases the defendant was charged with manslaughter, and four were the result of vehicular manslaughter. In the 14 cases that did not result in death of the victim, 10 involved various degrees of assault and battery. There were two cases of attempted murder and one each of kidnapping, arson, and disorderly conduct. In only one of the 75 cases was an epilepsy defense used successfully, and in this case (Matter of Torsney) there was no evidence that the defendant actually had epilepsy.

EPILEPTIC AUTOMATISMS AND ICTAL VIOLENCE

Although, as outlined above, there have been a number of reports in the medical literature and in the appellate legal literature of violent events that allegedly were the result of ictal automatisms, most of these cases are poorly documented. However, there have been several studies that have attempted to evaluate a possible relationship between epileptic seizures and violence and to answer the question of whether or not directed aggression can be a manifestation of an ictal event.

One of the first studies was done by Rodin (25). Between 1959 and 1964 most epileptic patients admitted to the Lafayette Clinic had a seizure induced in the EEG laboratory using bemegride as part of their routine evaluation. The seizure was recorded on the electroencephalogram, and the behavior of the patient was photographed using equipment that advanced the film automatically after each exposure. Photographs were satisfactory in 150 patients, 57 of whom had complex partial seizures. None of the patients exhibited significant violent or aggressive behavior. King and Ajmone-Marsan (42) directly observed a minimum of six complex partial seizures in each of 199 patients with EEG temporal lobe foci. Nine exhibited violent ictal behavior on one or more occasions. Seven of these nine showed resistive violence during the immediate postictal period at the end of the seizure; one had episodes of beating on her chest, and one picked up objects and threw them during automatic behavior. In none of these patients was interictal violence confirmed in the hospital. Delgado-Escueta et al. (43,44) recorded 691 complex partial seizures on CCTV–EEG in 79 patients. Seven exhibited resistive violence while fighting restraints. Three had stereotyped automatic motions such as thrashing and flailing of arms and kicking of legs. Six walked or ran away during the early part of the seizures and knocked down objects or tried to break open a door as part of the ambulatory automatism. None exhibited directed aggression.

Two studies have directly addressed the question of whether violence may occur in association with complex partial seizures. Ramani and Gumnit (45) selected 19 patients with a history of episodic aggressive behavior for intensive behavioral and electrophysiological monitoring for an average of 6 weeks. Ictal episodes were recorded on CCTV in 15 of the patients. None of them showed directed aggression during their seizures, but one exhibited nondirected resistive aggressive behavior postictally. Two of the patients exhibited repetitive aggressive behavior, not thought to be ictal, on the ward.

The most comprehensive study to address the question of whether crimes of violence can be committed during epileptic attacks was reported by Delgado-Escueta et al. (46). Physicians from 16 epilepsy programs in the United States, Canada, Germany, and Japan reviewed CCTV-EEG recording of approximately 5400 patients with epilepsy who had been studied in their laboratories. From this pool they selected 19 patients who exhibited aggressive behavior during recorded seizures. A total of 33 attacks were identified as possibly showing violent behavior. A panel of 18 epileptologists then convened in a workshop to review the case histories and the CCTV–EEG recordings of this group. The panel thought that a clinical diagnosis of epilepsy was incontestable in 13 of these 19 patients. Five of these 13 patients have been described in greater detail in individual reports (47–49).

The panel agreed on the definition of violence: the directed exertion of extreme and aggressive physical force that, if unrestrained, would result in injury, destruction, or abuse. A rating score of 0–6 was used to analyze the degree of violence in each recorded seizure. A rating of 0 represented no violence or aggressive behavior, 1 represented no directed aggressive behavior, 2 represented violence to property, 3 denoted threatening violence to a person, 4 denoted mild actual violence to a person, 5 represented moderate violence to a person, and 6 indicated severe violence to a person such as the use of physical force that resulted in serious injury or death. On the basis of this rating scale, six of the patients exhibited minimal or no aggression. The remaining seven patients exhibited violent ictal behavior that was rated 2–4. In most cases, spontaneous nondirected stereotyped aggressive movements, violence to property, shouting or spitting at persons, and mild to moderate violence toward another person were observed during the height of epileptogenic paroxysms. Nondirected aggression was observed at the end of a complex partial seizure in one case and after a tonic-clonic seizure in two patients. In these two patients, aggression appeared to be a reaction to being helped or restrained. All aggressive behavior rated 2–4 on the scale occurred during complex partial seizures. Amnesia for aggressive acts was present in all cases. The acts of aggression usually occurred at the beginning of a seizure and lasted an average of 29 seconds, whereas complete complex partial seizures lasted an average of 145 seconds in this series. Aggressive acts were stereotyped, simple, unsustained, and never supported by a consecutive series of purposeful movements.

DIFFERENTIAL DIAGNOSIS

The evidence from the studies discussed in the previous section suggests that directed aggression is unlikely to occur as an ictal manifestation, particularly not at the beginning of a complex partial seizure. Violence and aggressive behavior that does occur at the time of an ictal event is most likely to be nondirected "resistive" violence while the patient is exhibiting reactive automatisms or is in a postictal confusional state at the end of a complex partial or generalized tonic-clonic seizure. Before considering the details of the procedures that should be carried out in the evaluation of a patient who is alleged to have exhibited a violent ictal event, it would be worthwhile to consider other conditions that may give rise to episodic violent events that could be confused with an epileptic seizure.

EPISODIC DISCONTROL SYNDROME

"Episodic discontrol syndrome" is a term applied to a behavioral disorder in which there are paroxysmal outbursts of violence and rage of a magnitude far in excess of that of the precipitating stimulus. Frequently, there is an alleged loss of contact with the environment during the outbursts. Following the outbursts, the patient may exhibit remorse and may express feelings of depression and fatigue or need to sleep. Many of the features of the syndrome were described first by Karl Menninger (50), and the term "episodic discontrol syndrome" was first used by Monroe in a monograph published in 1970 (51). Subsequently, a number of other investigators have published studies of episodic discontrol syndrome (52–58). Four types of behavior have been included in the syndrome: (i) physical assault, especially wife and child beating; (ii) pathologic intoxication resulting in senseless violence; (iii) impulsive sexual behavior including sexual assaults; and (iv) a history of many traffic violations and serious automobile accidents (4).

A number of authors have suggested that episodic discontrol syndrome represents a type of complex partial seizure. However, the violent outbursts are almost always provoked, although the provoking stimulus is frequently so mild as to be discounted by the examining physician unless specifically sought while evaluating the patient's history. There have been no reports of such violent outbursts in these patients associated with ictal changes on the electroencephalogram even though a number of these patients have been studied on epilepsy monitoring units. The behavioral sequence observed in violent rage reactions is not that which has been described by Delgado-Escueta and colleagues for complex partial seizures (43,44).

Patients with episodic discontrol syndrome frequently tend to have a history of past head injuries, childhood seizure disorders, electroencephalogram with nonspecific abnormalities, and a variety of "soft" neurological signs. They may have evidence of frontal lobe dysfunction. Such patients appear to lack the capacity to sustain the normal inhibition of violent impulses which is exhibited by most of the population. It is likely that their poor impulse control is related to structural or (in the case of pathological intoxication) metabolic abnormalities, particularly of frontal lobe function, which impair the patients' impulse control so that minor provoking stimuli induce a violent reaction.

POSTICTAL PSYCHOSIS

Some patients, particularly those with medically intractable seizures, may exhibit a transient psychosis after a prolonged cluster of seizures or status epilepticus. This phenomenon is most frequently seen after a period of frequent repetitive complex partial seizures and may represent an impairment of normal function of the limbic system. The patient may become floridly psychotic, may experience hallucinations, and may be capable of directed aggression as may occur in other forms of psychosis. However, such aggressive acts are not ictal events but appear to be due to altered psychological function in which the patient has a marked impairment of his/her contact with reality. As mentioned above in the section on neurobiology, Engel et al. (59) have recently described an animal model in cats in which, during the interictal period between frequent seizures, kainic-acid-kindled cats become difficult to handle and display exaggerated defensive responses to mild threat. This model may be useful for the study of aggression or violence associated with postictal psychosis following frequent complex partial seizures.

DIAGNOSIS

Because of the continuing belief by many physicians that there is a proven relationship between epilepsy and violence, epileptologists are frequently called on to evaluate patients with paroxysmal episodes of behavioral outbursts for the possibility that such outbursts represent complex partial epilepsy. Most patients referred for such an evaluation do not have complex partial seizures. Such patients probably have a form of episodic discontrol syndrome. This diagnosis can be made on the basis of a detailed history and close observation of the patient during a violent outburst. Particular attention should be paid to the search for possible precipitating events even when such provocations seem trivial to the examiner. The fundamental characteristic of episodic discontrol syndrome is that the behavior represents a pathological behavioral response to a minor provoking stimulus.

The behavioral characteristics of complex partial seizures are now well understood. Delgado-Escueta and his colleagues (43,44,60) have suggested that complex partial seizures can be divided into three distinct electroclinical types. The first and most common type, which is now thought to be of hippocampal or hippocampal–amygdalar origin, has three predictable clinical phases. These consist of an initial motionless stare followed by stereotyped oral–alimentary automatisms (lip smacking, swallowing, mastication), followed by reactive quasipurposeful automatisms during periods of impaired consciousness. Type II seizures have no stare but start with complex quasipurposeful motor automatisms that tend to be characterized by movements of the extremities (such as flailing, bicycling movements of the legs, or karate-like movements) and sometimes by ambulatory behavior. Type II seizures are now thought to be extratemporal in origin (61). Type III complex partial seizures, what Caffi (62) originally termed "temporal lobe syncope," consist of drop attacks during which the patient remains flaccid and totally unresponsive for 2–3 minutes. The flaccid phase is then followed by a period of reactive automatisms which usually lasts several minutes before full recovery. All of the complex partial seizures thus far studied by Delgado-Escueta and his group have exhibited the characteristics of one of these three seizure types. Thus, to the extent that these observations can be extended to all patients with complex partial seizures, it can be concluded that if ictal violence does occur as part of a complex partial seizure it must occur in the context of one of these observed patterns of behavior. Furthermore, because patients are totally unresponsive during the stereotyped automatism phase of complex partial seizures, it is unlikely that organized and directed aggression, especially aggression involving complex acts, can truly be part of a complex partial seizure. Clearly, a paroxysmal behavioral change should not be called a complex partial seizure unless the pattern of behavior is fully consistent with modern concepts of the natural history and patterns of complex partial seizures.

What then should be the criteria for determining whether a violent crime was a result of an epileptic seizure? The 18 epileptologists who participated in the International Workshop of Aggression and Epilepsy suggested five relevant criteria for consideration (46): (i) The diagnosis of epilepsy should be established by at least one neurologist with special competence in epilepsy. (ii) The presence of epileptic automatisms should be documented by the case history and CCTV–EEG. (iii) The presence of aggression during epileptic automatisms should be verified by a video-recorded seizure in which ictal epileptiform patterns are also recorded on the electroencephalogram. (iv) The aggressive or violent act should be characteristic of the patient's habitual seizures as elicited in the history. (v) A clinical judgment should be made by the neurologist attesting to the possibility that the act was part of a seizure.

Epilepsy should not be used as a defense for interictal violence, even if the defendant has a well-documented history of epileptic seizures. Although a number of studies suggest that violence may occur more frequently in epileptics than in control populations, this is probably due to associated brain lesions or to adverse social factors rather than to the epilepsy directly. Although epilepsy and violence may occur in the same individual and share common etiologies, one does not necessarily cause the other. Therefore, even well-documented epilepsy should not be considered in the defense of criminal aggression unless the aggressive episode indeed occurred during an unequivocal epileptic seizure with characteristics such as those outlined above.

ACKNOWLEDGMENT

This chapter was based, in part, on an address entitled "Epilepsy and Violence: Medical and Legal Issues," presented at the Fifth Annual Merritt–Putnam Symposium, December 5, 1985, and published in *Epilepsia* 1986;27(Suppl 2):S77–S104.

REFERENCES

1. Maudsley H. *Body and mind*. London: Macmillan, 1873.
2. Kolb LC, Brodie HKH. *Modern clinical psychiatry*, 10th ed. Philadelphia: WB Saunders, 1982.
3. Griffith N, Engel J, Jr, Bandler R. Ictal and enduring interictal disturbances in emotional behaviour in an animal model of temporal lobe epilepsy. *Brain Res* 1987;400:360–364.
4. Goldstein M. Brain research and violent behavior. *Arch Neurol* 1974;30:1–26.
5. Pinel JPJ, Terit D, Rovner LI. Temporal lobe aggression in rats. *Science* 1977;197:1088–1089.
6. Caldecott-Hazard S, Ackermann RF, Engel R Jr. Opioid involvement in postictal and interictal changes in behavior. In: Morselli PL, Lloyd K, Quesney LF, Engel J Jr, eds. *Neurotransmitters in seizures and epilepsy III*. New York: Raven Press, 1984;305–314.
7. Stafford-Clarke D, Taylor FH. Clinical and electroencephalographic studies of prisoners charged with murder. *J Neurol Neurosurg Psychiatry* 1949;12:325–330.
8. Hill D, Pond DA. Reflections on 100 capital cases submitted to EEG. *J Ment Sci* 1952;98:23–43.
9. Hodge R, Walter V, Walter W. Juvenile delinquency: an electrophysiological, psychological and social study. *Br J Delinq* 1953:155–173.
10. Williams D. Neural factors related to habitual aggression: consideration of differences between those habitual aggressives and others who have committed crimes of violence. *Brain* 1969;92:503–520.
11. Pedley TA. EEG patterns that mimic epileptiform discharges but have no association with seizures. In: Henry CE, ed. *Current clinical neurophysiology*. Amsterdam: Elsevier/North-Holland, 1980; 307–336.
12. Riley T, Niedermeyer E. Rage attacks and episodic violent behaviour: electroencephalographic findings and general consideration. *Clin Electroencephalogr* 1978;9:113–139.
13. Gunn J. *Epileptics in prison*. London: Academic Press, 1977.
14. Gunn J, Bonn J. Criminality and violence in epileptic prisoners. *Br J Psychiatry* 1971;118:337–343.
15. College of General Practitioners. A survey of the epileptics in general practice. *Br Med J* 1960; ii:416–422.
16. Novick LF, Penna RD, Schwartz MS, Remmlinger E, Loewenstein R. Health status of the New York City prison population. *Med Care* 1977;15:205–216.
17. *Epilepsy in North Carolina: resources and recommendations*. Raleigh, NC: Chronic Disease Branch, Department of Human Resources, 1977.
18. King LM, Young QD. Increased prevalence of seizure disorders among prisoners. *JAMA* 1978;239:2674–2675.
19. Hauser WA, Kurland LT. The epidemiology of epilepsy in Rochester, Minnesota, 1935 through 1967. *Epilepsia* 1975;16:1–66.
20. Whitman S, Coleman TE, Patmon C, Desai BT, Cohen R, King LN. Epilepsy in prison: elevated prevalence and no relationship to violence. *Neurology* 1984;141:651–656.
21. Ounsted C. Aggression and epilepsy rage in children with temporal lobe epilepsy. *J Psychosom Res* 1969;13:237–242.
22. James IP. Temporal lobectomy for psychomotor epilepsy. *J Ment Sci* 1960;106:543–558.
23. Serafetinides EA. Aggressiveness in temporal lobe epileptics and its relations to cerebral dysfunction and environmental factors. *Epilepsia* 1965;6:33–42.
24. Taylor DC. Aggression and epilepsy. *J Psychosom Res* 1969;13:229–236.
25. Rodin EA. Psychomotor epilepsy and aggressive behaviour. *Arch Gen Psychiatry* 1973;28:210–213.
26. Currie S, Heathfield KWG, Henson RA, Scott DF. Clinical course and prognosis of temporal lobe epilepsy. *Brain* 1971;94:173–190.
27. Guerrant J, Anderson WW, Fischer A, Weinstein MR, Jaros RM, Deskins A. *Personality in epilepsy*. Springfield, IL: Charles C Thomas, 1962.
28. Mignone RJ, Donnelley EF, Sadowsky D. Psychological and neurological comparisons of psychomotor and non psychomotor epileptic patients. *Epilepsia* 1970;11:345–359.
29. Small JG, Milstein V, Stevens J. Are psychomotor epileptics different? *Arch Neurol* 1962;7:187–194.
30. Small JG, Small IF, Hayden MP. Further psychiatric investigations of patients with temporal and non-temporal lobe epilepsy. *Am J Psychiatry* 1966;123:303–310.
31. Juul-Jensen P. Epilepsy: a clinical and social analysis of 1020 adult patients with epileptic seizures. *Acta Neurol Scand* 1964;5(Suppl):S1–136.

32. Hermann BP, Schwartz MS, Whitman S, Karnes WE. Aggression and epilepsy: seizure type comparisons and high risk variables. *Epilepsia* 1980;22:691–698.
33. Hermann BP, Riel P. Interictal personality and behavioral traits in temporal lobe and primary generalized epilepsy. *Cortex* 1981;17:125–128.
34. Bear DM, Fedio P. Quantitative analysis of interictal behavior in temporal lobe epilepsy. *Arch Neurol* 1977;34:454–467.
35. Whitman S, Hermann BP, Black RB, Chhabria S. Psychopathology and seizure type in children with epilepsy. *Psychol Med* 1982;12:843–854.
36. Hermann BP. Neuropsychological functioning and psychopathology in children with epilepsy. *Epilepsia* 1982;23:545–554.
37. Treiman DM, Delgado-Escueta AV. Violence and epilepsy: a critical review. In: Pedley TA, Meldrum BS, eds. *Recent advances in epilepsy*, vol 1. London: Churchill Livingstone, 1983;179–209.
38. East WN. *An introduction to forensic psychiatry in the criminal courts*. New York: Williams Wood, 1927.
39. Gunn J, Fenton G. Epilepsy, automatism and crime. *Lancet* 1971;1:1173–1176.
40. Knox SJ. Epileptic automatism and violence. *Med Sci Law* 1968;8:96–104.
41. Treiman DM. Epilepsy and violence: medical and legal issues. *Epilepsia* 1986;27(Suppl 2):S77–S104.
42. King DW, Ajmone-Marsan C. Clinical features and ictal patterns in epileptic patients with EEG temporal lobe foci. *Ann Neurol* 1977;2:138–147.
43. Delgado-Escueta AV, Kunze U, Waddell G, Boxley J, Nadel A. Lapse of consciousness and automatisms in temporal lobe epilepsy: a videotape analysis. *Neurology* 1977;27:144–155.
44. Delgado-Escueta AV, Bascal FE, Treiman DM. Complex partial seizures on closed-circuit television and EEG: a study of 691 attacks in 79 patients. *Ann Neurol* 1982;11:292–300.
45. Ramani V, Gumnit RJ. Intensive monitoring of epileptic patients with a history of episodic aggression. *Arch Neurol* 1981;38:570–571.
46. Delgado-Escueta AV, Mattson RH, King L, et al. Special report. The nature of aggression during epileptic seizures. *N Engl J Med* 1981;305:711–716.
47. Saint-Hilaire JM, Gilbert M, Bouvier G, Barbeau A. Epilepsy and aggression: two cases with depth electrode studies. In: Robb P, ed. *Epilepsy updated: causes and treatment*. Miami, FL: Symposia Specialists, 1980;145–176.
48. Ashford JW, Schulz SC, Walsh GO. Violent automatism in a partial complex partial seizure. Report of a case. *Arch Neurol* 1980;37:120–122.
49. Treiman DM, Delgado-Escueta AV. Aggression during fear and flight in complex partial seizures: a CCTV–EEG analysis. *Epilepsia* 1981;22:243.
50. Menninger K. *The vital balance*. New York: Viking Press, 1963.
51. Monroe RQ. *Episodic behavioral disorder: a psychodynamic and neurophysiological analysis*. Cambridge, MA: Harvard University Press, 1970.
52. Bach-y-Rita, Lion JR, Climent CE, et al. Episodic dyscontrol: a study of 130 violent patients. *Am J Psychiatry* 1971;127:1473–1478.
53. Lion JR, Bach-y-Rita G, Ervin FR. The self-referred violent patient. *JAMA* 1968;205:503–505.
54. Lion JR, et al. Teaching the violent to recognize themselves. *JAMA* 1968;206:2221–2222.
55. Lion JR, Bach-y-Rita G, Ervin FR. Violent patients in the emergency room. *Am J Psychiatry* 1969;125:1706–1711.
56. Lion JR, Bach-y-Rita G. Group psychotherapy with violent outpatients. *Int J Group Psychother* 1970;20:185–191.
57. Lion JR. *Evaluation and management of the violent patient*. Springfield, IL: Charles C Thomas, 1972.
58. Elliott FA. The episodic dyscontrol syndrome and aggression. *Neurol Clin* 1984;2(1):113–125.
59. Engel J Jr, Caldecott-Hazard S, Bandler R. Neurobiology of behavior: anatomic and physiological implications related to epilepsy. *Epilepsia* 1986;27(Suppl 2):S3–S13.
60. Delgado-Escueta AV, Walsh GO. Type I complex partial seizures of hippocampal origin: excellent results of anterior temporal lobectomy. *Neurology* 1985;35:143–154.
61. Walsh GO, Delgado-Escueta AV. Type II complex partial seizures: poor results of anterior temporal lobectomy. *Neurology* 1984;34:1–13.
62. Caffi J. Zur Frage Klinischer Anfallformen bie psychomotorischer Epilepsie. *Schweiz Med Wochenschr* 1973;103:469–475.

Epilepsy: Current Approaches to Diagnosis and Treatment,
edited by Dennis B. Smith,
Raven Press, Ltd., New York © 1990.

13

Epilepsy

A Molecular and Cellular View

J. Kim Harris and Robert J. DeLorenzo

*Department of Neurology, Medical College of Virginia,
Richmond, Virginia 23298*

Epilepsy is clinically defined as recurrent seizures produced by paroxysmal neuronal discharges. Many conditions are known to cause epilepsy, but the cellular mechanisms underlying the excessive neuronal activity associated with seizures and epilepsy are only beginning to be clarified (1,2). The pace of investigation in this area is rapid and is accelerating. No single approach through pharmacologic, biochemical, biophysical, or anatomical research appears completely adequate to elucidate the causes of the excessive neuronal behavior underlying epileptic disorders. Nonetheless, highlighting several of the classical recent significant scientific advances in basic neuronal behavior related to epilepsy is a valuable way to understand a molecular view of epilepsy and is also helpful in determining how advances in molecular and cellular biology affect the development of new diagnostic and therapeutic approaches to epilepsy. Although it is not possible to cover all the advances in molecular neurobiology that relate to the regulation of neuronal excitability, several major areas have reached the stage where they can provide a clearer understanding of some of the clinical phenomena that are observed in seizure disorders.

The following research and basic neurobiologic topics and their relationship to clinical problems in epilepsy will be discussed in this chapter: (a) neuronal ion channels and seizure activity; (b) synaptic modulation and neurotransmitter effects in epilepsy; (c) functional anatomy of epilepsy; and (d) research models of epilepsy.

NEURONAL ION CHANNELS

The molecular mechanisms underlying epilepsy are complex. A thorough study of neuronal excitability requires a systematic examination of many separate cell functions. Medical and ethical limitations of using patients or human tissue have led to the use of animal models and simpler neuronal networks in vertebrate and invertebrate preparations. Cellular observations in these simpler systems have allowed the characterization of specific molecular events that can be extrapolated to neuronal behavior in humans.

In these experimental systems, membrane electrical properties and ion currents have been studied by use of voltage-clamp techniques and the more recently developed patch-clamp techniques (3–5). These elaborate biophysical techniques have allowed characterization of several neurotransmitter-dependent and voltage-dependent ion channels in a variety of experimental systems that relate to epilepsy.

VOLTAGE- AND PATCH-CLAMP RECORDING

Although many biochemical techniques are used to study ion channels, the voltage- and patch-clamp methods are particularly well suited to study the electrochemical responsiveness of membrane ion channels. The voltage-clamp technique monitors whole-cell transmembrane voltage and allows the ionic current effects on this voltage to be interrupted. This is accomplished by applying an outside voltage potential to the cell membrane through microelectrodes. This technique "clamps" the cell's transmembrane voltage to an experimentally desired level (5). When a cell is voltage-clamped, voltage-sensitive channels open or close, depending on the transmembrane potential. Varying ion concentrations in the bathing medium or selective use of channel-blocking agents allows dissection of the individually acting channels.

Patch-clamp techniques are an advance on the voltage-clamp methodology. Single, transmembrane ion channels are isolated by a glass micropipet. These micropipets are fire-drawn from glass tubing and have extremely fine internal conductive diameters that form highly resistant seals against membranes of living cells or isolated pieces of membrane (3). By suction manipulations, an isolated membrane patch can be removed from cells and then placed into test solutions. By altering the method of membrane patch preparation, the patch can be presented with either the cytosolic side to the test solution ("inside-out patch") or the extracellular side to the test solution ("outside-out patch"). This technique is very useful in observing single-channel opening and closing behavior in a variety of experimental paradigms.

Experiments using the voltage- and patch-clamp techniques as electrophysiological tools, coupled with mathematical–computer modeling, have significantly advanced our understanding of the behavior of specific ion channels. Further characterization of cell and membrane behavior may lead to keener insights into channel functions and the role they play in epilepsy.

SPECIFIC MEMBRANE ION CURRENTS

The specific ions that contribute to the major membrane currents in neurons are sodium (Na), potassium (K), calcium (Ca), and chloride (Cl) (4). The voltage potential (or transmembrane potential) of the cell depends on different ion concentra-

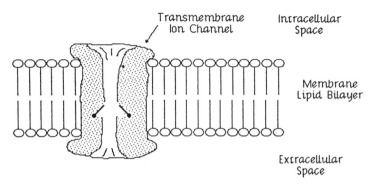

FIG. 1. Schematic model of a transmembrane ion channel forming an aqueous pore that is gated by voltage or other neurochemical mechanisms.

tions on each side of the cell membrane. Many mechanisms control or modulate the gating channels that govern ion movement into and out of the cell (5). Reviewing selected research findings concerning the function of these channels provides some insight into mechanisms underlying excitability in neurons. A schematic model of a transmembrane ion channel is shown in Figure 1.

Sodium Channels

Voltage-dependent Na^+ channels are a major site for Na^+ entry into cells. Molecular neurobiologists have obtained a detailed understanding of the Na^+ channel. The major channel protein has been identified, purified, and even sequenced for amino acid composition (6). Na^+ ions are responsible for the generation of the rapid depolarization of the action potential as described by Hodgkin and Huxley (7). A major portion of the action potential is created by the passage of Na^+ through specific channels in axonal membrane. Na^+ channels are located in neuronal cell bodies and synaptic areas as well, but in these locations, their opening and closing behavior is less well characterized than in the axon (8).

Recent advances characterizing the Na^+ channel involve identification and purification of the major channel protein (6), the elucidation of the Na^+ channel subunit–structural characteristics (6), and the influence of anticonvulsant drugs (such as phenytoin) on some aspects of channel activity (9).

Na^+ channels are glycoproteins that form an aqueous pore as they span across the membrane. There are two separate sites within the molecular substructure where voltage-dependent gating functions occur. Voltage affects these sites separately in altering channel-opening or channel-closing (5). Isolated Na^+ channels are estimated to measure $40\,\text{Å} \times 170\,\text{Å}$ and have an approximate molecular weight of 260–300 kilodaltons (kd). Ionic-channel biophysical characteristics appear to play a key role in limiting other cation passage through this channel.

Phenytoin (PHT), an anticonvulsant, affects Na^+ channels. It has been proposed that one mechanism of action of PHT is to block the Na^+ channel. This channel-inhibitory effect is quite complex. In contrast to the effects of tetrodotoxin (TTX), an irreversible Na^+-channel blocker, PHT exerts a cumulative and depressive, yet reversible, action on the Na^+ spike mechanism during repeated firing of the neuron. This channel inhibition is related to the use and firing frequency of the channel (9). PHT is thought to filter out sustained, high-frequency neuronal bursting. This cellular effect is probably partly responsible for the anticonvulsant property of PHT. This type of Na^+-channel modulation may limit interneuronal spread of cellular, electrical bursting behavior and diminish the clinical expression of epilepsy (9).

Isolation and purification of Na^+-channel proteins in several species demonstrates a copurifying phosphate donor identified as thiamine phosphate (11). In a recently developed experimental system, the major component of the Na^+ channel is associated with phosphate derivatives of thiamine (11). This protein is also identified as the major TTX-binding site (11). Phosphorylation of the protein has been studied in this system, and it demonstrates alterations in the presence of TTX, PHT, veratridine, and local anesthetics. These agents are all known to modulate or block the Na^+ channel itself. TTX and veratridine have different effects on the configuration of the Na^+ channel. Both inhibit channel protein phosphorylation, and it is proposed that channel activity is modulated by the net state of protein phosphorylation (12). Thus, by various means, regulation of Na^+ channels by PHT may represent a major site of activity of this important antiepileptic agent (9,12).

In addition to structural protein changes in the channel protein, it is also possible that differences in post-translational modulation of Na^+ channels may shed light on molecular alterations in ion channels postulated in epileptic patients. With Na^+-channel protein amino acid sequencing also available, a more focused evaluation of Na^+-channel genetics can be conducted comparing tissue from epileptic patients with that from nonepileptic controls. It is hoped that studies in this area will continue to accelerate our understanding of how alterations in Na^+-channel function may influence neuronal excitability and even epilepsy.

Potassium Channels

Since K^+ carries a positive charge, K^+ exiting the cell generates a positive, outward-going current that drives the transmembrane potential to a more negative value. This current acts to limit the cell's excitability as it moves the transmembrane potential away from the activation potential of the Na^+ channels. The balancing effect of the K^+ current is one key factor that limits the number of action potential spikes a neuron may fire in response to excitatory synaptic stimulation (13).

"Neuronal bursting" is a term used when neurons rapidly fire repeated action potentials. Neuronal bursting activity or bursting activity in cells that normally do not have long bursts may be one type of abnormal behavior that underlies epileptic pathophysiology. Because K^+ currents appear to play such a key role in bursting activity, much interest has been focused on these channels.

Several cell types have been effectively used to study K^+ channels. One well-characterized neuronal cell type in which potassium currents have been studied is the bullfrog ganglion cell (13). One of the desirable qualities facilitating studies in this system is that these cells are geometrically simpler than many mammalian cells, easing some of the technical difficulties of voltage- and patch-clamp analysis. Five separate K^+ currents have been differentiated in these cells by comparing characteristics of current size, voltage threshold, and response to blocking agents. K^+ currents have been given a variety of names, but a useful nomenclature for these five major channel types is I_A, I_K, I_M, $I_{K(Ca)}$, and I_{AHP} potassium currents (4) (see Table 1). Transmembrane voltage affects these different K^+ currents in the range of the action potential or in the subthreshold voltage regions. Identifying these different types of K^+ currents has been very useful in studying their role in specific models of neuronal excitability that might relate to epilepsy.

A brief characterization of specific K^+ currents can provide an insight into their regulation of neuronal excitability (13). $I_{K(Ca)}$ is a large, fast, voltage-dependent K^+ current. Calcium influx during the action potential affects this channel to maximize its K^+ conductance. I_{AHP} is another Ca-dependent K^+ current that is active even at negative potentials and leads to prolonged membrane hyperpolarization. The I_K current, also called the *rectifier current*, is a large, fast-acting K^+ current whose axonal function appears to repolarize the membrane following the peak of the action potential. The I_A and I_M currents are smaller currents that activate at more negative transmembrane potentials than does I_C, I_K, or I_{AHP}. The I_A current appears to influence voltage depolarization rate (trajectory) following hyperpolarization. I_M appears to be blocked by putative neurotransmitters such as acetylcholine and nucleotides.

In rapidly firing cells, such as bursting cells, and in experimentally induced bursting behavior, the cellular processes that arise to limit continuous firing are termed

TABLE 1. *Potassium channels*

Potassium channels	Channel characteristics	Activation	Inactivation
K channel	Delayed rectifier current, rapidly returns voltage toward resting state following Na^+ spike	Slow	Slow
A channel	Activates rapidly in subthreshold range; may have more significant representation in membrane areas involved in signal encoding	Fast	Fast
$K_{(Ca)}$ channel	Activity may be largely responsible for long hyperpolarizing pauses in bursting cells; Ca-dependent	Complex	?
M channel	Hormone/neurotransmitter-sensitive with inactivation	Slow	?
AHP channel	Also Ca-dependent; selective blockers of this channel may enhance repetitive firing	Slow	?

spike frequency adaptation (SFA) or *limitation of sustained high-frequency repetitive firing* (SRF) (14). Although SFA is not fully understood, K^+ channels are felt to be ideal candidates to hyperpolarize cells and limit excitability. Thus, K^+ channels may play an important role in limiting sustained neuronal firing in excited neuronal circuits.

Clinical epilepsy's excessive neuronal firing raises the possibility of a failure of cellular inhibitory processes. These types of events may occur because of an abnormality of the K^+ stabilizing effects on neuronal excitability. It is also possible that excessive, repetitive firing of this sort may recruit neuronal networks with broader clinical expression. It becomes clear that study of K^+-channel function is important in the attempt to seek answers to molecular events underlying epilepsy.

Calcium Channels

Calcium-ion channels have been known since Koketsu and Nishi (15) examined Ca-dependent action potentials. Cellular Ca^+ entry has two major effects: It produces voltage change as it travels down its concentration gradient, and it acts as a second messenger in intracellular processes. This calcium signal is received by specific Ca^{2+}-receptor proteins, such as calmodulin and the C kinase system, and is tied to a multitude of cellular processes (16).

Ca^{2+} concentration in the extracellular space is roughly 10,000 times its neuronal intracellular concentration. This Ca^{2+} gradient is maintained by (a) ATP-dependent Ca^{2+} pump activities in the plasma membrane, (b) mitochondrial buffering, and (c) sequestration in intracellular organelles such as the endoplasmic reticulum.

One of the major routes of Ca^{2+} entry into neurons is through voltage-dependent calcium channels (VDCCs). Calcium channels were first characterized in cardiac tissue and probed by many synthetic drugs called *organic calcium-channel blockers*. Currently, there are at least three neuronal VDCC subtypes (17) (see Table 2). The distinguishing characteristics between these subtypes include: voltage sensitivity; inactivation rates; and sensitivities to ions, drugs, and toxins. The nomenclature of these channels is not universally agreed upon, but one useful scheme identifies "long-lasting" (L), "transient" (T), and "neither T nor L" (N) channels (18).

L channels are activated by strong depolarizations, are resistant to inactivation, and are highly sensitive to Cd^{2+} blockade as well as to Ca^{2+}-channel agonists or antagonists. T channels are activated by weak depolarizations, are transiently open, and are less affected by Cd^{2+} or antagonist drugs. The N channels are activated by strong depolarizations and are resistant to drug modulation, but they are highly sensitive to Cd^{2+}. These observations suggest that the functional characteristics of VDCC are extremely complex and leave open the possibility that different channel characteristics may be defined in future investigations.

Ca^{2+}-channel agonists and antagonists effect certain neuronal groups more than others. Predicting the cumulative behavior of these agents can thus be problematic.

TABLE 2. *Calcium channels[a]*

Properties	T	N	L
Activation range	Pos[b] to -70 mV	Pos to -10 mV	Pos to -10 mV
Inactivation range	-100 to -60 mV	>-100 to -40 mV	-60 to -10 mV
Relaxation rate	Moderate	Moderate	Very slow
Conductance,			
single channel	8–10 pS[c]	11–15 pS	23–27 pS
Cd[2+] block	Resistant	Sensitive	Sensitive
Ca[2+] block	Sensitive	Less sensitive	Less sensitive
W-CGTx[d] block	Weak, reversible	Persistent	Persistent
Dihydropyridine			
sensitivity	No	No	Yes

[a]From ref. 68.
[b]Pos, positive values.
[c]pS, picosiemens.
[d]Snail (*Conus geographigus*) toxin.

Ca^{2+}-channel receptors and antagonist drugs also seem to exhibit a voltage-dependent interaction. In addition, there may be local concentrations of the different VDCCs at specific areas of the neuron (17). This type of subcellular VDCC localization may explain Ca^{2+}-channel antagonist effects on neurotransmitter release. Neurotransmitter release primarily occurs at synaptic zones. The VDCCs in the synaptic areas are primarily of the N type (relatively drug-effect resistant). Antagonist drugs may not block Ca^{2+}-activated neurotransmitter release because of the resistance of the represented VDCC. Conversely, if Ca^{2+}-channel agonists (enhancers of VDCC Ca^{2+} entry) are added to experimental systems, enough additional Ca^{2+} may be added to the synaptic environment to enhance neurotransmitter release. This additional Ca^{2+} is thought to gain access through L channels located in the membrane adjacent to synaptic neurotransmitter release zones. Many observations and experiments will be needed to more fully characterize Ca^{2+} channels and their heterogeneous effects on cell responses. These difficulties will not interfere with the exploration of drugs classified as Ca^{2+}-channel blockers, nor will they interfere with the potential use of these blockers in the treatment of epilepsy.

Modulating the Calcium Signal in Controlling Neuronal Excitability

The widespread second messenger effects of calcium on neuronal and other cell functions have intrigued scientists for many decades. However, it was only over the last 10 years that significant advances have been made in understanding the molecular mechanisms mediating the effects of calcium on neuronal function. The importance of understanding how calcium regulated neuronal excitability after its entry into the cell has been a focus of neuroscience research over the last decade. The discovery of a calcium-binding protein, calmodulin, was the first major breakthrough in understanding molecular mechanisms underlying some of the effects of calcium on cell function (19,20). An overwhelming body of evidence has now accumulated which suggests that many of the effects of calcium on cell function are mediated by calmodulin. The role of calmodulin in modulating nerve transmission and neuronal excitability has been extensively investigated and reviewed (21–25). Several important calcium-regulated processes have been shown to be mediated by calmodulin and by a major calmodulin target enzyme system, calmodulin kinase II (26–28). Figure 2 schematically demonstrates a hypothetical model for the role of calmodulin in synaptic excitability. Evidence from multiple laboratories has now confirmed the role of calmodulin in mediating some of the effects of calcium on neuronal excitability. Anticonvulsant drugs have been shown to antagonize calcium-mediated effects. Phenytoin, carbamazepine, and the benzodiazepines have all been shown to inhibit calmodulin activation of calmodulin kinase II (29,30). Concentrations required to inhibit CaM kinase II are in the low micromolar concentration ranges for anticonvulsant drug effects on the protein kinase. This enzyme plays an important role in mediating calcium-dependent protein phosphorylation of membrane and soluble proteins. CaM kinase II has been implicated by several investigators to be a major molecular mechanism mediating some of the second messenger effects of calcium in the cell. Thus, regulation of this important calcium-mediated event by phenytoin, carbamazepine, and diazepam provides a major regulatory site for these anticonvulsant drugs in regulating neuronal excitability. The precise relationship between this effect and the anticonvulsant activity of these compounds or their related side effects must still be further investigated.

The importance of calmodulin kinase II in regulating neuronal excitability has been widely recognized. Injection of CaM kinase II into identified invertebrate neurons has been shown to regulate potassium and calcium currents (31). In addition, CaM kinase II levels in hippocampal neurons have been shown to be chronically altered during long-term alteration of neuronal excitability in kindling (32). CaM kinase II activity is inhibited by specific anticonvulsants (23,29), and the subunits of CaM kinase II have been shown to be a major protein component of the postsynaptic density localizing this important enzyme system directly at the synapse (33–35). This growing body of evidence firmly establishes that CaM kinase II is a major enzyme regulating neuronal excitability and may have important correlations with the pathogenesis of epilepsy. Understanding the role of CaM kinase II in the pathophysiology of epilepsy and neuronal excitability is an important area for further investigation.

Another major molecular mechanism regulating the effects of calcium on neuronal excitability and cell function is the major enzyme system, protein kinase C. Protein kinase C has been implicated in regulating many of the effects of calcium on cell function and also has been implicated in mediating some of the effects of calcium in regulating specific ion conductances (16). Although no direct studies have been performed to investigate the effects of anticonvulsant drugs on the protein kinase C system, this is an important area for investigation. Both the protein kinase C and the CaM kinase II are important enzyme systems that have been implicated in

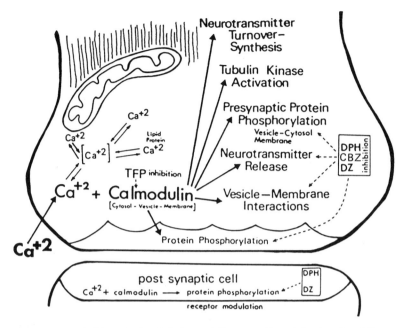

FIG. 2. The roles of Ca^{2+} and calmodulin in regulating synaptic protein phosphorylation, neurotransmitter release and turnover, and vesicle–membrane interactions, and the inhibitory effect of phenytoin (DPH), carbamazepine (CBZ), and diazepam (DZ) on these Ca^{2+}–calmodulin-stimulated processes. The inhibitory effects of these anticonvulsants on protein phosphorylation in synaptic membrane may also modulate the depolarization-dependent entry of Ca^{2+} into the nerve terminal. The importance of calmodulin in mediating the effects of Ca^{2+} on synaptic activity is becoming more evident, and the effects of major anticonvulsant compounds on Ca^{2+}–calmodulin systems provide an exciting area for further investigation. TFP, trifluoperazine (29).

regulating neuronal excitability. The modulation of these calcium target enzyme systems by anticonvulsant drugs is an important area to explore in the development of new anticonvulsant compounds.

Chloride Channels

Chloride (Cl^-) is the most abundant physiologic anion. The ion is 30 times more concentrated in the extracellular space than in the intracellular space. Although Cl^- contributes to membrane potential, its channel properties are less thoroughly studied than those of Na^+, K^+, or Ca^+. What is more widely explored is the coupling of the Cl^- channel with the receptor sites for GABA, benzodiazepines (BZs), and barbiturates. This relationship will be explored in the next section.

SYNAPTIC MODULATION AND NEUROTRANSMITTERS

GABA and Epilepsy

Gama-aminobutyric acid (GABA) is the major central nervous system inhibitory neurotransmitter. GABA exerts a major inhibitory effect on neuronal excitability, primarily through receptor sites that are linked to chloride channels (36). GABA effects are inhibitory because binding increases Cl^- permeability with resultant hyperpolarization. GABA-receptor–chloride-channel sites are known to bind barbiturates and BZs (37,38) (see Fig. 3). Classical GABA-receptor antagonists, picrotoxin and bicuculline, are potent convulsant agents. Interest in inhibitory neurotransmission has stimulated much work on the potential role of GABA in epilepsy. Some propose that a functional deficiency in GABA may be involved in human epilepsy.

Neurochemical markers for GABA synapses have been reported to be altered in animal models of epilepsy as well as in human epileptic temporal lobe tissue removed during epilepsy surgery (39). Other neurochemical markers for the GABA–BZ receptor may also shed some light on clinical epilepsy.

BZs are potent anticonvulsant agents. They are known to have several receptor subtypes that may be associated with different clinical effects. Seizures induced by pentylenetetrazol (PTZ) are blocked by BZs in nanomolar concentrations (38). This type of effect is reversible and saturable, and it demonstrates stereospecificity. GABA potentiates BZ binding to the nanomolar receptor site. The ability of BZs to regulate the Cl^- channel has been proposed as one of the molecular mechanisms mediating some of the neuronal stabilizing effects of the BZs (38). BZs in this concentration range, however, do not correlate with inhibition of maximal electroshock-induced seizures, and another BZ-binding site that may play a role in this effect is under study (38).

GABA–BZ receptors have also been studied in epileptic gerbils, a genetic model of generalized epilepsy. A 30% decrease in BZ binding in midbrain areas was demonstrated in these animals. The specific sites affected are primarily the substantia nigra and periaqueductal gray nuclear groups. The decrease in membrane receptors for BZs linked to GABA receptors in such a crucial region as the substantia nigra may add to seizure susceptibility in some forms of epilepsy (39). The idea of a functional anatomy subserving seizure propagation has reached expanded understanding and is discussed below. These results further indicate that the GABA–BZ–chloride-channel complex is important in maintaining neuronal stability and that alterations in function or distribution of this system may be involved in the pathogenesis of seizure disorders.

Excitatory Amino Acids and Receptors

L-Glutamate was proposed as an excitatory neurotransmitter 30 years ago (40). However, it was only recently that the study of excitatory amino acids (EAAs) grew

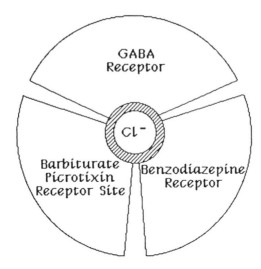

FIG. 3. Proposed chloride-channel–GABA/barbiturate/benzodiazepine receptor. This model illustrates the numerous receptor sites for modulatory channel function.

to include information on their involvement in epilepsy as well as information on neurobiologic development, learning, and cell injury (40).

The two main excitatory neurotransmitters are glutamate and aspartate (41). Many pathways in the brain utilize these neurotransmitters, including hippocampal afferents and major cortical output tracts that are widely activated during convulsions.

EAAs are thought to act through membrane receptors. Currently, the major types of EAA receptors are grouped as the N-methyl-D-aspartate (NMDA) receptor and the three non-NMDA receptors. NMDA is a synthesized glutamate analog found during early studies to be 10–1000 times more potent than L-glutamate. Non-NMDA receptors bind EAAs but are not receptors for NMDA. In the non-NMDA receptor category are kainate receptors, quisqualate receptors, and 2-amino-4- phosphonobutyrate (2-APB) receptors (42).

The excitatory transmission with NMDA receptors appears to be distinct from classical, fast-acting, synaptic transmission. NMDA receptors activate relatively long currents and allow Ca^{2+} as well as Na^+ entry. NMDA-receptor activation is also voltage-dependent, allowing complex synaptic modulation with these unique properties (42).

EEA Receptors

Characterization of the EAA receptors has not only involved electrophysiologic approaches but has also involved the use of an increasing number of substances that antagonize receptor activation (41). Some of these substances such as diaminopimelate (DAP), 2-amino-7-phosphonoheptanoate (2-APH), 2-amino-5-phosphonopentanoic acid (5AP), and aminoadipate act as competitive inhibitors. NMDA-receptor characteristics also involve antagonism by Mg^{2+}. This ion does not block kainate- or quisqualate-receptor-associated channels as effectively (43).

Initial studies evaluating noncompetitive EAA-receptor blockers characterized chlorpromazine and the experimental compound HA-966 as effective inhibitors (42). Other substances, now widely investigated, include a series of dissociative anesthetics and opiates such as ketamine and phencyclidine that also block EAA receptors in a noncompetitive fashion (40).

EAA and Epilepsy

Intense interest has been focused on the potential role of excitatory amino acids in the pathophysiology of epilepsy (44). Kainate, a potent epileptogenic agent (45), applied in low concentrations to hippocampal slices depresses GABA-mediated, inhibitory, postsynaptic potentials (46). A strong relationship between the phenomenon of long-term potentiation (LTP) and epilepsy led to evaluation of the role of NMDA receptors in these processes (47).

NMDA-receptor antagonists block the development of LTP and also act as potent anticonvulsants (47). This type of anticonvulsant effect was demonstrated by suppression of sound-induced seizures in DBA/2 mice (48). When tested in this system, the NMDA antagonists are as potent as diazepam. 2-APH injection into the inferior colliculus inhibits sound-induced seizures in rats (47). Limbic seizures in amygdala-kindled rats (49) and systemic pilocarpine-induced seizures (50) are also potently suppressed by 2-APH.

Studies using 2-APH indicate that an anticonvulsant effect can be achieved in many seizure models. These studies are extremely encouraging and indicate that a new family of anticonvulsant agents may be available for use in patients with epilepsy. This potential therapeutic action is an exciting area at present for the development of new anticonvulsant agents.

FUNCTIONAL ANATOMY OF EPILEPSY

Previous sections have dealt with ion channel function, ion currents, and neurotransmitter effects in relation to epilepsy. A molecular approach dealing with integrated cell processes associated with epileptic conditions must also take into account the neural network interactions that participate in convulsions. A focus on neural network effects has been explored for many years. Penfield (51) proposed the concept of centrencephalic centers coordinating generalized convulsions. This particular line of reasoning has stimulated significant interest in subcortical structures that may subserve epilepsy. Yakovlev (52) reported that epileptic patients who developed Parkinson's disease had a reduction in their seizure frequency. Reports such as these have suggested the role of the substantia nigra as an important structure participating in generalized convulsions.

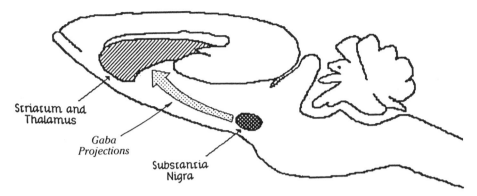

FIG. 4. The GABA projections from the substantia nigra project to several forebrain areas and appear to have a facilitatory effect on seizure propagation. (Redrawn from ref. 39.)

Substantia Nigra and Epilepsy

The search for centrencephalic centers subserving epileptic phenomena led to the biochemical evaluation of many deep gray structures. Using the 2-deoxyglucose method of Sokoloff in evaluating neuronal metabolism, the substantia nigra was found to be the deep-gray nuclear group whose metabolism was most dramatically stimulated in mice which were given PTZ and which subsequently suffered generalized convulsions (53). Thus, attention was turned to the substantia nigra as a major site regulating neuronal excitability.

With GABA representing the major inhibitory neurotransmitter in the central nervous system, it was postulated that local enhancement of GABA concentration in the substantia nigra may affect elements in seizure mechanisms (see Fig. 4). In an effort to expand these theories, the maximal electroshock (MES) model of seizure initiation was used. Investigations were initiated to study the effects of increased or decreased concentrations of GABA in the substantia nigra. GABA transaminase, an enzyme responsible for GABA's metabolic deactivation, is irreversibly inhibited by the GABA analog gamma-vinyl-GABA (GVG). GVG injections into ventral mesencephalic structures enhanced GABA concentration there and impaired seizure production in the MES model (39). GABA measurements in GVG-injected sites reflect the increased local GABA concentration. Local GVG injections in the substantia nigra produced several days of seizure protection (39).

Increased local GABA effects were also evaluated by injection of a GABA agonist bilaterally into midbrain regions. Muscimol, a GABA agonist, was injected bilaterally into midbrain areas, resulting in decreased MES seizure activity. Similar use of this agent also suppressed PTZ seizures in a duration- and dose-dependent fashion (53). Bilateral substantia nigra injections of muscimol decreased the duration of kindled seizures (39). Fluorothyl-inhalation-induced seizures, another convulsive model, was inhibited by GABA-agonist administration bilaterally into the substantia nigra, reflecting the resultant elevated seizure threshold (39).

With compartmental GABA concentration increases and local GABA-agonist administration both demonstrating similar inhibition in kindling, maximal electroshock, and other models of epilepsy, experiments evaluating destructive lesions in the substantia nigra were performed. Focal electrocoagulation and local kainic acid administration were employed to lesion the substantia nigra. Bilateral destructive lesioning attenuated bicuculline-induced tonic–clonic seizures. This decreased seizure expression indicated a protective shift in bicuculline dose–response rather than a purely motor phenomenon such as one might see with interruption of upper-motor-neuron tracts. The substantia nigra area most implicated in these experimental studies is the pars reticulata (39).

Efferent projections from pars reticulata are mainly GABAergic and directed at many cortical and thalamic areas. Local increases of GABA in the pars reticulata decrease the projected GABAergic activity. These projections may represent a common denominator for regulating seizure propagation (39,53). The dopaminergic structures of the substantia nigra within pars compacta do not appear to affect the alteration in seizure production. The substantia nigra's GABAergic pathways are strongly implicated and may act as a gating mechanism regardless of the mechanism of seizure onset in this experimental model (53). These pathways may act with a facilitatory effect on seizure propagation and may represent one of several brain areas that play a key role in epilepsy.

Mamillothalamic Pathway and Epilepsy

Recent research has provided another possible anatomic area that may support the centrencephalic theory of seizure generation. This line of investigation has used PTZ as a model for generalized absence seizures (54,55). Using the 2-deoxyglucose method to evaluate PTZ effects, a thalamic–midbrain circuit involving the mamillary bodies and their rostral and caudal connections have been characterized. This circuit seems critical in the early expression of PTZ-induced seizures (56). Ethosuximide, a drug that is clinically useful in absence seizures, blocks PTZ-stimulated convulsions. Phenytoin, known to be relatively ineffective in most absence seizures, is relatively ineffective in the PTZ epilepsy model. The experimental model of PTZ-induced seizures is useful to explore possible mechanisms of this seizure type, which is characteristic of a centrencephalic model of epilepsy.

Using this experimental model, PTZ infusion leads to synchronous, high-voltage discharges representing epileptiform activity on the electroencephalogram (EEG). This generalized, spike-and-wave activity is also seen with clinical seizure activity in humans. Large areas of increased 2-deoxyglucose in many brain areas are demonstrated during the seizure activity. The increased metabolism is especially prevalent in the cortex, thalamus, hippocampus, globus pallidus, and substantia nigra. Administration of ethosuximide in this PTZ seizure model modifies the seizure activity by decreasing discharges and aborting seizure activity. Also, ethosuximide causes a significant decrease in the 2-deoxyglucose measurements, reflecting a corresponding decrease in metabolic rate. A significant finding in this model, utilizing ethosuximide, is the selective continuation of significant 2-deoxyglucose uptake in the mamillary body nuclei, mamillothalamic tract, anterior nucleus of the thalamus, mamillary peduncle, and the dorsal and ventral tegmental nuclei in the mesencephalon. These results suggest that these localized anatomic structures were the main or most sensitive neuronal substrates in this type of seizure activity (57).

This experimental finding led to the characterization of specific alterations of subcortical structures in an epilepsy model that may modulate generalized convulsive activity. The observations were subsequently confirmed by lesioning the mamillothalamic tract, thereby producing a significant decrease in mortality, seizure duration, and clinical seizure activity. This evidence supports the suspected importance of this functional anatomic pathway subserving convulsive discharge and suggests that it may play an important role in the genesis of generalized absence seizures (57).

Forebrain Region Associated with Generalized Epilepsy

Systemically administered convulsants can stimulate generalized seizures. Although many regions (e.g., hippocampus and amygdala) are very sensitive to local convulsants, as demonstrated by electrographic or metabolic findings, the site of seizure initiation in generalized seizures is unknown. The search for areas responsible for generalized seizure initiation has recently been stimulated by the finding of a prefrontal region with striking convulsant sensitivity (58). This area is defined as the deep prepiriform cortex (DPC) site that elicits generalized seizures with picogram amounts of injected bicuculline, a GABA-receptor antagonist (58). This anatomic region does not correspond to a previously defined anatomic structure.

The DPC site is active in generalized seizure initiation from kainic acid or carbachol administration even when the convulsant is delivered unilaterally. The EEG also demonstrates bilateral spiking with unilateral injections. Muscimol (a GABA agonist), if injected locally before the convulsant, prevented seizures produced in this model from bicuculline or picrotoxin. Preadministration of atropine prevented carbachol-induced seizures but was ineffective against other convulsants (58).

When excitatory amino acids were delivered to the DPC, generalized convulsions were produced. However, this response could be blocked by pretreatment with the NMDA-receptor blocker, 2-APH. 2APH also blocked kainic acid-induced seizures. Because kainic acid receptors are poorly blocked by 2APH, it is suggested that NMDA receptors may be partly responsible for kainic acid seizure propagation (39).

This functional anatomic site participating in generalized seizure propagation in these various experimental paradigms may be a key neural structure involved in generation of some types of generalized epilepsy. Further characterization of this anatomic region may provide further insights into the regulation of neuronal excitability.

MODELS OF EPILEPSY

Kindling

With the publication of Goddard's findings in 1967 that introduced the kindling phenomenon (59), a new avenue of neuronal investigation was opened. This neuro-behavioral model is analogous to the process of using many small twigs to start a large fire (i.e., "kindling"). Kindling is initiated by small electrical or chemical stimulations of brain tissue that initially have no direct excitatory effect on the brain. With various patterns of repeated stimulus delivery, an intensified response occurs in the animal over time. This enhanced response to the unaltered stimulation culminates in a clinical behavior representing convulsive activity in the animal. Once the animal exhibits the full convulsive response, it is described as being effectively kindled. This process represents an excellent example of neuronal plasticity. Many separate sites within the brain have been kindled, but much emphasis has been placed specifically on the olfactory–limbic system, since it is these sites that have proven to be the best areas to produce kindling. A characteristic enhanced or intensified full convulsive response appears to last indefinitely in the electrically kindled animal despite long stimulus-free intervals. This change is considered an excellent model for a long-term plasticity such as memory.

The characteristic clinical behavior in kindling is graded according to the extent of behavioral effects following the stimulus. The first clinical stage in the rat model involves facial clonus; subsequently, stage 2 involves head nodding; stage 3, fore-limb clonus; stage 4, rearing; and stage 5, full convulsive discharge with rearing and falling. These clinical stages have been described with several different patterns and intensities of electrical pulsing sequences (60).

This predictable animal model is useful for several types of analysis in epilepsy research. It also has provided a rational basis supporting the hypotheses of the development of mirror foci in humans.

Despite the importance of the kindling phenomena, very little is known regarding the underlying cause of the kindling response. Morphologic assessment of kindled foci has been negative (32). Understanding the fundamental mechanisms of kindling may prove to be valuable to epilepsy research.

Metabolic Activity in Kindling

In a chemically kindled animal model using the drug carbachol, whose receptor-mediated effects occur through muscarinic receptors, focal 2-deoxyglucose uptake was increased following carbachol injection. This effect was blocked by atropine (49). Repeated drug administration results in electrical after-discharges even without demonstrable behavioral changes with the first injections. Full kindling behavior eventually results in most animals. The enhanced focal glucose uptake in the site of carbachol injection reveals a habituation process during the repeated stimulation (51). Demonstration of focal 2-deoxyglucose metabolic changes allows speculation that specific biochemical processes will be defined in different stages of kindling. These changes may be similar to processes occurring in epileptic foci in humans (61).

Pharmacologic Interactions in Kindling

Chemical kindling like that described with carbachol is blocked by atropine, a blocker of muscarinic receptors (61). One implication of this result is that a receptor-mediated process is at work in chemical kindling. Kindling is enhanced with reserpine preadministration, suggesting that a decrease in noradrenaline concentration may promote the kindling phenomenon (62). This area of research may provide some insight into the pharmacological manipulation of seizures.

Network Interactions in Kindling

The ability of the kindling phenomenon to represent a model of neuronal plasticity affecting large areas of cells is supported by several lines of observation. Animals that have been previously kindled in one brain site have been shown to be much easier to kindle when other kindling sites are attempted (59). This enhancement of seizure development with new kindled sites may have relevance to mirror focus development in human epileptic patients. Certainly, this evidence reflects the changes that can occur in distant sites away from the specific area of initial kindling (63).

The role of substantia nigra in the kindling phenomenon has been intensively investigated. Recent experiments have found that bilateral substantia nigra injection of muscimol (a GABA-receptor agonist), given to previously kindled rats, results in suppression of seizure activity (53). This finding would present further evidence of the importance of network interactions in the kindling phenomena and suggests that the substantia nigra represents an important brain area modulating the development of kindled seizures (53).

These experiments that develop and explore the kindling phenomenon may have direct bearing on progress in epilepsy research. The kindling model may provide insights into basic mechanisms controlling neuronal excitability and the development to mirror foci in humans.

Biochemical Changes in Kindling

Although kindling represents a long-lasting effect on the animal model, prolonged biochemical changes have only recently been observed. Septal kindling produces a persistent, measurable biochemical change in the phosphorylation of hippocampal membranes (32). The pattern reflects decreased phosphorylation occurring in a calcium–calmodulin-dependent fashion. Altered phosphoproteins fall within several size ranges, but two major endogenous phosphoproteins affected are in the 50,000- to 60,000-dalton range (32). Further resolution of the identity of these proteins suggests that they represent the autophosphorylated subunits of the enzyme calmodulin kinase II (32). The decrease in calcium–calmodulin-dependent phosphorylation of these enzyme subunits may reflect a molecular mechanism underlying neuronal plasticity. This enzyme has been implicated in neurotransmitter release (16) and has been identified as a major protein component of the postsynaptic density (PSD) (33), making it an ideal candidate to modulate synaptic activity (64).

This biochemical avenue of research may be one mechanism to understand the changes occurring in epileptic patients that result in recurrent seizures. One provocative postulate related to the kindling model suggests that convulsions may result from recurrent, subconvulsive neuronal discharges with a kindling-like effect on relevant neural structures. Understanding more of the biochemical alterations in kindling may allow therapeutic intervention in the development of epilepsy in humans.

BRAIN-SLICE TECHNIQUES

Historical Development

Studies of epileptic phenomena have developed rapidly with the realization that unanswered questions can be explored *in vitro* with brain-slice techniques. The development of this methodology began with the search for thin, respiring, neural tissue for metabolic measurements. The retina was widely used in the 1920s. Soon, comparisons were made to razor-cut sections of rat brain. Small, voltage-gradient electrical stimulations of brain slices revealed increased respiration and glycolysis. It began to be widely expected that brain slices could perform in relative isolation and that the slice could display aspects of its functioning *in vitro*, as it does in the intact brain (65).

Drugs such as barbiturates and phenothiazines were administered to the slice bath and were found to oppose the electrical stimulation effects (66). Control of slice environment also allowed analysis of neurotransmitter elaboration concurrent with measurements of metabolic and electrical parameters (54). Collaboration with electrophysiologists provided electrical measurements similar to those found *in situ*, and this continued to support the development of this laboratory technique.

Advantages of Brain-Slice Methodology

Brain-slice techniques have allowed the study of intrinsic neuronal and synaptic properties that underscore the generation of burst activity and other hyperexcitable neuronal behavior thought to be important in epilepsy. The slice has been ideal for exploration of potassium and calcium conductances as well as for analysis of channel-blocking drugs that modulate neuronal firing patterns (68). Analogues of both ictal and interictal spikes can be produced in hippocampal slice tissue treated with convulsive agents (69,70). Prepared slices often have 10^3 to 10^4 cells allowing preservation of 10^3 to 10^5 synaptic contacts, thereby enhancing the insight into synaptic modulated events.

Brain-Slice Experimental Overview

Brain slices from many brain areas have been studied. Because of space limitations, hippocampal brain-slice data will be emphasized. The use of slice preparations covers broad areas of interest in neurophysiology, neurochemistry, and neuropharmacology. The following sections will function as a highlighted view of brain-slice utility in neurophysiology and neuropharmacology as related to epilepsy.

Bursting Phenomenon and Paroxysmal Depolarizing Shifts

Repetitive, high-frequency discharges from a cell are termed a "burst." Bursting behavior has been most extensively studied in invertebrate neurons (71) but has also been characterized in vertebrates, such as in the CA_3 region of the hippocampus. Bursting is a normal behavior in certain cells and can be seen as an endogenous activity of both isolated cells and whole cellular networks (72).

In invertebrates, endogenous bursts consist of a slow depolarization with triggered, rapid action potentials in series of variable duration. Experimentally, strings of action potentials can be blocked by the Na^+-channel-blocking drug TTX (73), but the slow depolarizing phase appears to remain. This persistence suggests that it is influenced by or related to calcium currents (74).

The CA_3 region in hippocampal slice preparation appears to have bursting neurons whose effects spread very minimally during normal behavior. With application of convulsants, burst discharges generate broad network bursting behavior. The network appears to follow these bursting pacemaker cells (72). This population behavior appears to represent an experimental equivalent of the electroencephalographic hallmark of epilepsy: the interictal spike. The network processes that allow change from that of the normal cell bursting behavior to network bursting behavior are a major focus of research efforts. A major electrophysiological process evaluated in brain-slice systems that relates to bursting behavior is the paroxysmal depolarizing shift (PDS).

PDS in Brain

The PDS is a depolarization of relatively long duration within a cell. The PDS usually triggers a burst of action potentials as described above. This may spread to include coincident activity of large networks of cells (75). Convulsant treatment is thought to generate the PDS phenomenon by modulating excitatory synaptic currents (76). Some have characterized this as a giant excitatory postsynaptic potential (EPSP). Because bursting behavior is described also as a normal cellular behavior that does not invoke seizures, inhibitory synaptic and network mechanisms are thought to be an important regulator of network organization. GABA serves as a major inhibitory neurotransmitter in the hippocampus. It has been observed that agents that block GABA and are delivered to the slice preparation are powerful convulsants and give rise to synchronous epileptiform discharges (77).

Slice experimentation represents a convenient and powerful method to study potential epileptogenic mechanisms. Other, associated studies with brain-slice techniques have gained great interest. These include kindling and long-term potentiation in slices.

Kindling in Slices

The generation of kindling phenomena in hippocampal slices has been achieved by delivery of trains of electrical stimuli (78). The stimulation is delivered along known pathways, and field recordings are often examined at the CA$_3$ hippocampal section by extracellular electrodes.

Single stimuli to slices typically elicited a response of two prominent negative deflections and a positive slow wave. With stimulus trains, three types of epileptiform activity were seen: after-discharges, spontaneous bursts, and stimulus-triggered bursts (78).

A useful, descriptive name for this process of hippocampal activation is "stimulus-train-induced bursting" (STIB). It is unclear whether STIB-like activity occurs during kindling. It is known that hippocampal after-discharges are found with STIB. These after-discharges are an associated finding in whole-brain kindling (61). The molecular processes underlying STIB are still being characterized, but this model is a viable electrical-stimulation alternative to *in vitro* chemical convulsant models of hippocampal slice epileptiform generation. Another process that has received intense interest using hippocampal slice techniques is that of long-term potentiation.

Long-Term Potentiation in Hippocampal Slice

Learning, whether it be ideational information or a motor skill, implies retention of a long-lasting change within the nervous system. The search for long-lasting physiologic changes in neural systems that may represent learning led to observations by Bliss and Gardner-Medwin (79) in slice preparations. They found that synaptic efficiency could be greatly increased following tetanic stimulation of the perforant path to the dentate gyrus. The increased synaptic amplitude (a definition of synaptic efficiency) was shown to last up to 16 weeks in an experimental model. This process has been termed "long-term potentiation" (LTP), and available evidence suggests that LTP also occurs in behavioral learning models. The neural changes resulting in LTP in experimental models may shed new insight on the biochemical basis of learning, but it may also reflect alterations in neuronal pathophysiology associated with epilepsy.

Similarities exist between the effects of kindling and those of LTP. Recent investigations have included examinations of the role of excitatory neurotransmitters on the long-term effects seen in kindled and LTP models (80).

As described above, glutamate is a putative excitatory neurotransmitter. Glutamate-receptor characterization in both LTP and kindling in brain-slice models reveals increased glutamate membrane-binding sites. These membrane sites may be one lasting type of biochemical change that underlies the long-lasting qualities of LTP (80).

These models demonstrate biochemical elements of neuronal plasticity and serve important roles. They also allow biochemical characterization of complex processes. They serve as models in the experimental analysis of neuronal physiology and pathophysiology in processes as complex as learning and epilepsy.

SUMMARY

It is suggested from investigations into cellular and molecular neuronal activity that epilepsy represents a complex coupling of ion channel function, neurotransmitter action, and functional cellular anatomy. Continued study in these areas should elucidate the myriad of factors that result in the clinical expression of epilepsy. It is firmly expected that patients will directly benefit from these avenues of study as a more clear picture emerges from the research directed at characterizing neuronal excitability and understanding the pathogenesis of epilepsy.

REFERENCES

1. Delgado-Escueta AV, Ward AA, Woodbury DM, Porter RJ, eds. *Advances in neurology*, vol 44. New York; Raven Press, 1986;3–55.
2. Nistico G, Morselli P, Lloyd K, Fariello R, Engel J, eds. *Neurotransmitters, seizures, and epilepsy III*. New York: Raven Press, 1986.
3. Jackson M, Lecar H, Morris C, Wong B. Single channel current recording in excitable cells. In: Barker I, McKelvy J, eds. *Current methods in cellular neurobiology*. New York: John Wiley & Sons, 1980;61–99.
4. Hille B. *Ionic channels in excitable membranes*. Sunderland, MA, Sinauer Associates, 1984.
5. Koestlere J. Voltage-gated channels and the generation of the action potential. In: Kendel E, Schwartz J, eds. *Principles of neural science*, 2nd ed. New York: Elsevier, 1985.
6. Agnew WS, Levinson SR, Brabson JS, Raffery MA. Purification of the tetrodotoxin-binding component associated with the voltage-sensitive sodium channel from *Electrophorus electricus electroplax* membranes. *Proc Natl Acad Sci USA* 1978;75:2606–2610.
7. Hodgkin A, Huxley A. Action potentials recorded from inside a nerve fibre. *Nature* 1939;144:710–711.
8. Narahashi T. Modulators acting on sodium and calcium channels: patch-clamp analysis. In: Delgado-Escueta AV, Ward AA, Woodbury DM, Porter RJ, eds. *Advances in neurology*, vol 44. New York: Raven Press, 1986;211–224.

9. Yaari Y, Selzer M, Pincus J. Phenytoin: mechanisms of its anticonvulsant action. *Ann Neurol* 1986; 201:171–184.

10. Schoffeniels E. Protein phosphorylation and nerve conduction. In: Lahlou B, ed. *Epithelial transport in lower vertebrates*. 1979;295–297.

11. Schoffeniels E, Dandrifosse G, Bettendorff I. Phosphate derivatives of thiamine and Na$^+$ channel in conducting membranes. *J Neurochem* 1984;43:269–271.

12. Schoffeniels E. Thiamine phosphorylated derivatives and bio-electrogenesis. *Arch Int Physiol Biochim* 1983;91:233–242.

13. Adams P, Galvan M. Voltage-dependent currents of vertebrate neurons and their role in membrane excitability. In: Delgado-Escueta AV, Ward AA, Woodbury DM, Porter RJ, eds. *Advances in neurology*, vol 44. New York: Raven Press, 1986; 137–170.

14. McLean M, MacDonald R. Limitation of sustained high frequency repetitive firing: a common anticonvulsant drug mechanism of action? In: Nistico G, Morselli P, Lloyd K, Fariello R, Engel J, eds. *Neurotransmitters, seizures, and epilepsy III*. New York: Raven Press, 1986;23–38.

15. Koketsu K, Nishi S. Calcium and action potentials of bullfrog sympathetic ganglion cells. *J Gen Physiol* 1969;53:608–623.

16. Rasmussen H. The calcium messenger system. *N Engl J Med* 1986;314(17):1094–1101.

17. Miller, RJ. Multiple calcium channels and neuronal function. *Science* 1987;235:46–52.

18. Tsien R. Calcium currents in heart cells and neurons. In: Kaczmarek L, Levitan I, eds. *Neuromodulation: the biochemical control of neuronal excitability*. New York: Oxford University Press, 1987;206–242.

19. Cheung WY. Calmodulin role in cellular regulation. *Science* 1980;207:19–27.

20. Klee CB, Crouch TH, Richmand PG. Calmodulin. *Annu Rev Biochem* 1980;49:489–515.

21. DeLorenzo RJ, Freedman SD, Yohe WB, Maurer SC. Stimulation of Ca^{2+}-dependent neurotransmitter release and presynaptic nerve terminal protein phosphorylation by calmodulin and a calmodulin-like protein isolated from synaptic vesicles. *Proc Natl Acad Sci USA* 1979;76:1838–1842.

22. DeLorenzo RJ. Role of calmodulin in neurotransmitter release and synaptic function. *Ann NY Acad Sci* 1980;356:92–109.

23. DeLorenzo RJ. The calmodulin hypothesis of neurotransmission. *Cell Calcium* 1981;2:365–385.

24. DeLorenzo RJ. Calmodulin in neurotransmitter release and synaptic function. *Fed Proc* 1982; 41:2275.

25. DeLorenzo RJ. Calcium-calmodulin protein phosphorylation in neuronal transmission: a molecular approach to neuronal excitability and anticonvulsant drug action. In: Delgado-Escueta AV, Wasterlain CG, Treiman DM, Porter RJ, eds. *Advances in neurology*, vol 34: *status epilepticus*. New York: Raven Press, 1983;325–338.

26. Goldenring JR, Gonzalez B, McGuire JS Jr, DeLorenzo RJ. Purification and characterization of a calmodulin-dependent kinase from rat brain cytosol able to phosphorylate tubulin and microtubule-associated proteins. *J Biol Chem* 1983;258:12632–12640.

27. Bennett MK, Erondu NE, Kennedy MB. Purification and characterization of a calmodulin-dependent protein kinase that is highly concentrated in brain. *J Biol Chem* 1983;258:12735–12744.

28. Schulman H, Greengard P. Stimulation of brain membrane protein phosphorylation by calcium and an endogenous heat-stable protein. *Nature* 1978;271:478–479.

29. DeLorenzo RJ. A molecular approach to the calcium signal in brain: relationship to synaptic modulation and seizure discharge. *Adv Neurol* 1986;44:435–464.

30. DeLorenzo RJ, Burdette S, Holderness J. Benzodiazepine inhibition of the calcium–calmodulin protein kinase system in brain membrane. *Science* 1982;213:546–649.

31. Sakakibara M, Alkon DL, DeLorenzo RJ, Goldenring JR, Neary JT, Heldman E. Modulation of calcium-mediated inactivation of ionic currents by Ca^{2+}/calmodulin-dependent protein kinase II. *J Biophys* 1986;50:319–327.

32. Goldenring JR, Wasterlain CG, Oestreicher A, et al. Kindling induces a long-lasting change in the activity of a hippocampal membrane calmodulin-dependent protein kinase system. *Brain Res* 1986;377:47–53.

33. Goldenring J, McGuire J, DeLorenzo R. Identification of the major postsynaptic density protein as homologous with the major calmodulin-binding subunit of a calmodulin-dependent protein kinase. *J Neurochem* 1984;42:1077–1084.

34. Kennedy MR, Bennett MK, Erondu NE. Biochemical and immunochemical evidence that the "major PSD protein" is a subunit of a calmodulin-dependent protein kinase. *Proc Natl Acad Sci USA* 1983;80:7357–7361.

35. Kelly PT, McGuinness TL, Greengard P. Evidence that the major postsynaptic density protein is a component of a Ca^{2+}/calmodulin-dependent protein kinase. *DNAS* 1984;3:945–949.

36. Ticku M, Rastogi S. Convulsant/anticonvulsant drugs and GABAergic transmission. In: Nistico G, Morselli P, Lloyd K, Fariello R, Engel J, eds. *Neurotransmitters, seizures, and epilepsy III*. New York: Raven Press, 1986;163–177.

37. Ticku M, Maksay G. Convulsant depressant site of action at the allosteric benzodiazepine–GABA receptor–ionophore complex. *Life Sci* 1983;33:2636–2675.

38. DeLorenzo R, Dashefsky L. Anticonvulsants. In: Lajtha A, ed. *Handbook of neurochemistry*, vol 9. New York: Plenum Press, 1985;363–403.

39. Gale K. Role of the substantia nigra in GABA-mediated anticonvulsant actions. In: Delgado-Escueta AV, Ward AA, Woodbury DM, Porter RJ, eds. *Advances in neurology*, vol 44. New York: Raven Press, 1986;343–364.

40. Rothman S, Olney J. Excitotoxicity and the NMDA receptor. *Trends Neurosci* 1987;10(7):299–301.

41. Czuczwar S, Frey H, Loscher W. *N*-Methyl-D, L-aspartic acid-induced convulsions in mice and their blockade by antiepileptic drugs and other agents. In: Nistico G, Morselli P, Lloyd K, Fariello R, Engel J, eds. *Neurotransmitters, seizures, and epilepsy III*. New York: Raven Press, 1986;235–246.

42. Watkins J, Olverman H. Agonists and antagonists for excitatory amino acid receptors. *Trends Neurosci* 1987;10(7):265–272.

43. Meldrum B, Chapman A. Excitatory amino acid antagonists and anticonvulsant agents: receptor subtype involvement in different seizure models. In: Nistico G, Morselli P, Lloyd K, Fariello R, Engel J, eds. *Neurotransmitters, seizures, and epilepsy III*. New York: Raven Press, 1986;223–245.

44. Rothman S, Olney J. Glutamate and the pathophysiology of hypoxic–ischemic brain damage. *Ann Neurol* 1986;19:105–111.

45. Albala B, Moshe S, Okada R. Kainic acid induced seizures: a developmental study. *Dev Brain Res* 1984;13:139–148.

46. Fonnum F. Glutamate: a neurotransmitter in mammalian brain. *J Neurochem* 1984;42:1–11.

47. Croucher M, Collins J, Meldrum B. Anticonvulsant action of excitatory amino acid antagonists. *Science* 1982;216(4548):899–901.

48. Loscher W, Frey H. Aminooxyacetic acid: correlation between biochemical effects, anticonvulsant action and toxicity in mice. *Biochem Pharmacol* 1978;27:103–108.

49. Peterson D, Collins J, Bradford H. The kindled amygdala model of epilepsy: anticonvulsant action of amino acid antagonists. *Brain Res* 1983;275:169–172.

50. Turski L, Cavalheiro E, Turski W, Meldrum B. Excitatory neurotransmission within substantia nigra pars reticulata regulates threshold for seizures produced by pilocarpine in rats: effects of intranigral 2-amino-7-phosphonoheptanoate and *N*-methyl-D-asparate. *Neuroscience* 1986;18(1):61–77.

51. Penfield W. Epileptic automatisms and the centrencephalic integrating system. *Res Publ Assoc Res Nerv Ment Dis* 1952;30:513–528.

52. Yakovlev P. Epilepsy and Parkinsonism. *N Engl J Med* 1928;198:620.

53. McNamara J, Rigsbee L, Galloway M. Evidence that substantia nigra is crucial to the neural network of kindled seizures. *Eur J Pharmacol* 1983;86:485–486.

54. Rodin E, Onuma T, Wasson S, Porzak J, Rodin M. Neurophysiological mechanisms involved in grand mal seizures induced by Metrazol and Megimide. *Electroencephalogr Clin Neurophysiol* 1971;30(1):62–72.

55. Velasco F, Velasco M, Estrada-Villaneuva F, Machado J. Specific and nonspecific multiple unit activities during the onset of pentylenetetrazol seizures. I. Intact animals. *Epilepsia* 1975;16:207–214.

56. Miroki M, Ferrendelli J. Interruption of the mamillothalamic tract prevents seizures in guinea pigs. *Science* 1984;226:72–74.

57. Ferrendelli J, Miski M. Functional anatomy of experimental generalized seizures. In: Nistico G, Morselli P, Lloyd K, Fariello R, Engel J, eds. *Neurotransmitters, seizures, and epilepsy III*. New York: Raven Press, 1986;355–367.

58. Gale K, Piredda S. Identification of a discrete forebrain site responsible for the genesis of chemically induced seizures. In: Nistico G, Morselli P, Lloyd K, Fariello R, Engel J, eds. *Neurotransmitters, seizures, and epilepsy III*. New York: Raven Press, 1986;205–217.

59. Goddard G. Development of epileptic seizures through brain stimulation at low intensity. *Nature* 1967;214:1020–1021.

60. Bonhaus D, Walters J, McNamara J. Investigation of mechanism by which substantia nigra propagates kindled seizures. In: Nistico G, Morselli P, Lloyd K, Fariello R, Engel J, eds. *Neurotransmitters, seizures, and epilepsy III*. New York: Raven Press, 1986;189–202.
61. Wasterlain C, Farber D, Fairchild D. Synaptic mechanisms in the kindled epileptic focus: a speculative synthesis. In: Delgado-Escueta AV, Ward AA, Woodbury DM, Porter RJ, eds. *Advances in neurology*, vol 44. New York: Raven Press, 1986;411–434.
62. McNamara J. Neurobiology general principles related to epilepsy. In: Glaser G, Perry J, Woodbury D, eds. *Antiepileptic drugs: mechanisms of action*. New York: Raven Press, 1980;185–197.
63. McNamara J. Kindling model of epilepsy. In: Delgado-Escueta AV, Ward AA, Woodbury DM, Porter RJ, eds. *Advances in neurology*, vol 44. New York: Raven Press, 1986;303–318.
64. Fujisawa H, Yamauchi T, Okumo S, Nakata H. Possible role of calmodulin-dependent protein kinase in nerve functions. In: Ebashi S, Endo M, Imahori K, Kakiuchi S, Nishizuka K, eds. *Calcium regulation in biological systems*. New York: Academic Press, 1984;129–140.
65. McIlwain H. Introduction: cerebral subsystems as biological entities. In: Dingledine R, ed. *Brain slices*. New York: Plenum Press, 1984;1–7.
66. Greengard O, McIlwain H. Anticonvulsants and the metabolism of separated mammalian cerebral tissues. *Biochem J* 1955;61:61–68.
67. McIlwain H, Snyder S. Stimulation of piriform and neocortical tissues in an *in vitro* flow-system: metabolic properties and release of putative neurotransmitters. *J Neurochem* 1970;17:521–530.
68. Anderson W, Swartzwelder S, Wilson W. The NMDA receptor antagonist 2-amino-5-phosphonovalerate blocks stimulus train-induced epileptogenesis but not epileptiform bursting in the rat hippocampal slice. *J Neurophys* 1987;57:1–21.
69. Miles R, Wong R, Maub R. Synchronized after discharges in the hippocampus: contributions of local synaptic interactions. *Neuroscience* 1984;12:1179–1189.
70. Schwartzkroin P, Prince D. Penicillin-induced epileptiform activity in the hippocampal *in vitro* preparation. *Ann Neurol* 1977;1:463–469.
71. Lewis D, Huguenard J, Anderson W, Wilson W. Membrane currents underlying bursting pacemaker adaptation in invertebrates. In: Delgado-Escueta AV, Ward AA, Woodbury DM, Porter RJ, eds. *Advances in neurology*, vol 44. New York: Raven Press, 1986;235–261.
72. Johnston D, Brown T. The synaptic nature of the paroxysmal depolarizing shift in hippocampal neurons. *Ann Neurol* 1984;16(Suppl):S65–S71.
73. Strumwasser F. Membrane and intracellular mechanisms governing endogenous activity in neurons. In: Carlson F, ed. *Physiological and biochemical aspects of nervous integration*. Englewood Cliffs, NJ: Prentice-Hall, 1968;329–342.
74. Gorman A, Hermann A, Thomas M. Intra-cellular calcium and the control of neuronal pacemaker activity. *Fed Proc* 1981;40:2233–2239.
75. Ayala G, Dichter M, Gumnit R. Genesis of epileptic interictal spikes. New knowledge of cortical feedback systems suggests a new physiological explanation of brief paroxysms. *Brain Res* 1973; 52:1–18.
76. Johnston D, Brown T. Giant synaptic potential hypothesis for epileptiform activity. *Science* 1981; 211:294–297.
77. Prince D, Connors B. Mechanisms of epileptogenesis in cortical structures. *Ann Neurol* 1984; 16(Suppl):S59–S64.
78. Stasheff S, Bragdon A, Wilson W. Induction of epileptiform activity in hippocampal slices by trains of electrical stimuli. *Brain Res* 1985;344:296–302.
79. Bliss T, Gardner-Medwin A. Long-lasting potentiation of synaptic transmission in the dentate area of the unanesthetized rabbit following stimulation of the perforant path. *J Physiol* 1973;23:357–374.
80. Collingridge G, Bliss T. NMDA receptors—their role in long-term potentiation. *Trends Neurosci* 1987;6:288–293.

Appendix I

Interplay of Economics, Politics, and Quality in the Care of Patients with Epilepsy: The Formation of the National Association of Epilepsy Centers

Robert J. Gumnit

National Association of Epilepsy Centers,
Minneapolis, Minnesota 55416

The goal for epilepsy treatment today is complete seizure control without toxicity. This goal can be achieved for most patients.

Patients with epilepsy present with different degrees of severity, requiring different combinations of resources. A family practitioner might see 20 different patients with epilepsy each year and none of them might be truly difficult cases. A neurologist probably sees 400 different cases of epilepsy per year and 40 or more will be severely afflicted.

Seizures are very common. Nine percent of the population will have a seizure at some time in their life. About a third of them have simple febrile seizures that usually do not present major problems. Another third will have only one seizure and are easily managed. The remaining third will have more than one seizure on two or more occasions, thus qualifying for the diagnosis of epilepsy. On any given day, 0.5–1% of the population of the United States is actively having seizures and requires medical care. Many of these people will respond to average doses of almost any of the anticonvulsants and can be treated by their primary care physician. Some require the attention of a neurologist. At least one-tenth of the people with active epilepsy (or 0.1% of the population of the United States, i.e., 2.25 million people) have seizures that are difficult to control and require specialized care. Care for patients with a chronic disease such as epilepsy can be stratified into four levels:

1. At the primary care level, the diagnosis is easily made and the patient can be treated satisfactorily in a typical office setting.
2. At the secondary care level, the attention of a specialist such as a neurologist is required. Often the patient requires a thorough evaluation in the hospital.
3. Patients with more complex seizure disorders need to be referred to a tertiary-level center, where more comprehensive care is available. Many university hospitals and private tertiary referral centers are equipped to handle such cases.

4. A small number of cases require referral to a fourth-level center. These people require prolonged intensive neurodiagnostic monitoring, specialized pharmacokinetic evaluation, and highly specialized surgery.

The present situation in medical care reimbursement in this country is extraordinarily complex. Actions by the federal government and private insurers in the last 10 years have created a situation in which many who need care lack access to a physician who can provide it. Payment is not readily available or is inadequate for certain highly specialized services. Intensive neurodiagnostic monitoring [e.g., simultaneous combined video and electroencephalographic (EEG) recording], the prolonged hospitalization needed to evaluate complex treatment issues in epilepsy, and the work-up for epilepsy surgery are cases in point.

Electroencephalography is necessary for the proper diagnosis of seizures. In the early years of electroencephalography, the economic, financial, and political situation regarding patient care was rather simple. The capital expense involved in setting up an EEG laboratory was relatively high, and therefore most laboratories were operated by hospitals. The physician received an interpretation fee, or a salary, and was free to worry about quality. While the income of individual practitioners varied, and no one got very rich, the physician did all right if the fee was reasonable. Because the hospital could easily recapture its cost, it usually gave the electroencephalographer whatever he wanted in the way of facilities and technical personnel.

Some physicians recognized that there was the potential for greater profit in the technical component of the charge than in the professional component. This situation is ethically neutral. Thieves could operate under either system, and honest work could be done under either system. There was, however, the issue of control over resources and income, depending upon who took the risk of making the capital investment and hired the technologists. Taking responsibility for the technical component did increase the complexity of (a) the physician's job and (b) the relationship between the physician and the hospital. Since very few people had insurance for outpatient care at that time, nearly all of the work was done in the hospital.

The more complex the equipment and the studies, the more serious the issues. Certainly, magnetic resonance imaging (MRI) and positron emission tomography (PET) scanning are far more complex than a routine electroencephalogram. However, setting up an appropriate intensive neurodiagnostic monitoring program introduces a large amount of complexity.

Up to this point, the economic and quality issues could be handled by the existing scientific professional societies. The American EEG Society could issue guidelines, and the question of accreditation could be raised. None of these activities violated the charitable role of a scientific society organized as a 501(c)(3). However, in the 1980s a number of major laws were passed that have altered the situation significantly.

The federal government passed the TEFRA Act, which affects (a) Medicare reimbursement for capital investment and (b) payment for technical costs in hospitals. Under that law, only the hospital will be reimbursed for the technical component of most tests. The Medicare prospective payment, or DRG, system states that hospitals will be paid a lump sum for each admission, based on discharge diagnoses and procedures performed. Taken together, these two laws greatly restrict the amount of money available for hospital services and capital investment, placing major constraints on new developments.

In many states, Medicaid programs have adopted prospective payment plans and other Medicare-style regulations. In all states, Medicaid programs have greatly reduced the reimbursement to hospitals for capital and operating expenses and have similarly reduced the fees paid to physicians.

Since many patients with intractable seizures are permanently disabled, and thus have their care paid for by Medicare and/or Medicaid, these changes place a particular burden on epilepsy centers. Other prepaid plans (HMOs, PPOs, etc.) place similar pressures on the hospitals and doctors.

Private insurance companies also face major problems. Major cost-shifting occurred as hospitals shifted costs to the private insurance companies to make up for the reductions made by Medicare, Medicaid, and the HMOs. As a result, private insurance companies have adopted a number of tactics to reduce their expenditures. They began invoking long-existing clauses in their contracts stating they would not pay for experimental services or for services that were "medically unnecessary." In practice, this means that anything unusual is denied, placing a major burden on those who are providing new services and treatments. Since the field of epilepsy has been experiencing significant developments in recent years, epilepsy centers have suffered more than most.

Entrepreneurs have developed so-called managed care services to sell to the insurance companies. Managed care arrangements have led to all kinds of subtle and not so subtle pressures on physicians to deny services or to discharge patients from the hospital early. In that way, the managed care companies can demonstrate that they are saving money for the insurance company or for the industrial firm that, after all, is paying the health insurance premiums.

Managed care, preadmission screening, concurrent review, and so on, use a lot of manpower. A huge bureaucracy has developed, consisting primarily of personnel who are largely ignorant of the treatment of uncommon conditions. If something is not obvious and is not listed on their tic sheets, denial is routine.

These aforementioned factors create several problems:

1. A tussle has developed between the doctor and the hospital for scarce resources. The physician, in his role of patient advocate, must become more aggressive if patients are to get the resources they need.

2. Arbitrary decisions result in denial of reimbursement for the care of many patients. Since difficult cases of epilepsy require unusual treatments, this is a particular problem for the epilepsy center.

3. Since the average physician's bill is rather small, the insurance companies get away with many arbitrary denials because the physician chooses not to fight. If the amount of money at issue is $50 or even $500, the average physician will think

several times over before spending thousands of dollars on attorneys' fees to fight the insurance company.

What are the implications for the treatment of epilepsy? It is proven that a substantial number of patients fail to respond to usual treatment. A comprehensive medical, psychological, and social approach has been demonstrated to be effective in the care of these complex patients. However, this approach requires expensive, high-tech care [including intensive neurodiagnostic monitoring (INDM), especially video/EEG diagnostic services] and long stays in the hospital.

The surgical treatment of epilepsy has become safer and more effective than ever before. Many more patients can now benefit from surgical treatment. This requires even more high-tech intensive neurodiagnostic monitoring such as implanted electrodes, as well as long hospital stays and rehabilitation services.

If we are to bring about improved quality of care for patients with intractable seizures in this complex political and economic environment, certain forces have to be brought together:

1. We need agreed-upon standards of care so that it is clear that patients are receiving appropriate services.

2. Extensive lobbying must be carried out in Congress and in state legislatures, with various regulatory authorities within federal and state governments, with national insurance groups, and with individual insurance companies. We are clearly in an era of groups negotiating with groups. The individual physician is not heard; the physician representing a national association *is* heard.

3. To have an adequate number of epilepsy centers, we need to help new centers grow into comprehensive treatment programs. This requires helping each other and sharing information.

4. We need to develop mutual self-help mechanisms to deal with the business aspects of practice. If each epilepsy center has to learn how to do it on its own, it will take forever to develop adequate resources for the nation.

The established scientific societies have major limitations in dealing with these problems:

1. They are limited by law on how much they can spend on lobbying activities.

2. Scientific organizations cannot engage in activities that relate to the business aspects of providing care, and they have been sued in the past for restraint of trade.

3. The scholarly societies are set up to organize scientific meetings, to publish journals, and so on. They are not organized for effective political action.

4. The officers of these societies are selected because they can give wise scientific counsel, have participated actively in the functions of the society, have published a lot of papers, and so on. These are very valuable attributes, but they do not necessarily prepare one for dealing with the government and insurance companies.

5. The dues structures of these societies do not generate enough money to do the job. To be effective, lobbying has to be done by qualified professionals. This costs a lot of money. If one needs legal advice, it cannot be obtained on a *pro bono* basis or

sought from the least expensive attorney. These are complex subjects that require the best corporate attorneys, and they are very expensive.

These factors led to the creation of the National Association of Epilepsy Centers (NAEC). The NAEC was organized by physicians who are active in all of the scientific societies. However, it was organized for economic and political purposes, which must be kept separate from charitable activities.

The NAEC was incorporated as a 501(c)(6) trade association. Under IRS rules, a trade association is permitted to carry on certain activities that would be disqualified as lobbying for a charitable 501(c)(3). The NAEC is primarily an organization of facilities. Comprehensive care of patients with difficult seizure disturbances is not an individual activity but, instead, requires a well-organized group.

Development of health care policy today is a highly visible political activity. The people who make the decisions are politicians, although they don't always run for office. Politicians, by the nature of their jobs, are less interested in providing care than in the *appearance* of providing care. The lesson for us is that one must deal with a political situation with political techniques. The NAEC works effectively in this area.

The NAEC has recently approved a series of criteria or "guidelines" by which specialized epilepsy centers can measure themselves. The working hypothesis is that epilepsy centers can be divided into tertiary- and fourth-level medical and surgical centers. Tertiary-level centers can manage many of the cases of epilepsy that are complex, but they do not have a large team of highly specialized physicians to deal with the most difficult cases. At the present time, approximately ten centers in the United States qualify as fourth-level centers. The criteria for tertiary- and fourth-level centers are described in the NAEC's "Recommended Guidelines for Diagnosis and Treatment" (Appendix II).

The purpose of the NAEC is to help make it possible for people with epilepsy who require highly specialized care to obtain it. If you would like information about the facilities that make up the membership of the Association, more information about specialized care for epilepsy, or information about the NAEC itself, please write to the Association at 5775 Wayzata Blvd., Suite 255, Minneapolis, Minnesota 55416, or call (612) 525-1160.

Appendix II

The National Association of Epilepsy Centers

Recommended Guidelines for Diagnosis and Treatment

INTRODUCTION

The National Association of Epilepsy Centers has established as one of its foremost objectives the development of guidelines for the services, personnel and facilities appropriate for specialty epilepsy centers. The guidelines also include recommendations for referral of patients to such centers. The following document is the result of that effort. It involved many months of work and discussion by committee members from epilepsy centers across the United States.

These Guidelines are intended to assist existing and developing epilepsy centers and purchasers of services in evaluating appropriateness and quality of care. A comprehensive approach to the care of patients with intractable seizures is the most compassionate, medically appropriate and cost-effective approach. Differences will naturally exist among epilepsy centers in the range of services provided. These Guidelines seek to establish basic definitions of the scope and quality of services which any specialty epilepsy center should achieve.

A specialty epilepsy center is a program providing comprehensive diagnostic and treatment services primarily or exclusively to patients with intractable epilepsy; that is, patients whose

Prepared and distributed by:

The National Association of Epilepsy Centers
5775 Wayzata Blvd., Suite 255
Minneapolis, MN 55416
(612) 525-1160

seizures have not been brought under acceptable control using the resources available to the family physician or general neurologist. Such a program is staffed by physicians, nurses, technologists, psychologists and others with specialized training and experience in the field. "Tertiary" medical centers should provide the basic range of medical, neuropsychological, and psychosocial services needed in an epilepsy referral center. Surgical services are generally not provided except on a referral or emergency basis. Tertiary centers will eventually be found in many university and some large community hospitals.

"Fourth level" *medical* epilepsy centers serve as regional or national referral facilities providing services to populations of tens of millions of people. They should provide the more complex forms of intensive neurodiagnostic monitoring (INDM) and other diagnostic procedures, more extensive neuropsychological and psychosocial services, and limited neurosurgical services for epilepsy treatment. A more sophisticated staffing mix should also be found in a fourth level center.

A "fourth level" *surgical* epilepsy center should be capable of conducting complete surgical evaluations, as well as having staff with the expertise to perform a broad range of surgery procedures for epilepsy. A fourth level center may consist of separate medical and surgical programs, or there may be one combined medical and surgical program.

It is important that these highly specialized resources be used appropriately. While they are not needed routinely by the majority of the patients with epilepsy, they must be available to those whose epilepsy cannot be effectively treated at the primary or secondary care level. Early intervention is most likely to achieve the best results, and these services should be provided to the appropriate patients without undue delay.

This document was developed by the members of the Medical Diagnosis and Treatment Committee and the Surgical Treatment Committee of the National Association of Epilepsy Centers, and was adopted by the Board of the National Association of Epilepsy Centers on October 17, 1988. The Guidelines may be reviewed and updated as considered necessary by the Board.

Medical Diagnosis and Treatment Committee

John R. Gates, M.D., Chair	Minneapolis, MN
Fritz E. Dreifuss, M.D.	Charlottesville, VA
Donald W. King, M.D.	Augusta, GA
Dennis Smith, M.D.	Portland, OR
Susan Spencer, M.D.	West Haven, CT

Surgical Treatment Committee

Hans Lüders, M.D., Chair	Cleveland, OH
Jerome Engel, Jr., M.D.	Los Angeles, CA
Robert E. Maxwell, M.D.	Minneapolis, MN
George A. Ojemann, M.D.	Seattle, WA
Dennis Spencer, M.D.	New Haven, CT

THE NATIONAL ASSOCIATION OF EPILEPSY CENTERS RECOMMENDED GUIDELINES FOR DIAGNOSIS AND TREATMENT

I. TERTIARY LEVEL EPILEPSY REFERRAL CENTER

A. Services Provided
1. Electrodiagnostic

   a. A minimum of eight-hour video/EEG with surface/sphenoidal recording with supervision by EEG technologist and assistance by epilepsy staff nurse or monitoring technician if necessary.

2. Epilepsy Surgery
   a. Emergency or elective neurosurgery including removal of incidental lesions; e.g., tumors, hematomas.
   b. Management of complications.
   c. An established referral agreement with a fourth level epilepsy surgical center for surgical procedures for epilepsy, when indicated.

3. Imaging
   a. Magnetic Resonance Imaging.
   b. Computerized Axial Tomography.
   c. Cerebral Angiography.

4. Pharmacological Expertise
   a. Quality assured antiepileptic drug levels.
   b. 24-hour antiepileptic drug level service.
   c. Pharmacokinetic expertise by at least one member of team.

5. Neuropsychological/Psychosocial Services
   a. Comprehensive neuropsychological test batteries for evaluation of cerebral dysfunction for vocational and rehabilitative purposes.
   b. An established referral agreement for comprehensive psychogenic seizure management.
   c. Clinical psychological services.
   d. Social services.
   e. School services for children as required.

6. Rehabilitation (Inpatient and Outpatient)
   a. Sufficient physical therapy, occupational therapy, and speech therapy for managing the complications of simple lesional excisions.

7. Consultative Expertise
   a. Neurosurgery (if a neurosurgeon is not Program Director).
   b. Internal Medicine.
   c. Pediatrics.
   d. General Surgery.
   e. Obstetrics/Gynecology.

B. Personnel

1. Physicians
   Neurologist(s) with board certification in Neurology and Clinical Neuro-

physiology and/or neurosurgeon with board certification in Neurosurgery. He/she should also have training in the pharmacology of antiepileptic drugs. A second such individual would also be desirable. Board certification by the American Board of Clinical Neurophysiology (ABCN) would be required of only one neurologist or neurosurgeon.

Any licensed physician could be Program Director, but ordinarily a neurologist with special expertise in epilepsy and training in neurodiagnostic techniques would serve in this role.

2. Neuropsychologist/Neuropsychometrist
    a. Neuropsychologist—Ph.D. in Clinical Psychology with specialization in Clinical Neuropsychology as evidenced by pre- or post-doctoral training and/or work experience; or, a Ph.D. in Psychology with post-doctoral training from an APA-approved Clinical Neuropsychology Program.
        Responsibilities: Supervision of neuropsychological evaluations and assessments. May also supervise the interventional psychologists.
    b. Psychometrist—a bachelor's degree in a behavioral science plus supervised experience in test administration and scoring under the direction of a qualified neuropsychologist. This individual will administer and score neuropsychological tests.

3. Psychosocial
    a. Clinical Psychologist/Counseling Psychologist—Ph.D from an APA-approved Clinical or Counseling Psychology Program, and with a special interest in epilepsy.
    b. Social Worker—ACSW preferred with experience coordinating case services for epilepsy patients in an outpatient setting.
    c. School services for children.

4. Nursing
    a. Clinical Nurse Specialist/Nurse Clinician—Qualifications to include nursing with experience in epilepsy (MSN desirable).
        Responsibilities: Provide patient and family education and coordinate nursing services for epilepsy center.
    b. Head Nurse/Staff Nurse—Qualifications include R.N. with experience in epilepsy.
        Responsibilities: Coordinate nursing functions for inpatient service.

5. EEG Technologist(s)
    When intensive neurodiagnostic monitoring of patients is performed, an EEG technologist, monitoring technician, or epilepsy staff nurse must observe the patient and maintain recording integrity. (A monitoring technician is defined as an individual trained in seizure observation capable of maintaining recording integrity in the temporary absence of an EEG technologist.)

    All technologists and technicians should be certified in basic life support. All technologists preferably would be board eligible or certified by ABRET. All technologists should meet AEEG Society long term monitoring qualifications. The chief technologist should be ABRET registered and have special training in long term monitoring.

6. Rehabilitation Services
   a. Registered Occupational Therapist.
   b. Physical Therapist supervised by M.D.
   c. Speech Therapist and Vocational Counselor also desirable.

7. Support Services available on a consultative basis
   a. Psychiatrist, board certified (ABPN) with special interest and expertise in treatment of epileptic patients with psychiatric disorders, who has made a significant time commitment to the program.
   b. Neurosurgeon (if neurosurgeon is not Program Director).
   c. Internist.
   d. Pediatrician.
   e. General Surgeon.
   f. Obstetrician/Gynecologist.
   g. Biomedical Engineer.

II. FOURTH LEVEL—MEDICAL CENTER FOR EPILEPSY

A. Services Provided

1. Electrodiagnostic
   a. 24-hour video/EEG with surface/sphenoidal electrodes with supervision by EEG technologist or epilepsy staff nurse, supported when appropriate by monitoring technician or automated ictal and interictal activity detection program.
   b. Intracarotid amobarbital (Wada) testing.
   c. Pharmacological activation/suppression of EEG.

2. Epilepsy Surgery
   a. Emergency neurosurgery.
   b. Complications management.
   c. Open biopsy.
   d. Stereotactic biopsy.
   e. Excision of incidental lesions.
   f. An established referral arrangement with a fourth level surgery center for epilepsy.

3. Imaging
   a. Magnetic Resonance Imaging.
   b. Computerized Axial Tomography.
   c. Cerebral Angiography.

4. Pharmacological Expertise
   a. Quality assured antiepileptic drug levels.
   b. 24-hour antiepileptic drug level service.
   c. Pharmacokinetic analysis for each patient.

5. Neuropsychological/Psychosocial Services
   a. Comprehensive psychogenic inpatient treatment services.
   b. Interventive/supportive inpatient psychological and social services.

    c. Comprehensive neuropsychological test batteries for evaluations and localization of cerebral dysfunction as well as complete assessment of characterological and psychopathological issues.

    d. Supervision of the neuropsychological testing component of the intracarotid amobarbital test.

    e. Vocational counseling capabilities.

    f. School services for children as required.

6. <u>Rehabilitation (Inpatient and Outpatient)</u>
    a. Physical Therapy.
    b. Occupational Therapy.
    c. Speech Therapy.
    d. Vocational Education.

7. <u>Support Services</u> available on a consultative basis
    a. Internal Medicine.
    b. Pediatrics.
    c. General Surgery.
    d. Obstetrics/Gynecology.
    e. Rehabilitation Medicine.

B. Personnel

1. <u>Physicians</u>
    a. <u>Medical Director</u> with board certification in Neurology, or board certification in Neurosurgery with special training in epilepsy and intensive neurodiagnostic monitoring techniques.
    b. <u>Neurologist</u> with board certification in Neurology and special training in the pharmacology of antiepileptic drugs.
        Both of these individuals should have specific training in prolonged EEG recording with video monitoring capability (per AEEG Society guidelines for monitoring in epilepsy). At least one of these physicians should be certified by the American Board of Clinical Neurophysiology (ABCN).
    c. <u>Neurosurgeon</u> board certified with special interest in epilepsy.
    d. <u>Psychiatrist</u> board certified (ABPN) with special interest in treatment of epileptic patients with psychiatric disorders.
    e. <u>Pharmacologist or Pharm.D.</u> with special interest and training in epilepsy.
    f. Other long-term monitoring electroencephalographers per AEEG guidelines.

2. <u>Neuropsychology</u>
    a. <u>Neuropsychologist</u>—Ph.D. in Clinical Psychology with specialization in Clinical Neuropsychology as evidenced by pre- or post-doctoral training and/or work experience; or, a Ph.D. in Psychology with post-doctoral training from an APA-approved Clinical Neuropsychology Program.
        Responsibilities: Supervision of neuropsychological evaluations and assessments. May also supervise interventional psychologists.
    b. <u>Psychometrist</u>—M.S. in Psychology with training in Neuropsycho-

metrics or a minimum of a bachelor's degree and two years experience in Neuropsychometrics. This individual will perform neuropsychometric examinations.

3. Psychosocial
   a. Clinical Psychologist/Counseling Psychologist—Ph.D. from an APA-approved Clinical or Counseling Psychology Program, and with a special interest in epilepsy.
   b. Social Worker—ACSW preferred with experience coordinating case services for epilepsy patients in an outpatient setting.
   c. School services for children.

4. Nursing
   a. Clinical Nurse Specialist/Nurse Clinician—Qualifications to include nursing with experience in epilepsy (MSN desirable).
      Responsibilities: Provide patient and family education and coordinate nursing services for epilepsy center.
   b. Head Nurse/Staff Nurse—Qualifications include R.N. with experience in epilepsy.
      Responsibilities: Coordinate nursing functions for inpatient service.

5. EEG Technologist(s)
   When intensive neurodiagnostic monitoring of patients is performed, an EEG technologist, monitoring technician, or epilepsy staff nurse must observe the patient and maintain recording integrity. (A monitoring technician is defined as an individual trained in seizure observation and capable of maintaining recording integrity in the temporary absence of an EEG technologist.)
   All technologists and technicians should be certified in basic life support. All technologists preferably would be board eligible or certified by ABRET. All technologists should meet AEEG Society long-term monitoring qualifications. The chief technologist should be ABRET registered and have special training in long-term monitoring.

6. Rehabilitation Services
   a. Registered Occupational Therapist.
   b. Physical Therapist supervised by M.D.
   c. Speech Therapist and Vocational Counselor also preferred.

7. Support Services
   a. Internist.
   b. Pediatrician.
   c. General Surgeon.
   d. Obstetrician/Gynecologist.
   e. Rehabilitation Medicine (Physiatrist).
   f. Biomedical Engineer.

III. FOURTH LEVEL—SURGICAL CENTER FOR EPILEPSY

A. Services Provided

   1. Electrodiagnostic

    a.   24-hour video/EEG with surface and sphenoidal electrodes with supervision by EEG technologist or epilepsy staff nurse, supported when appropriate by monitoring technician or automated seizure and interictal activity detection program.

    b.   Invasive 24-hour recording with subdural electrodes, depth electrodes, or epidural electrodes under continual supervision and observation.

    c.   Intracarotid amobarbital (Wada) testing.

    d.   Functional cortical mapping utilizing subdural electrodes or intraoperative stimulation.

    e.   Evoked potential recording, capable of being used safely with implanted electrodes.

    f.   Electrocorticography.

2.   Epilepsy Surgery
    a.   Emergency neurosurgery.
    b.   Complication management.
    c.   Open biopsy.
    d.   Stereotactic biopsy.
    e.   Lesional excision.
    f.   Intracranial electrodes and cortical resection.
    g.   Corpus callosotomy.
    h.   Cortical resection, including hemispherectomy.
    i.   Clinical experience of greater than 25 cases per year.

3.   Imaging
    a.   Magnetic Resonance Imaging.
    b.   Computerized Axial Tomography.
    c.   Cerebral Angiography.

4.   Pharmacological Expertise
    a.   Quality assured antiepileptic drug levels.
    b.   24-hour antiepileptic drug level service.
    c.   Pharmacokinetic consultative services.

5.   Neuropsychological/Psychosocial Services
    a.   Comprehensive neuropsychological test batteries for localization of cerebral dysfunction as well as complete assessment of characterological and psychopathological issues.
    b.   Interventive and supportive inpatient psychological and social services.
    c.   School services for children.

6.   Rehabilitation (Inpatient and Outpatient)
    a.   Physical Therapy.
    b.   Occupational Therapy.
    c.   Speech Therapy.
    d.   Vocational Education.

7.   Consultative Expertise
    a.   Psychiatrist board certified (ABPN) with special interest in treatment of epileptic patients with psychiatric disorders.
    b.   Internal Medicine.

      c. Pediatrics.

      d. General Surgery.

      e. Obstetrics/Gynecology.

B. Personnel

    1. Physicians

        a. Neurologist with board certification in Neurology and special training in invasive intensive neurodiagnostic monitoring (per AEEG Society guidelines for monitoring in epilepsy).

        b. Neurosurgeon with board certification, special interest in epilepsy, and experience in resection of epileptogenic tissue and invasive monitoring techniques.

           At least one of these physicians should be certified by the American Board of Clinical Neurophysiology (ABCN).

        c. Other long-term monitoring electroencephalographers per AEEG Society guidelines.

           "a" or "b" would ordinarily serve as Program Director.

    2. Neuropsychology

        a. Neuropsychologist—Ph.D. in Clinical Psychology with specialization in Clinical Neuropsychology as evidenced by pre- or post-doctoral training and/or work experience; or, a Ph.D. in Psychology with post-doctoral training from an APA-approved Clinical Neuropsychology Program.

           Responsibilities: Supervision of neuropsychological evaluations and assessments. May also supervise interventional psychologists.

        b. Psychometrist—M.S. in Psychology with training in Neuropsychometrics or a minimum of a bachelor's degree and two years experience in Neuropsychometrics. This individual will perform neuropsychometric examinations.

    3. Psychosocial

        a. Clinical Psychologist/Counseling Psychologist—Ph.D. from an APA-approved Clinical or Counseling Psychology Program, and with a special interest in epilepsy.

        b. Social Worker—ACSW preferred with experience coordinating case services for epilepsy patients in an outpatient setting.

        c. School services for children.

    4. Nursing

        a. Clinical Nurse Specialist/Nurse Clinician—Qualifications to include nursing with experience in epilepsy (MSN desirable).

           Responsibilities: Provide patient and family education and coordinate nursing services for epilepsy center.

        b. Head Nurse/Staff Nurse—Qualifications include R.N. with experience in epilepsy.

           Responsibilities: Coordinate nursing functions for inpatient service.

    5. EEG Technologist(s)

        When intensive neurodiagnostic monitoring of patients is performed, an EEG technologist, monitoring technician, or epilepsy staff nurse must observe the patient and maintain recording integrity. (A monitoring technician is defined as an individual trained in seizure observation and capable of maintaining recording integrity in the temporary absence of an EEG technologist.)

All technologists and technicians should be certified in basic life support. All technologists preferably would be board eligible or certified by ABRET. All technologists should meet AEEG Society long-term monitoring qualifications. The chief technologist should be ABRET registered and have special training in long-term monitoring.

6. Rehabilitation Services
    a. Registered Occupational Therapist.
    b. Physical Therapist supervised by M.D.
    c. Physiatrist with special interest in neurological dysfunction.
    d. Speech Therapist and Vocational Counselor also preferred.

7. Support Services
    a. General Internist.
    b. Pediatrician.
    c. General Surgeon.
    d. Obstetrician/Gynecologist.
    e. Rehabilitation Medicine (Physiatrist).
    f. Biomedical Engineer.

IV. FACILITIES

Continuous observation of patients undergoing intensive neurodiagnostic monitoring is mandatory. This is particularly critical for patients with indwelling electrodes. Observation must be by qualified health care providers such as EEG technologists, or epilepsy staff nurses, as defined under Personnel. Such observation is, of course, in addition to ongoing medical and nursing care.

Facilities for the management of epilepsy should in general include:

★ An inpatient recording suite with access to full resuscitative capabilities.
★ A dedicated unit with a nursing staff whose sole function is to care for individuals with epilepsy. The unit's design and furnishings should minimize risk of injury to patients subject to seizures and falls.
★ 24-hour medical coverage on site.
★ Availability of the full spectrum of imaging services on site.

Fourth level surgical programs which perform monitoring of patients with indwelling electrodes must assure electrical safety and must meet the standards of the American EEG Society's recommendations for intensive neurodiagnostic monitoring.

A separate outpatient recording unit may be acceptable in a tertiary or fourth level facility if appropriate care can be assured for patients with medical emergencies. This can be accomplished through contractual arrangements with a nearby hospital to provide such emergency services. There must also be ready access to emergency resuscitative equipment in the outpatient monitoring suite itself. Medication reduction to increase seizure yield is not recommended in an outpatient setting.

PATIENT REFERRAL TO SPECIALTY EPILEPSY CARE

Sophisticated diagnostic procedures and surgical treatment must be available for those patients who are likely to benefit from such care. It is essential that persons experiencing seizures be seen and treated at the appropriate level of care. It is important not only that the most difficult cases of epilepsy be referred for specialty care, but also that patients who can be successfully treated at the primary or secondary care level are not inappropriately referred for specialty care. The flowsheet which follows is an integral part of these Guidelines. It details the progression of a patient from first seizure through possible referral to a specialty epilepsy center.

The first step for individuals experiencing an initial seizure or seizures is to consult their primary care physician in their own community. This may involve hospitalization, or if the

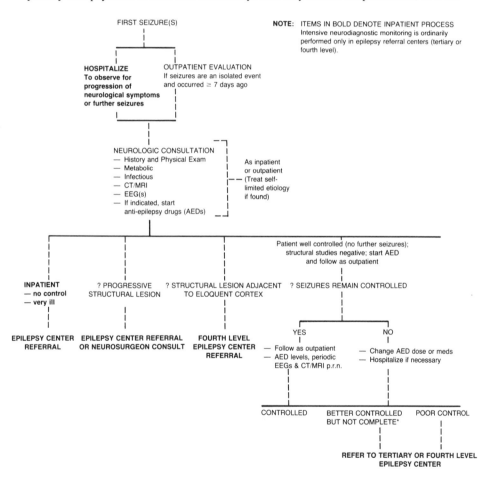

*At any point where the patient continues to have an unacceptable seizure frequency after two or more AEDs in six or more months.

first seizure was an isolated event and took place more than a week prior to the physician visit, an outpatient evaluation may be sufficient. The primary care physician may choose to begin a treatment program, or refer the individual to a general neurologist for a consultation. In any event, if seizure control cannot be achieved at the primary care level within approximately three months, a referral to a general neurologist is indicated. The neurologic consultation should include a history and physical examination, metabolic studies and various other studies including routine EEG examinations as described in the flow sheet. If the patient's seizures are well-controlled the patient can be followed on an outpatient basis with follow-up visits to the neurologist as needed.

If seizure control is not achieved by the general neurologist within another nine months, referral to a tertiary or fourth level epilepsy center should be made without further delay. The referral may be to an epilepsy center with or without epilepsy surgery capability, depending on the seizure type and availability of consultants. Referral from a tertiary to a fourth level center should be based on the need for one or more of these specific requirements:

1. Invasive intracranial video/EEG recording.
2. Inpatient psychological or psychiatric intervention and/or milieu therapy.
3. Difficult pharmacological problems.
4. Possible psychogenic seizures likely to require inpatient treatment.
5. Patient likely to require epilepsy surgery, especially if intensive post-operative rehabilitation will be needed after aggressive topectomy, lobectomy, or corpus callosotomy.

ABOUT THE NATIONAL ASSOCIATION OF EPILEPSY CENTERS

The National Association of Epilepsy Centers was founded in 1987 as a non-profit organization whose goals are complementary to those of existing scientific and charitable organizations such as the American Epilepsy Society and the Epilepsy Foundation of America. Its original members were directors of ten prominent epilepsy centers across the country. It has since grown to include the majority of specialized epilepsy centers in the United States.

NAEC's activities are based on four overall goals:

1. To provide information about issues relevant to the care of patients with epilepsy to appropriate government and industry officials.
2. To exchange information among its members about the business aspects of providing such services.
3. To participate in the development of standards for facilities and programs for providing these services.
4. To assist in the development of standards for the provision of medical and surgical treatment of epilepsy.

Please direct inquiries about the Guidelines or the Association to: Robert J. Gumnit, M.D., President, National Association of Epilepsy Centers, 5775 Wayzata Blvd., Suite 255, Minneapolis, MN 55416. Phone (612) 525-1160.

Subject Index

A

Absence seizures
    automatisms, 8, 10
    in childhood, 18–19, 100–102
    classification, 10, 18–19
    and myoclonus, 21
    positron emission tomography, 86
Acceptable blood levels, 129–130, 134
Acetylsalicylic acid, 147
Acquired epileptic aphasia, 22
Action myoclonus, 10
Adrenocorticotropic hormone, 96
Age of onset, 92
Aged. *See* Elderly
Aggression, 211–226
    diagnosis, 221–224
    EEG studies, 214
    legal literature, 219–220
    neurobiology, 212–213
Agranulocytosis, 119–120
Aicardi syndrome, 21
Ambulatory cassette recording, 62–63, 69
2-Amino-7-phosphonohetanoate, 238
Amygdalar seizures, 16
Amygdalohippocampectomy, 178–179
Amytal test, 177
Anger, 189, 197
Anterior frontal epilepsies, 15
Anticoagulants, 146
Antidepressants, 199–200
Antidiuretic hormone, 146–147
Antiepileptic drugs. *See* Drug treatment
Anxiety, 197
Aspartate, 237
Astatic seizures, 21
Astrocytoma, 81, 83
Asymmetries, EEG, 40
Asymmetry index, 84
Atonic seizures, 11
Attenuation EEG pattern, 66, 68
Audio EEG recording, 64–65
Aura. *See also* Partial epilepsy
    definition, 9

mental changes, 196
Autoinduction, 104, 132–133
Automatisms
    complex partial seizures, 8
    and violence, 218–221
Autonomic symptoms, 7
Awareness, 4

B

Barbiturates, 47
Benign childhood epilepsy with centro-
    temporal spikes, 12–14
Benign epileptiform transients of sleep,
    34–35
Benign focal epileptiform discharges of
    childhood, 46–47, 52
Benign myoclonic epilepsy in infancy, 18,
    97
Benign neonatal convulsions, 18
Benign neonatal familial convulsions, 18
Benign partial epilepsy of childhood, 102
"Benign rolandic spikes," 31–32
Benzodiazepine receptor, 236–237
Benzodiazepines, EEG, 47
BETS (benign epileptiform transients of
    sleep), 34–35
Blitz-Nick-Salaam Krampfe, 20
Blood levels
    and dosage, 133–134
    drug interactions, 129–130
Bone marrow suppression, 119
Brain damage, 194
Brain-slice techniques, 244–247
Breach rhythm, 38
Breastfeeding, 136
Bursting cells, 230–231, 245–246

C

CA3 region, 245–246
Cable telemetry, 60–62
Calcium-channel blockers, 232–233

obtain free PHT when on VPA: PHT toxicity
   because of ↑ free (binding affected) p.113

CBZ best control for partial Sz (monotherapy)
   vs PB, PHT, PRD   p.116

CBZ: less behavior toxicity p.118
   than PB, PHT, PRD

CBZ less effective than PB, used in primary
   gen TC Sz   p. 119

CBZ measure platelets + WBC before Rx
   & q 3 month for 1 year
   (if < 3000 stop CBZ)   p.119

PHT dosing: if HS, draw level 10-12 hr & 18-20 hr
   post dose (= early am & late afternoon)
                p 121
   if a great a morning peak or too low
   a late afternoon trough, bc AM + HS
lowers Tq previously (how do you decide) p 122
   Ask Calvin Gorman
give folic acid & Vit D   p. 122 (some give not
   D unless Radiology evidence of osteomalacia
   but I would give before this)
hyperglycemia & glycosuria due to inhibit
   secretion of insulin   p 122
Primidone
   125 mg HS for 3 d & ↑ gradual p.126
VPA: displaces most binding of other AED (obtain
   free level of other drugs); may cause toxicity
   related to free level of other AED   p.128
take VPA c̄ meals or after to prevent nausea
   (less c̄ divalproex Na
check NH3
   ↑ aminotransferase   p.128-9
divalproex Na given BID
VPA alone 1-1½ gm (c̄ PHT, give 3-4 g)   p129
   total PHT low but toxicity due to unbound p

Course on monitoring
photo of fig 1, 2, 3